Essentials of Pediatric Surgery

Edited by

Sultan Mohsen Ghanem

Faculty of Medicine
University of Kufa
Iraq

Najah Hadi

Faculty of Medicine
University of Kufa
Iraq

&

Nada Al-Haris

Faculty of Medicine
University of Kufa
Iraq

Essentials of Pediatric Surgery

Editors: Sultan M. Ghanem, Najah R. Hadi & Nada Al-Haris

ISBN (Online): 978-981-4998-84-0

ISBN (Print): 978-981-4998-85-7

ISBN (Paperback): 978-981-4998-86-4

need for a court order if at any point you breach any terms of this License Agreement. In no event will any delay or failure by Bentham Science Publishers in enforcing your compliance with this License Agreement constitute a waiver of any of its rights.

3. You acknowledge that you have read this License Agreement, and agree to be bound by its terms and conditions. To the extent that any other terms and conditions presented on any website of Bentham Science Publishers conflict with, or are inconsistent with, the terms and conditions set out in this License Agreement, you acknowledge that the terms and conditions set out in this License Agreement shall prevail.

Bentham Science Publishers Pte. Ltd.
80 Robinson Road #02-00
Singapore 068898
Singapore
Email: subscriptions@benthamscience.net

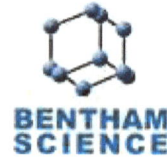

BENTHAM SCIENCE

CONTENTS

PREFACE

The ongoing struggle with coronavirus has resulted in a forced distance between the professor and his students. Moreover, we lost our loved ones and colleagues. The importance of pediatric surgery has been compromised due to the neglect of this delicate specialized field, resulting in the loss of many cases due to the loss of the correct written curriculum. I decided with my students, at the final stage of studying medicine, that we would have a hand that writes and a hand that works to save children with surgical problems that require surgical intervention. It might be simple at first, but we believe it is more than that. For a child with the slightest trace of a birth defect, to live for decades would be a blessing. Therefore, we started to communicate, consult, summarise, disagree, and agree through the closed electronic circuit; accordingly, the result of these efforts is the book titled "Essentials of Pediatric Surgery" that we are now putting in the hands of our students and our dear colleagues to serve as the best guide in the field of pediatric surgery. We have summarized the important chapters of the international references related to pediatric surgery that benefit medical students and trainees to enter the field of specialization in pediatric surgery. All thanks and appreciation to those who contributed, participated, and gave their time. We are full of happiness and joy because we did not succumb to the coronavirus epidemic and its repercussions, and we hope that the earth will be free of coronavirus. We stand a minute of silence in respect of those who have passed. It is necessary to note the great effort made by Dr. Houreleen H. Salman in following up the book step by step and all those who contributed and participated in it. I do not forget the continuous support of the Dean of the College of Medicine, Professor Raed Reda Omran; I give them all my love and respect.

Sultan M. Ghanim
Faculty of Medicine
University of Kufa
Iraq

List of Contributors

Asalah T. Gumer	6th Grade Medical College, Faculty of Medicine, University of Kufa, Iraq
Assalah T. Gumer	6th Grade Medical College, Faculty of Medicine, University of Kufa, Iraq
Fatima H. Naeima	6th Grade Medical College, Faculty of Medicine, University of Kufa, Iraq
Hiba A. Mirza	6th Grade Medical College, Faculty of Medicine, University of Kufa, Iraq
Houreleen H. Salman	6th Grade Medical College, Faculty of Medicine, University of Kufa, Iraq
Hayder D. Abbas	5th Grade Jabir Ibn Hayyan Medical University, University of Kufa, Iraq
Karrar K. Abdulsahib	6th Grade Medical College, Faculty of Medicine, University of Kufa, Iraq
Karrar Z. Sadoun	5th Grade Jabir Ibn Hayyan Medical University, Iraq
Nada R. Alharis	Faculty of Medicine University of Kufa, Iraq
Najah R. Hadi	Faculty of Medicine University of Kufa, Iraq
Noor Al-Huda I. Khalaf	6th Grade Medical College, Faculty of Medicine, University of Kufa, Iraq
Sultan M. Ghanim	ME Uint, Medical College, Faculty of Medicine, University of Kufa, Iraq
Sarah N. Ahmed	6th Grade Medical College, Faculty of Medicine, University of Kufa, Iraq
Zainab H. Ibrahim	6th Grade Medical College, Faculty of Medicine, University of Kufa, Iraq

Senior Editor

Sultan M. Ghanim
General Surgery Board
Supspicialty Pediatric Surgery board
Professor
ATLS Instuctor, ME Uint
Medical College,
Faculty of Medcine,
University of Kufa
Iraq

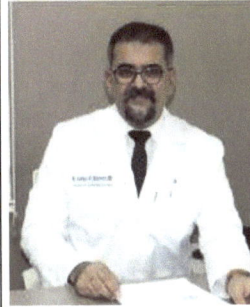

Editor

Najah R. Hadi
Najah Hadi,PhD, FRCP, FACP
Professor and Consultant
Faculty of Medicine
University of Kufa,
Iraq

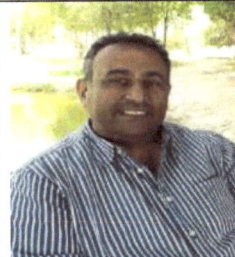

Nada R. Alharis
Professor of Diagnostic Radiology
Faculty of Medicine
University of Kufa
Iraq

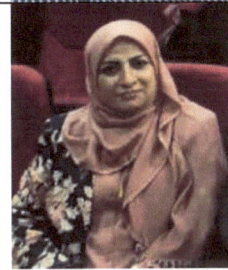

Contributors

Houreleen H. Salman
6th Grade Faculty of Medicine,
University of Kufa
Iraq

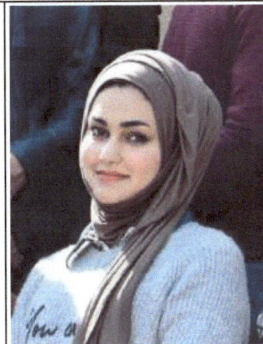

Hayder D. Abbas 5th Grade Jabir Ibn Hayyan Medical University, Najaf, Iraq	
Assalah T. Gumer 6th Grade Faculty of Medicine, University of Kufa Iraq	
Karrar K. Abdulsahib 6th Grade Faculty of Medicine, University of Kufa Iraq	
Karrar Z. Sadoun 6th Grade Collage of Medicine, Jabir Bin Hayyan Medical University, Najaf, Iraq	

Noor Al-Huda I. Khalaf 6th Grade Faculty of Medicine, University of Kufa Iraq	
Zainab H. Ibrahim 6th Grade Faculty of Medicine, University of Kufa Iraq	
Sarah N. Ahmed 6th Grade Faculty of Medicine, University of Kufa Iraq	
Fatima H. Naeima 6th Grade Faculty of Medicine, University of Kufa Iraq	

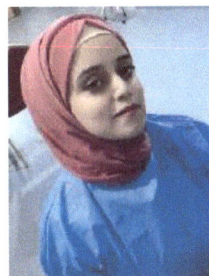

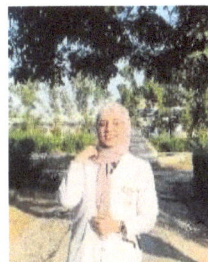

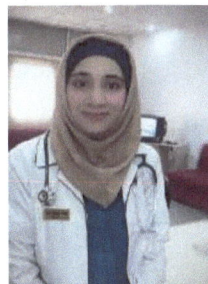

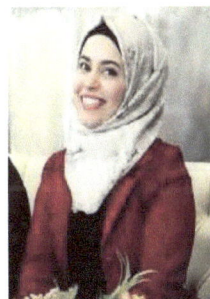

CHAPTER 1

Physiology of the Newborn

Sultan M. Ghanim[1,*] and **Najah R. Hadi**[2]

[1] *ME Unit, Medical College, Faculty of Medicine, University of Kufa, Iraq*
[2] *Faculty of Medicine, University of Kufa, Iraq*

Abstract: The survival of the neonates is dependent on the physiological charac-teristics that enable them to adapt themselves initially to the placenta and then to the extra uterine environment. Of all the pediatric patients, neonates exhibit the most distinguishing physiological features that ensure their rapid development. This chapter focuses on the physiological characteristics exhibited by the neonates in the intrauterine as well as the extra uterine environment.

Keywords: Growth, Neonate, Physiology.

PHYSIOLOGY OF NEWBORN

Newborns are classified based on gestational age *vs.* weight, and gestational age *vs.* head circumference and length. Preterm infants are those born before 37 weeks of gestation. Term infants are those born between 37 and 42 weeks of gestation. Post-term infants have a gestation that exceeds 42 weeks [1]. Small for-gestational-age (SGA): Babies whose weight is below the 10th percentile for age. Large for-gestational - age (LGA): Those at or above the 90th percentile for age. The babies whose weight falls between these extremes are appropriate-for-gestational-age (AGA). Premature infants are characterized as moderately low birth weight (1501_2000g) Very low birth weight (1001_1500g) extremely low birth weight (less than 1000g). SGA newborns are thought to suffer intrauterine growth retardation (IUGR) as a result of placental, maternal, or fatal abnormalities, conditions associated with IUGR are shown in Fig. (**1.1**) [2].

Although SGA infants may weigh the same as premature infants, they have different physiologic characteristics. Due to intrauterine malnutrition, bodyfat levels are frequently below 1% of the total bodyweight. This lack of body fat increases the risk of Hypothermia in SGA infants. Hypoglycaemia is the most

---

[*] **Corresponding author Sultan M. Ghanim:** ME Unit, Medical College, Faculty of Medicine, University of Kufa, Iraq; Tel: +9647816669997; E-mail: sultanmalsaadi@uokufa.edu.iq

common metabolic problem for neonates and develops earlier in SGA infants due to higher metabolic activity and reduced glycogen stores. The red blood cell (RBC) volume and the total blood volume are much higher in the SGA infant compared with the preterm AGA or the non-SGA full-term infant. Infants born before 37 weeks of gestation, regardless of birth weight, are considered premature. The physical exam of the premature infant reveals many abnormalities.

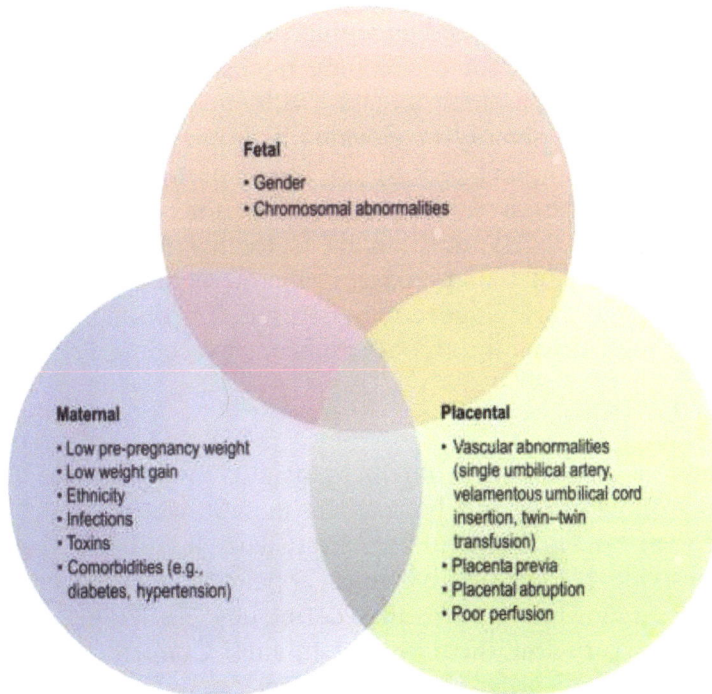

Fetal
- Gender
- Chromosomal abnormalities

Maternal
- Low pre-pregnancy weight
- Low weight gain
- Ethnicity
- Infections
- Toxins
- Comorbidities (e.g., diabetes, hypertension)

Placental
- Vascular abnormalities (single umbilical artery, velamentous umbilical cord insertion, twin–twin transfusion)
- Placenta previa
- Placental abruption
- Poor perfusion

Fig. (1.1). Diagram of conditions associated with deviations in intrauterine growth. (Adapted from Simmons R. Abnormalities of fatal growth, in: Gleason CA, Devaskar SU, Eds. Avery's Diseases of the Newborn. Philadelphia: Saunders; 2012. p. 51.

Special problems with the preterm infant include the following:

- Weak suck reflex
- Inadequate gastrointestinal absorption
- Hyaline membrane disease (HMD)
- Intraventricular hemorrhage
- Hypothermia

- Patent ductus arteriosus
- Apne
- Hyperbilirubinemia
- Necrotizing enter colitis (NEC)
- Specific Physiologic Problems of the Newborn

HYPOGLYCAEMIA

Clinical signs of hypoglycaemia are nonspecific and subtle. Seizure and coma are the most common manifestations of severe hypoglycaemia. Neonatal hypoglycaemia is generally defined as a glucose level lower than 50 mg/dL [3]. Infants who are at high risk for developing hypoglycaemia are those who are premature; SGA; or born to mothers with gestational diabetes, severe preeclampsia, or HELLP (hemolysis, elevated liver enzymes, low platelet count). Newborns that require surgical procedures are at particular risk of developing hypoglycaemia; therefore, a 10% glucose infusion is typically started on admission to the hospital. Hypoglycaemia is treated with an infusion of 1–2 mL/kg (4–8 mg/kg/ min) of 10% glucose. If an emergency operation is required, concentrations of up to 25% glucose may be used. Traditionally, central venous access has been a prerequisite for glucose infusions exceeding 12.5%.

HYPERGLYCEMIAS

Hyperglycemias is a common problem associated with the use of parenteral nutrition in very immature infants born at less than 30 weeks' gestation and birth weight of less than 1.1 kg. These infants are usually less than 3 days of age and are frequently septic [4]. Hyperglycemias appear to be associated with both insulin resistance and relative insulin deficiency, reflecting the prolonged catabolism seen in very low birth weight infants. Congenital hyperinsulinism refers to an inherited disorder that is the most common cause of recurrent hypoglycaemia in infants. This group of disorders was previously referred to as nesidioblastosis. Nesidioblastosis is a term used to describe hyperinsulinemiahypoglycaemia attributed to dysfunctional pancreatic beta cells with a characteristically abnormal histological appearance.

CALCIUM

Calcium is actively transported across the placenta of the total amount of calcium transferred across the placenta, 75% is observed after 28 weeks' gestation, which partially accounts for the high incidence of hypocalcaemia in preterm infants. Neonates are predisposed to hypocalcaemia due to limited calcium stores, renal immaturity, and relative hypoparathyroidism secondary to suppression by high fetal calcium levels [5]. Hypocalcaemia is defined as an ionized calcium level of less than (1.22) mmol/L (4.9 mg/dL) [6]. At greatest risk for hypocalcaemia are preterm infants, newborn surgical patients, and infants born to mothers with complicated pregnancies, such as those with diabetes or those receiving bicarbonate infusions. Calcitonin, which inhibits calcium mobilization from the bone, is increased in premature and asphyxiated infants. Signs of hypocalcaemia are similar to those of hypoglycaemia and may include jitteriness, seizures, cyanosis, vomiting, and myocardial arrhythmias. Symptomatic hypocalcaemia is treated with 10% calcium gluconate administered intravenous at a dosage of 1–2 mL/kg (100–200 mg/kg) over 30 minutes while monitoring the electrocardiogram for bradycardia [4]. Asymptomatic hypocalcaemia is best treated with calcium gluconate in a dose of 50 mg of elemental calcium/kg/ day added to the maintenance fluid: 1 mL of 10% calcium gluconate contains 9 mg of elemental calcium.

MAGNESIUM

Magnesium is actively transported across the placenta. Half of total body magnesium is in the plasma and soft tissues. Hypomagnesaemia is observed with growth retardation, maternal diabetes, after exchange transfusions, and with hypoparathyroidism. Magnesium deficiency should be suspected and confirmed in an infant who has seizures that do not respond to calcium therapy. Emergent treatment consists of magnesium sulphate 25–50 mg/kg IV every 6 hours until normal levels are obtained.

BLOOD VOLUME

Total RBC volume is at its highest point at delivery. Estimations of blood volume for premature infants, term neonates, and infants are summarized in Table **1.1**. By about 3 months of age, total blood volume per kilogram is nearly equal to adult levels as infants recover from their postpartum physiologic nadir. A Hematocrit greater than 50% suggests placental transfusion has occurred. Although this effects on haemoglobin levels does not persist, iron stores are positively impacted up to 6 months of age by delayed cord clamping.

Table (1.1). Estimation of Blood Volume.

Group	Blood volume (ml/kg)
Premature infants	85-100
Term newborns	85
1 month <	75
3 months to adult	70

HAEMOGLOBIN

At birth, nearly 80% of circulating haemoglobin is fetal (a2Aγ2F), when infant Erythropoiesis resumes at about 2–3 months of age, most new haemoglobin is adult. When the oxygen level is 27 mmHg, 50% of the bound oxygen is released from adult haemoglobin (P50 = 27 mmHg) [7].

POLYCYTHEMIA

A central venous haemoglobin level greater than 22 g/dL or a Hematocrit value greater than 65% during the first week of life is defined as polycythemia. After the central venous Hematocrit value reaches 65%, further increases result in rapid exponential increases in blood viscosity. Neonatal polycythemia occurs in infants of diabetic mothers, infants of mothers with toxaemia of pregnancy, or SGA infants. Polycythemia is treated using a partial exchange of the infant's blood with fresh whole blood or 5% albumin.

ANEMIA

Haemolytic Anemia

Haemolyticanaemia is most often a result of placental transfer of maternal antibodies that are destroying the infant's erythrocytes. This can be determined by the direct Coombs test. The most common severe anaemia is Rh incompatibility. Haemolytic disease in the newborn produces jaundice, pallor, and hepato splenomegaly. ABO incompatibility frequently results in hyperbilirubinemia, but rarely causes anaemia. Congenital infections, Hemoglobinpathies (sickle cell disease), and thalassemia produce haemolyticanaemia. In a severely affected infant with a positive-reacting direct Coombs test result, a cord haemoglobin level less than 10.5 g/ dL, or a cord bilirubin level greater than 4.5 mg/dL, immediate exchange transfusion is indicated,for less severely affected infants, exchange transfusion is indicated when the total indirect bilirubin level is greater than 20 mg/dL.

Hemorrhagic Anemia

Significant anaemia can develop from hemorrhage that occurs during placental abruption. Internal bleeding (intraventricular, subgaleal, meditational, intra-abdominal) in infants can also often lead to severe anaemia. Usually, hemorrhage occurs acutely during delivery. Twin–twin transfusion reactions can produce polycythemia in one baby and profound anaemia in the other.

Anemia of Prematurity

Decreased RBC production frequently contributes to anaemia of prematurity. Erythropoietin is not released until a gestational age of 30–34 weeks has been reached. These preterm infants have large numbers of erythropoietin-sensitive RBC progenitors. Successful increases in Hematocrit levels using epoitin may obviate the need for blood transfusions and reduce the risk of blood born infections and reactions [8].

Jaundice

In the hepatocytes, bilirubin created by hemolysis is conjugated to glucuronic acid and rendered water soluble. Conjugated (also known as direct) bilirubin is excreted in bile. Unconjugated bilirubin interferes with cellular respiration and is toxic to neural cells. Subsequent neural damage is termed kernicterus and produces athletic cerebral palsy, seizures, sensor neural hearing loss, and, rarely, death. Even healthy full-term infants usually have an elevated unconjugated bilirubin level. This peaks about the third day of life at approximately 6.5–7.0 mg/dL and does not return to normal until the tenth day of life. A total bilirubin level greater than 7 mg/dL in the first 24 hours or greater than 13 mg/dL at any time in full-term newborns often prompts an investigation for the cause. Breast-fed infants usually have serum bilirubin levels 1–2 mg/dL greater than formula-fed babies [9, 10]. The common causes of prolonged indirect hyperbilirubinemia are listed in Table **1.2**.

Table (1.2). Causes of indirect hyperbilirubinemia.

Breast milk jaundice	Pyloric stenosis
Haemolytic disease	Crigler-Najjar syndrome
Hypothyroidism	Extra vascular blood

Pathologic jaundice within the first 36 hours of life is usually due to excessive production of bilirubin.Phototherapy is initiated for newborns:

1. Less than 1500 g, when the serum bilirubin level reaches 5 mg/dL.
    2.1500–2000 g, when the serum bilirubin level reaches 8 mg/dL.
    3.2000–2500 g, when the serum bilirubin level reaches 10 mg/dL.

Formula- fed term infants without haemolytic disease are treated by phototherapy when levels reach 13mg/dL. For haemolytic-related hyperbilirubinemia, phototherapy is recommended when the serum bilirubin level exceeds 10 mg/dL by 12 hours of life, 12 mg/dL by 18 hours, 14 mg/dL by 24 hours, or 15 mg/dL by 36 hours [11].

Retinopathy of Prematurity

Retinopathy of prematurity (ROP) develops during the active phases of retinal vascular development from the 16th week of gestation. In full-term infants the retina is fully developed and ROP cannot occur. The exact causes are unknown, but oxygen exposure (greater than 93–95%), low birth weight, and extreme prematurity are risk factors that have been demonstrated [12, 13]. Retro-lental fibroplasias (RLF) are the pathologic change observed in the retina and overlying vitreous after the acute phases of ROP subsides [14 - 16]. The American Academy of Paediatrics' guidelines recommend a screening examination for all infants who received oxygen therapy who weigh less than 1500 g and were born at less than 32 weeks' gestation, and selected infants with a birth weight between 1500 and 2000 g or gestational age of more than 32 weeks with an unstable clinical course, including those requiring cardio respiratory support [17].

Fluids and Electrolytes

At 12 weeks of gestation, the fetus has a total body water content that is 94% of body weight. This amount decreases to 80% by 32 weeks' gestation and 78% by term. A further 3–5% reduction in total body water content occurs in the first 3–5 days of life. Body water continues to decline and reaches adult levels (approximately 60% of body weight) by 11⁄2 years of age. Extracellular water also declines by 1–3 years of age [18].

Shock

Shock is a state in which the cardiac output is insufficient to deliver adequate oxygen to meet metabolic demands of the tissues. Cardiovascular function is determined by pre-load, cardiac contractility, heart rate, and afterload. Shock may be classified broadly as hypovolemic, Cardiogenic, or distributive (systemic inflammatory response syndrome [SIRS]) septic or neurogenic.

Hypovolemic Shock

In infants and children, most shock situations are the result of reduced preload secondary to fluid loss, such as from diarrhea, vomiting, or blood loss from trauma. Shock resulting from acute hemorrhage is treated with the administration of 20 mL/kg of Ringer's lactate solution or normal saline as fluid boluses. If the patient does not respond, a second bolus of crystalloid is given. Type-specific or cross-matched blood is given to achieve a SpO2 of 70%. In newborns with a coagulopathy, fresh frozen plasma or specific factors are provided as the resuscitation fluid.

Cardiogenic Shock

Myocardial contractility is usually expressed as the ejection fraction that indicates the proportion of left ventricular volume that is pumped. Myocardial contractility is reduced with hypoxemia and acidosis. Isotropic drugs increase cardiac contractility. Inotropes are most effective when hypoxemia and acidosis are corrected. In cases of fluid-refractory shock and cardiogenic shock, isotropic drugs are necessary. Traditionally, administration of Inotropes requires the adjunct of central venous access. However, initial administration of pressors through peripheral Ivs may be prudent.

Distributive Shock

Distributive shock is caused by derangements in vascular tone from endothelial damage that lead to end-organ hypotension and is seen in the following clinical situations: (1) septic shock, (2) SIRS, (3) anaphylaxis, and (4) spinal cord trauma. Septic shock in the paediatric patient is discussed in further detail.

Septic Shock

Septic shock is a distributive form of shock that differs from other forms of shock. Cardiogenic and hypovolemic shock lead to increased SVR and decreased cardiac output. Septic shock results from a severe decrease in SVR and a generalized maldistribution of blood and leads to a hyper dynamic state [19]. The pathophysiology of septic shock begins with a nidus of infection. Organisms may invade the blood stream, or they may proliferate at the infected site and release various mediators into the blood stream. Substances produced by microorganisms, such as lipopolysaccharide, end toxin, exotoxin, and lipid moieties, and other products can induce septic shock by stimulating host cells to release numerous cytokines, Chemokines, leukotrienes, and endorphins. Therapy has focused on developing antibodies to end toxin to treat septic shock. Antibodies to end toxin have been used in clinical trials of sepsis with variable results [20 - 22]. TNF is released primarily from monocytes and macrophages. It is also released from natural killer cells, mast cells, and some activated T-lymphocytes.IL-1 is produced primarily by macrophages and monocytes. IL-1, previously known as the endogenous progeny, plays a central role in stimulating a variety of host responses, including fever production, lymphocyte activation, and endothelial cell stimulation, to produce pro- coagulant activity and to increase adhesiveness. IL-2, also known as T-cell growth factor, is produced by activated T-lymphocytes and strengthens the immune response by stimulating cell proliferation. It's clinically apparent side effects include capillary leak syndrome, tachycardia, hypotension, and increasedcardiac index, decreased SVR, and decreased left ventricular ejection fraction. Preterm and term newborns have poor responses to various antigenic stimuli, reduced gamma globulin levels at birth, and reduced maternal immunoglobulin supply from placental transport [23]. The use of intravenous immunoglobulin's (IVIGs) for the prophylaxis and treatment of sepsis in the newborn, especially the preterm, low birth weight infant, has been studied in numerous trials with varied outcomes [24]. PC Based on the marginal reduction of neonatal sepsis without a reduction in mortality, routine use of prophylactic IVIG cannot be recommended. Patients with severe septic shock often do not respond to conventional forms of volume loading and cardiovascular supportive medications. The administration of arginine vasopressin has been shown to decrease mortality in adult patients with recalcitrant septic shock (Table **1.3**).

Table (1.3). Vasoactive medications commonly used in newborn.

Vasoactive Agent	Principal Modes of Action	Major Hemodynamic Effects	Administration and Dosage	Indications
Epinephrine	α and β agonist	Increases heart rate and myocardial contractility by activating β1 receptors	0.1 mL/kg of 1:10,000 solution given IV intracranial, or endotrachea l0.05–1.0 µg/kg/min IV	Cardiac resuscitation; short-term use when severe heart failure resistant to other drugs
Norepinephrine	α and β agonist	Increases BP by vasoconstriction with its greater action on β receptors	20–100 ng/kg/min initially, up to 1.0 µg/kg/min as base	Shock state with high cardiac output and low systemic vascular resistance
Vasopressin	ADH agonist in arterioles	May replace basal vasopres-sin levels in cases of severe hypotension	0.018–0.12 units/kg/h used as a rescue treatment	Restoration of vascular tone in vasodilator shock
Dopamine, low dose	Stimulates dopamine receptors	Decrease in vascular resistance in splanchnic, renal, and cerebral vessels	<5 µg/kg/min IV	Useful in managing Cardiogenic or hypovolemic shock or after cardiac surgery
Dopamine, intermediate dose **High dose**	Stimulates β1 receptors; myocardial Stimulates α receptors	Isotropic response Increased peripheral and renal vascular resistance	5–10 µg/kg/min IV 10–20 µg/kg/min IV	Blood pressure unresponsive to low dose Septic shock with low systemic vascular resistance

Vasoactive Agent	Principal Modes of Action	Major Hemodynamic Effects	Administration and Dosage	Indications
Dobutamine	Synthetic β1 agonist in low doses; α and β2 effects in higher doses	Increased cardiac output, increased arterial pressure; less increase in heart rate than with dopamine	1–10 μg/kg/min IV	Useful alternative to dopamine if increase in heart rate undesirable
Isoproterenol	β1 and β2 agonist	Increased cardiac output by positive isotropic and chronotropic action and increase in venous return; systemic vascular resistance generally reduced; pulmonary vascular resistance generally reduced	0.5–10.0 μg/kg/min IV	Useful in low-output situations, especially when heart rate is slow
Sodium nitropruside	Direct-acting vasodilator that relaxes arteriolar and venous smooth muscle	After load reduction; reduced arterial pressure	1–10 μg/kg/min IV (for up to ten minutes); 0.5–2.0 μg/kg/min IV	Hypertensive crisis; vasodilator therapy
Milrinone	Phosphodiesterase inhibitor relaxes arteriolar and venous smooth muscle via calcium/cyclic adenosine monophosphate	Increased cardiac output, slight decreased BP, increased oxygen delivery	75 μg/kg bolus IV, then 0.75– 1.0 μg/kg/min IV	Useful as an alternative or in addition to dopamine (may act synergistically) if increased heart rate undesirable

ANESTHETIC CONSIDERATIONS FOR PAEDIATRIC SURGICAL CONDITIONS

Preoperative Anesthesia Evaluation

Patients undergoing anesthesia benefit from a thorough preanesthetic/preoperative assessment and targeted preparation to optimize any coexisting medical conditions. The ASA Physical Status (PS) score is a means of communicating the condition of the patient but is not intended to represent operative risk and serves primarily as a common means of communication among care providers Table **1.4**. Any child with an ASA PS of 3 or greater should be seen by an anaesthesiologist prior to the day of surgery.

Table (1.4). ASA physical status classifications.

ASA classification	Patient status
1	A normal healthy patient
2	A patient with mild systemic disease
3	A patient with sever systemic disease
4	A patient with sever systemic disease that is a constant threat to life
5	A moribund patient who is not expected to survive without the operation
6	A declared brain-dead patient whose organs are being removed for donor purposes
E	An emergency modifier for any ASA classification when failure to immediately correct a medical condition poses risk to life or organ viability

General Principles

In addition to the physical examination, the essential elements of the preoperative assessment in all patients are listed in Box **1.1**.

Box 1.1. Essential Elements of the Preoperative Assessment (in Addition to Physical Examination).

Vital signs
Height/weight
Heart rate
Respiratory rate
Blood pressure
Pulse oximetry (both in room air and with supplemental O2 if applicable)
Allergies
Medications
Cardiac murmur
history Previous subspecialty encounters
Past aesthetic history including any adverse per aesthetic
Events
Emergence
delirium
Postoperative nausea and vomiting
Difficult intubation
Difficult IV access
Past surgical history
Family history of pseudo cholinesterase deficiency or malignant hyperthermia

Patient History

Documentation of allergy status is an essential part of the preoperative evaluation, particularly because prophylactic antibiotics may be administered prior to the incision.Allergies to certain antibiotics (especially penicillin, ampicillin, and cephalosporin) are the most common medication allergies in children presenting for an operation. Anaphylactic allergic reactions are rare, but can be life threatening if not diagnosed and treated promptly.It has been well documented that prophylactic medications (steroids, H1 and H2 blockers) are ineffective in preventing aphylaxis in susceptible patients. If anaphylaxis occurs (hypotension, urticaria or flushing, bronchospasm), the mainstays of treatment are stopping the latex exposure: stopping the operation, changing to no latex gloves, and removing any other sources of latex; andresuscitation: fluids, intravenous (IV) epinephrine (bolus and infusion), steroids, Diphenhaydramine, and ranitidine. Family history should be reviewed for pseudo cholinesterase deficiency (prolonged paralysis after succinylcholine) or any first-degree relative who experienced malignant hyperthermia (MH).

MISCELLANEOUS CONDITIONS

Malignant Hyperthermia Susceptibility

The incidence of an MH crisis is 1:15,000 general anaesthetics in children, and 50% of patients who have an MH episode have undergone a prior general anaesthetic without complication. MH is an inherited disorder of skeletal muscle calcium channels, triggered in affected individuals by exposure to either inhalational anaesthetic agent (*e.g.*, isoflurane, desflurane, sevoflurane), succinylcholine, or both in combination, resulting in an elevation of intracellular calcium. However, many patients who develop MH have a normal history and physical examination. In the past, patients with mitochondrial disorders were thought to be at risk. Recent evidence suggests that the use of inhaled anaesthetic agents appears safe in this population, but succinylcholine should still be avoided, as some patients may have rhabdomyolysis (elevated CPK, hyperkalemia, myoglobinuria) with hyperkalemia without having MH (Box **1.2**).

Box 1.2. Muscle Diseases Associated with Malignant Hyperthermia.

Central core myopathy
Becker muscular dystrophy
Duchene muscular dystrophy
Myotonic dystrophy
King–Den borough syndrome

The resulting MH crisis is characterized by hyper metabolism (fever, hypercarbia, and acidosis), electrolyte derangement (hyperkalemia), arrhythmias, and skeletal muscle damage (elevated creatine phosphokinase [CPK]). This constellation of events may lead to death if unrecognized and/or untreated. Dantrolene, which reduces the release of calcium from muscle sarcoplasmic reticulum, when given early in the course of an MH crisis, has significantly improved patient outcomes. With early and appropriate treatment, the mortality is now less than 10%. Current suggested therapy can be remembered using the mnemonic "Some Hot Dude

Better Give Iced Fluids Fast" and is summarized in Box **1.3** [25].

Treatment of Malignant Hyperthermia Crisis

Box 1.3. Treatment of Malignant Hyperthermia Crisis.

"Some Hot Dude Better Give Iced Fluids Fast" **Stop all triggering agents, administer 100% oxygen Hyperventilate: treat Hypercarbia** **Dantrolene (2.5 mg/kg) immediately** **Bicarbonate (1 mEq/kg): treat acidosis** **Glucose and Insulin: treat hyperkalemia with 0.5 g/kg glucose, 0.15 units/kg insulin** **Iced Intravenous fluids and cooling blanket** **Fluid output: ensure adequate urine output: Furosemide and/or mannitol as needed** **Fast heart rate: be prepared to treat ventricular tachycardia**

Trisomy 21

Perioperative complications occur in 10% of patients with Trisomy 21 who undergo no cardiac surgery and include severe bradycardia, airway obstruction, difficult intubation, post-intubation croup, and bronchospasm. Patients may experience airway obstruction due to a large tongue and mid-face hyperplasia.The incidence of obstructive sleep apnea (OSA) may exceed 50% in these patients and may worsen after anesthesia and operation. Airway obstruction may persist even after adenotonsillectomy [26]. Many patients with Trisomy 21 have a smaller calibre trachea than children of similar age and size; therefore, a smaller Endotracheal tube (ETT) may be required. Some Trisomy 21 patients may have a longer segment of tracheal stenosis due to complete tracheal rings below the level of the cricoids.27Congenital heart disease (CHD) is encountered in 40–50% of patients with trisomy21. The most common defects are atrial and ventricular septal defects, tetralogy of Fallout, and atrioventricular (AV) canal defects. For children with a cardiac history, records from their most recent cardiology consultation and echocardiogram should be available for review at the time of preoperative evaluation.Patients with Trisomy 21 have laxity of the ligament holding the odontoid process of C2 against the posterior arch of C1, leading to atlantoaxial instability in about 15% of these patients. Cervical spine instability can potentially lead to spinal cord injury in the anaesthetic period. The need for and utility of preoperative screening for this condition is controversial.Even if the radiographic exam is normal, care should be taken preoperatively to keep the neck in as neutral a position as possible, avoiding extreme flexion, extension, or rotation, especially during tracheal intubation and patient transfer.

Preoperative Fasting Guideline

Research performed at our institution has demonstrated that intake of clear liquids (*i.e.*, liquids that print can be read through, such as clear apple juice or Pedialyte) up until 2 hours prior to the induction of anesthesia does not increase the volume or acidity of gastric contents [28]. Our policy is to recommend clear liquids until 2 hours prior to the patient's scheduled arrival time. Breast milk is allowed up to 3 hours before arrival for infants up to 12 months of age. Infant formula is allowed until 4 hours before arrival in infants <6 months old, and until 6 hours before arrival in babies 6–12 months old. All other liquids (including milk), solid food, candy, and gum are not allowed <8 hours before induction of anesthesia. Although these are the guidelines for our institution, the surgeon should be aware that NPO (nil per os) guidelines are variable and institutionally dependent.

Laboratory Tests

At the time of consultation, selected laboratory studies may be ordered, but routine laboratory work is usually not indicated. Policies vary among institutions regarding the need for preoperative haemoglobin testing. In general, for any patient undergoing a procedure with the potential for significant blood loss and need for transfusion a complete blood count (CBC) should be performed in the preoperative period. Certain medications, particularly anticonvulsants (tegretol, depakote), may be associated with abnormalities in blood components (white blood cells, red blood cells, platelets), making a preoperative CBC desirable. Although serum electrolytes are not routinely screened, electrolytes may be helpful in patients on diuretics. Preoperative glucose should be monitored in neonates, insulin- dependent diabetic patients, and also in any patient who has been receiving parenteral nutrition or IV fluids with a dextrose concentration >5% prior to surgery.Routine pregnancy screening in all females who have passed menarche is strongly recommended. An age-based guideline (at our institution, any female >11 years of age) may be preferable.The nature of the planned operation may also require additional studies, such as coagulation screening (Prothrombin time [PT], partial thromboplastin time [PTT], international normalized ratio [INR]) prior to craniotomy, tonsillectomy, or surgeries with anticipated large blood loss.

Post Anaesthetic Apnea

Even without the additional burden of anaesthetic/opioid- induced respiratory depression, the risk of apnea is increased in ex-premature infants due to the immaturity of the central and peripheral chemoreceptor, with blunted responses to hypoxia and hypercapnia.In addition, anaesthetic agents decrease upper airway, chest wall, and diaphragmatic muscle tone, thereby further depressing the ventilator response to hypoxia and hypercapnia. Also, although most apneic episodes occur within the first 2 hours after anesthesia, apnea can be seen up to 18 hours postoperatively. The increased risk of apnea impacts post anaesthetic care of infants born prematurely, mandating that those at high risk be admitted for cardio respiratory monitoring. A Hematocrit<30% was identified as an independent risk factor, with the recommendation that ex-premature infants with this degree of anaemia be hospitalized postoperatively for observation regardless of post conceptual age.

Anterior Meditational Mass

It has long been recognized that the anaesthetic management of the child with an anterior meditational mass (AMM) can be very challenging and fraught with the risk of sudden airway and cardiovascular collapse. Patients presenting with AMMs (*e.g.*, lymphoma) are at particularly high risk of airway compromise and cardiovascular collapse with the induction of general anesthesia due to compression of the trachea, great vessels, or right-sided cardiac chambers when intrinsic muscle tone is lost and spontaneous respiration ceases [29, 30]. The absence of signs and symptoms of airway compression and cardiovascular compromise does not preclude the possibility of life-threatening airway collapse or cardiovascular obstruction upon induction of anesthesia. Several studies have confirmed the lack of correlation between presenting cardiopulmonary symptoms and the presence of airway or vascular compression on computed tomography (CT) scan, emphasizing the importance of preoperative testing regardless of reported symptomatology in order to best assess Perioperative risk [31, 32]. The preoperative evaluation should begin with a careful history to elicit any respiratory symptoms that could indicate the presence of tracheal compression and/or tracheomalacia, including cough, dyspnea, wheezing, chest pain, dysphagia, orthopnea, and recurrent pulmonary infections. Symptoms may be positional, occurring when supine and improving when sitting. Chest CT is helpful in planning the anaesthetic technique and in evaluating the potential for airway compromise during anesthesia Echo-cardiograph is useful to assess the pericardial status, myocardial contractility, and compression of the cardiac chambers and major vessels, and should be performed in as supine a position as possible. Flow-volume loops and fluoroscopy can also provide a dynamic assessment of airway compression that other tests cannot assess. When possible, percutaneous biopsy of the mass using local anesthesia with or without judicious doses of sedative medication is often ideal and poses the least risk to the patient (Figs. **2** and **3**).

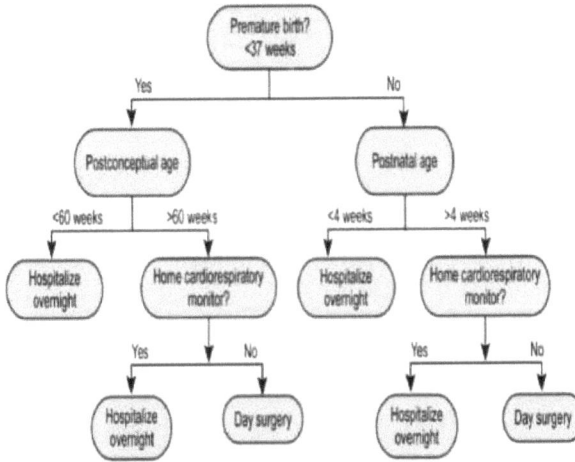

Fig. (2). This algorithm is useful for decision making regarding eligibility for outpatient surgery.

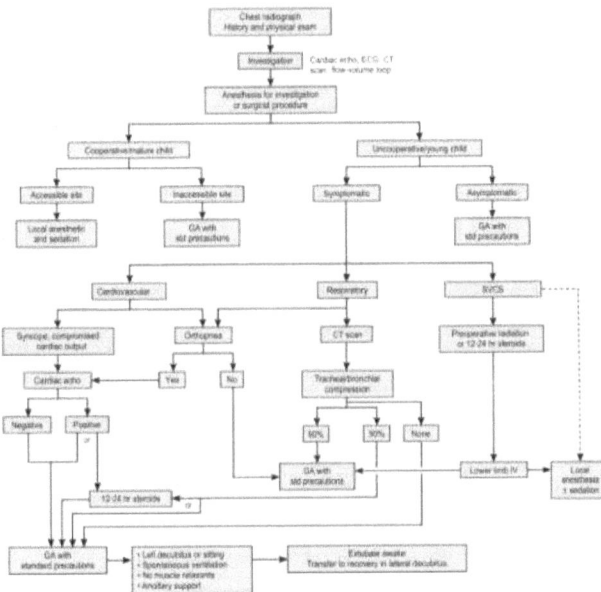

Fig. (3). This algorithm describes management of the patient with a large anterior meditational mass. GA, general anesthesia; SVCS, superior vena cava syndrome (Adapted from Cheung S, Lerman J. Meditational masses and anesthesia in children, in: Riazi J, editor, The Difficult Paediatric Airway. Anesthesiol Clin North Am 1998; 16:893–910).

Endocarditic Prophylaxis

Lesions associated with increased risk of infective endocarditic (IE) in children include cyanotic CHD, endocardium cushion defects, and left-sided lesions, with the relative risk of developing IE highest in the 6 months following cardiac surgery and in patients <3 years of age [33].

SPECIAL ISSUES IN PATIENTS WITH CONGENITAL HEART DISEASE

Pulmonary Hypertension

In children with CHD, prolonged exposure of the pulmonary vascular bed to high flows secondary to left-to-right shunting, pulmonary venous obstruction, or high left atrial pressures can lead to elevated pulmonary artery (PA) pressures and the development of pulmonary hypertension (PH). Other paediatric populations at risk for the development of PH include an increasing population of premature infants with BPD, and children with chemotherapy-induced PH, genetic conditions such as glycogen storage diseases and heritable PH, certain connective tissue diseases, and port pulmonary hypertension. Aesthetic management strategies are guided by three considerations: (1) appropriate manipulation of factors affecting pulmonary vascular resistance (PVR); theeffects of anaesthetic agents on PVR; and (3) maintenance of cardiac output (CO) and coronary perfusion pressures. Increases in PVR can potentially culminate in RV failure if excessive [34, 35]. Normal preload should be maintained and hypotension avoided in these patients in order to optimize CO, coronary artery flow, and oxygen supply to the RV. Dopamine, epinephrine, and Milrinone should be available to improve cardiac function if necessary, and inhaled nitric oxide should also be available intraoperative.

Cyanosis and Polycythemia

Cyanosis in patients with CHD can be the result of either right-to-left shunting with inadequate pulmonary blood flow (PBF) or admixture of oxygenated and deoxygenated blood in the systemic circulation. Severe, longstanding cyanosis causes a variety of systemic derangements including hematologic, neurologic, vascular, respiratory, and coagulation abnormalities. During preoperative evaluation, the child's baseline range of haemoglobin–oxygen saturation, heart rate, and blood pressure should be noted along with any history of stroke, seizure, or pre-existing neurologic defects. Care should be taken intraoperative to maintain normal fluid balance and cardiac function. The use of air filters in the IV lines and meticulous attention to air in volume lines without filters is essential to avoid the occurrence of paradoxical emboli in children with right-to-left shunts. Controlled ventilation is recommended for all but the shortest procedures due to the ventilator abnormalities in these patients. Preoperative phlebotomy is recommended only in patients who have Hematocrit $\geq$ 65%, are experiencing symptoms of hyper viscosity, and are not dehydrated. The acute onset of symptomatic hyper viscosity syndrome can be seen in cyanotic patients whose Hematocrit abruptly increases due to dehydration. In these patients, rehydration is recommended rather than phlebotomy (Box **1.4**).

Box 1.4. Cardiac Conditions for Which Antibiotic Prophylaxis with Dental, Respiratory Tract, Gastrointestinal, and Genitourinary Procedures is Indicated.

Congenital heart disease (CHD)
Unrepaired cyanotic CHD, including palliative shunts and conduits
Completely repaired congenital heart defect with prosthetic material or device, whether placed by surgery or by catheter intervention, during the first 6 months after the procedure
Repaired CHD with residual defects at the site or adjacent to the site of a prosthetic patch or prosthetic device (which inhibit endothelialization)
Cardiac transplantation recipients who develop cardiac valvulopathy
Prosthetic cardiac valves
Previous infective endocarditic

The Difficult Pediatric Airway

The patient with a "difficult airway" may require advanced airway management techniques in order to secure his or her airway including the lighted stylet, video laryngoscope, flexible fibber optic bronchoscope, direct laryngoscope with incubating stylet, fibber optic rigid laryngoscope, an anterior commissural scope, laryngeal mask airway (LMA) facilitated fibber optic intubation, cricothyrotomy, and tracheotomy. Anaesthesiologists and facilities do not need availability of all of the listed techniques (Table **1.5**).

Table 1.5. Syndromes and Craniofacial Abnormalities Associated With Difficult Intubation.

Syndrome	Associated Features
Arthrogryposis	Limited mouth opening and cervical mobility
Beckwith-wiedmann	Macroglossia
Freeman-Sheldon (whistling face)	Microsomal
Goldenhar syndrome (hemi facialmicrosomal)	Hemi facialmicrosomal, mandiblehyperplasia (uni-or bilateral)
Klippel–feil	Limited cervical mobility
Mucopolysaccharidoses (*e.g.*, hurler)	Macroglossia, limited cervical mobility, infiltration of tongue, supraglottis
Peirrerobin	Micrognathia, glossopteris, cleft palate
Treacher-collins	Maxillary, mandiblehyperplasia
Trisomy 21 (down)	Macroglossia, subglottic stenosis, atlantoaxial instability

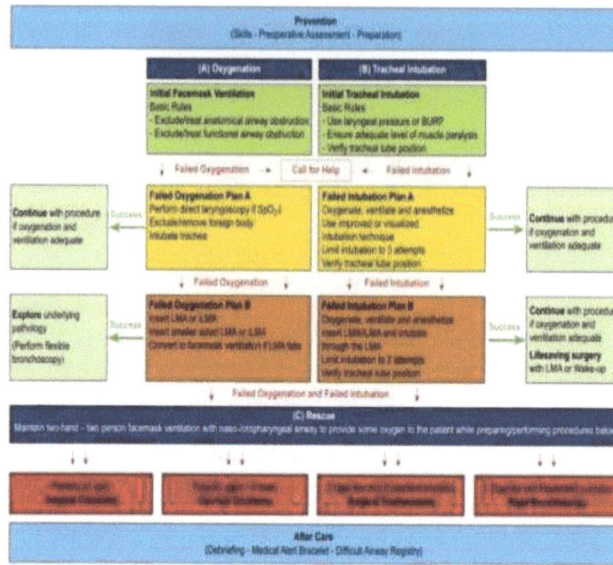

Fig. (4). This algorithm can be useful in the management of the infant/child who is difficult to ventilate and/or intubated (Adapted from Weiss M, Engelhardt T. Proposal for the management of the unexpected difficult paediatric airway. Paediatr Anaesth 2010; 20:454–464, used with the permission of the Difficult Airway Society (DAS).) LMA, Laryngeal Mask Airway.

Post Anesthesia Care

The recovery period for infants and children may be more crucial than for adult patients, with 3–4% of infants and children developing major complications in the recovery period, compared with only 0.5% of adults. Most of these complications occur in the youngest children (<2 years of age) and are most commonly respiratory in nature (Fig. **4**) [36].

Common Postanestheia Problems

Postoperative events can include pain, emergence delirium, nausea and/or vomiting, hypoxia, and stridor, which may be due to laryngospasm or subglottic edema. Persistence of these conditions can delay discharge. The most common minor adverse effects of anesthesia include throat pain or discomfort from airway tubes, and postoperative nausea and vomiting (PONV). These issues should be discussed with families preoperatively, along with assurances of prophylaxis and/or treatment if necessary.

Postoperative Nausea and Vomiting

PONV is the most common cause of delayed discharge from the postanestheia care unit (PACU) and the most common reason for unanticipated hospitalization following outpatient operations [37, 38]. Certain procedures, such as strabismus surgery, middle ear surgery, orchidopexy, and umbilical hernia repair, are associated with a >50% incidence of postoperative vomiting. Similarly, the perioperative use of any opioid is associated with a very high incidence of PONV, even when general anaesthetic drugs associated with a lower incidence of nausea, such as propofol, are used [39]. Common approaches to treat or prevent PONV include alteration of the anaesthetic technique Perioperative administration of an antiemetic (either pro-phylactically or as treatment), and limitation of postoperative oral intake [40, 41].

Respiratory Complications

Respiratory complications are the most serious of the common problems seen postoperatively in infants and children. All respiratory complications are more common in children with a recent history of respiratory tract infection.The incidence of post-intubation croup has decreased from 6% to 1% of all intubated children [42]. This reduction has occurred because of the development and use of sterile, implant-tested ETTs, routine humidification of anaesthetic gases, and the use of an appropriately sized (air leak pressure of <25 cm water) ETT. Laryngospasm, while potentially life threatening, is almost always transient and treatable by early application of continuous positive airway pressure (CPAP) by mask combined, if necessary, with a small dose of propofol (1–2 mg/kg). Rescue with succinylcholine is indicated if oxygen denaturation persists despite CPAP and propofol. Laryngospasm can also occur in the OR during anaesthetic induction or emergence from anesthesia. Patients at an increased risk of late go's patients include those with a recent history of a URI [43, 44]. Bronchospasm is more common in children with poorly controlled asthma and those exposed to secondhand smoke. It is most often managed with administration of nebulizer β-agonists such as albuterol [44].

Intraoperative Awareness

Intraoperative awareness is a rare but disturbing condition in which patients undergoing an operation and anesthesia can recall surroundings, sounds, events, and sometimes even pain. The definition of intraoperative awareness is: becomingconscious during a procedure performed under general anesthesia, with subsequent explicit memory of specific events that took place during that time. Certainly, the likelihood of a clear memory of a painful event during surgery is a much rarer event than the other events more commonly reported. However, there are multiple adverse consequences of intraoperative awareness, including post-traumatic stress disorder and medical legal implications.

Pain Management

The goal of postoperative pain management should be to achieve good pain relief with minimal adverse effects. Effective pain management is associated with early mobilization, more rapid recovery, and faster return to work, school, and play. The management of pain in infants and children is hampered by the difficult that exists in assessing pain. Many children may respond to pain by emotionally withdrawing from their surroundings, and this may be misinterpreted by the medical and nursing staff as evidence that they have no pain. In addition, when questioned as to their degree of pain, children may not volunteer useful information for fear of painful interventions (*e.g.*, "shots"). Examples of these pain scales include Crying, requires O$_2$, Increased vital signs, Expression, Sleepless (CRIES) for neonates (until 1 month of age), Face, Legs, Activity, Cry, Consol ability (FLACC) from 1 month to age 4 years, FACES for ages 5–9 years and in children who are developmentally appropriate, and a numerical scale for those older than 10 years of age [45, 46].

Opioid

Opioid remain the mainstay in pain control postoperatively, although regional analgesic techniques (epidural or peripheral nerve block) are being increasingly used in infants and children, resulting in a decrease in Perioperative opioid requirements. There are many opioid available for both IV and oral administration, but they all have common adverse effects. These include dose-dependent respiratory depression, dysphagia, somnolence, nausea and vomiting, pruritus, constipation, and urinary retention. Morphine remains the standard by which the potency of other opioid is measured morphine is best administered in a patient-controlled device (patient-controlled analgesia [PCA]) to allow self-titration of medication according to the level of pain experienced. Patients receiving PCA should be continuously monitored for cardiorespiratory depression by monitoring the echocardiogram, respiratory rate, and pulse oxeimetry [47]. When PCA devices are not used, the intermittent bolus administration of morphine to opioid-naive children should be started at 0.05–0.1 mg/kg every 2–4 hours. If the treatment of pain is initiated in the PACU or intensive care setting, similar doses may be administered every 5–10 minutes until the child is comfortable. Fentanyl is a synthetic opioid that usually has a relatively short duration of action as a result of its rapid distribution into fat and muscle due to its high lipid solubility. When compared with morphine, fentanyl is about 100 times more potent. Hydromorphone is a well-tolerated alternative to morphine and fentanyl, and is thought to cause less pruritus and sedation than morphine.

Nonsteroidal Anti-Inflammatory Drugs

Acetaminophen is an effective analgesic for mild to moderate pain and can be administered rectally in the Perioperative period, especially to infants. Rectal absorption is variable and bioavailability is lower, mandating a higher initial dose (30–40 mg/kg) than that administered orally (10–15 mg/kg) [48, 49]. A rectal dose of 30 mg/kg of acetaminophen has proved to have analgesic properties similar to 1 mg/kg of ketorolac. Ketorolac is a nonsteroidal anti-inflammatory drug (NSAID) with both oral and parenteral formulations that has been shown to have excellent pain control characteristics un-associated with PONV or respiratory depression. Dosage recommendations are 0.5 mg/kg IV (maximum dose 30 mg) every 6–8 hours for 48 hours. Due to its effects on renal blood flow and tubular function, ketorolac is contraindicated in patients with pre-existing impairment of renal function.

Discharge Criteria

In general, children should be comfortable, awake, and stable, on room air or back to baseline oxygen supplementation, have age-appropriate vital signs, and be well hydrated before discharge from outpatient surgery. These variables have been quantified with the modified Alderet score as in the Box **1.5**.

Box 1.5. Criteria for Discharge Home from the Post anesthesia Care Unit.

Return to preoperative level of consciousness
Normothermia (≥35.5°C)
No oxygen requirement (or return to baseline oxygen requirement)
Return to preoperative level of motor function (excepting expected effects of nerve block) Acceptable pain control
No ongoing vomiting, minimal nausea
Absence of surgical bleeding
At least 30 minutes after last administration of opioid
Discharge acceptable to surgeon
Oral intake (if required by surgeon)

Vascular Access

Obtaining vascular access of any kind is especially challenging in children. A peripheral intravenous (PIV) cannula is the most commonly used device for venous access. Placement of an intravenous catheter in children can be quite traumatic to the child, the parents, and the attendant health care providers. In some situations, it can be a fairly frustrating and time-consuming procedure, frequently requiring multiple attempts [1]. The specific vascular access device (VAD) and the site chosen for its placement to obtain venous access is based on the indications, urgency of need, and expected duration of use. In an emergency, other options should be considered after a few failed attempts at PIV cannula insertion. Historically, the only available options were a venous cutdown or an emergency central venous catheter (CVC). These options take considerable time and often require the services of a paediatric surgeon. Intraosseous (IO) needle placement is the most common contingency method of emergency vascular access in children. Mechanical IO introducer devices allow for easier training of emergency medical personnel and have improved the success rate of IO placement in the pre-hospital setting. With appropriate training, an IO needle can be placed more quickly than a PIV cannula [2]. In sick neonates, umbilical vessels are frequently cannulated but can be used for only a finite period (maximum of 5 days for an umbilical artery catheter [UAC] and 14 days for an umbilical venous catheter [UVC]) [3, 4]. Early placement of a peripherally introduced central catheter (PICC) is preferable in these infants. Persistence with using PIV cannula leads to higher complication rates and reduces the number of future PICC placement sites. Complications that are common to all types of VADs are extravasations of infuscate, hemorrhage, phlebitis, septicaemia, thrombosis, and thromboembolic. Multiple studies have shown that catheter-related blood stream infections can be prevented with appropriate education and training utilizing insertion and maintenance bundles [4 - 7].

Peripheral Venous Access

Insertion of a PIV is the most frequently used method of gaining vascular access. In infants and children, PIV access is usually achieved by using the veins on the dorsum of the hand, forearm, dorsum of the foot, medial aspect of the ankle, and the scalp. In infants, the median vein tributaries on the ventral aspect of the distal forearm and wrist and the lateral tributaries of the dorsal venous arch on the dorsum of the foot may be available, but typically allow cannulation of only the finest-diameter catheters. The location of the distal long saphenous vein (anterior to the medial malleolus) is fairly constant and is frequently palpable, making it one of the most popular veins used for PIV access, particularly in infants. It allows a larger catheter and excellent stabilization of the catheter as well. Scalp veins can be readily visible and accessible, but it can be difficult to maintain access for any length of time. Similarly, external jugular vein catheters tend to get dislodged promptly in a moving patient and may be useful for only a short time. Several techniques have been shown to be beneficial in cumulating a peripheral vein, including warming the extremity, transillumination [8] and epidermal vasodilators [9], Ultrasound (US) guidance has been used to obtain access to basilica and brachial veins in the emergency department [10, 11]. Devices utilizing near-infrared imaging of the veins up to a depth of 10 mm are being used routinely in the hospitals, as well as by emergency medical personnel in the field, to find and access peripheral veins in all age groups [8, 12].

Umbilical Vein and Artery Access

Neonates are often managed with catheters placed either in the umbilical vein and/ or one of the umbilical arteries. They can be used for monitoring central venous or arterial pressure, blood sampling, fluid resuscitation, medication administration, and total parenteral nutrition (TPN). To minimize infectious complications, the UVCs are usually removed after a maximum of 14 days [4, 13]. These catheters are typically placed by neonatal nurse practitioners or neonatologists and require dissection of the umbilical cord stump within a few hours of birth.It is possible for the paediatric surgeon to cannulated the umbilical vessels after the umbilical stump has undergone early desiccation. A small vertical skin incision is made above or below the umbilical stump to access the umbilical vein or artery, respectively. Once the fascia is incised, the appropriate vessel is identified, isolated, and cannulated. The tip of the UVC should be positioned at the junction of the inferior vena cava (IVC) and the right atrium (RA) [14] the xiphisternum is a good landmark for the RA/IVC junction. On the chest radiograph, the tip of the UVC should be at or above the level of the diaphragm (Fig. **1.5**). These umbilical vessel catheters have been associated with various complications. In addition to tip migration, sepsis and vessel thrombosis can occur. Additionally, UVCs have been associated with perforation of the IVC, extravasations of infuscate into the peritoneal cavity, and portal vein thrombosis [15] UACs are associated with aortic injuries, thromboembolic of the aortic branches, aneurysms of the iliac artery and/or the aorta, paraplegia, and gluteal ischemia with possible necrosis [14].

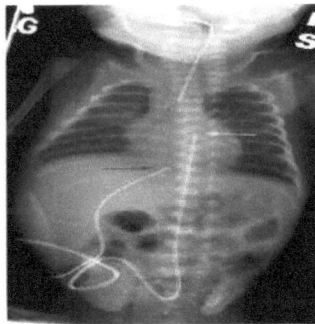

Fig. (1.5). Abdominal and chest film of a newborn shows the umbilical artery catheter at the level of the seventh thoracic vertebral body (yellow arrow) and the umbilical venous catheter (red arrow) at the level of the diaphragm, these are the recommended positions for these catheters.

Peripherally Introduced Central Catheter

PICC lines provide reliable central venous access in neonates and older children without the need for directly accessing the central veins. PICC lines are suitable for infusion of fluids, medications, TPN, and blood products. Many institutions caring for sick children have developed special teams and protocols for placement of PICC lines to reduce variations in practice and increase availability [16]. The modified Salinger technique is used most frequently. A small PIV catheter (about 24 gauges) is first placed, preferably with US guidance, in a suitable extremity vein such as the basilica, cephalic, or long saphenous vein. A fine guide wire is advanced through the catheter and into the vein, and the initial catheter is removed. The track is then dilated, and a peel-away PICC introducer sheath is advanced over the guide wire. The guide wire is then removed, and the PICC line is introduced through the sheath (Fig. **1.6**). The tip of the PICC should be placed at the superior vena cava (SVC)/RA junction or the IVC/RA junction. Tip locations peripheral to these are considered noncentral and are associated with higher complications [17] PICC lines are also eminently suitable for short- to medium-term (weeks) home intravenous therapy of antibiotics or TPN [18]. The most common complications associated with PICC lines are infections, occlusion, and dislodgement of the catheter [36].

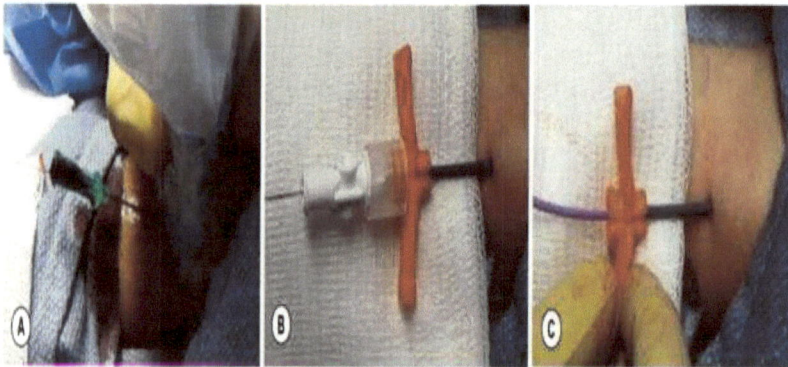

Fig. (1.6). This sequence of three photographs demonstrates peripherally inserted central venous catheter placement using Seldinger technique. (A) The cephalic vein is being accessed in the left antecubital fossa with real-time ultrasound guidance. (B) A vein dilator with peel-away sheath has been situated over the guide wire. (C) The catheter is being advanced through the peel-away sheath.

Central Venous Catheters

With the development of PICC teams and the increasing use of PICC lines, there has been a decline in the use of CVCs in neonates and older children [16]. Non-tunnelled CVCs are used for short- and medium-term indications, whereas surgically placed tunnelled CVCs are used for medium- and long-term indications. In premature neonates, if PICC placement is not successful, tunnelled CVCs are preferentially used because of their smaller size and durability as opposed to no tunnelled CVCs. The central veins accessed for placement of CVCs are the bilateral internal jugular veins, subclavian veins, and femoral vein. In older children and full-term neonates, the percutaneous Salinger technique is used. Use of US guidance for percutaneous central venous access is the standard of care for the internal jugular and femoral sites. The benefits of US assistance include a higher success rate, faster access, fewer needle passes, and fewer arterial punctures [20 - 25]. Real-time two- dimensional US guidance is recommended when placing a CVC into the internal jugular vein (IJV) in adults and children in elective situations [22]. The majority of blood stream infections in children are associated with the use of a vascular access device.

Tunnelled CVCs inserted in the neck veins in neonates have been associated with a higher rate of complications than those placed in the femoral region.

Totally Implanted Central Venous Catheter

Totally implantable intravascular devices (ports) are subcutaneous reservoirs attached to CVCs. The reservoirs are made of a metal or hard plastic shell with a central silicone septum that is penetrated for access. They provide a reliable, long-lasting solution for patients who need intermittent access to their central venous system. They are ideal for patients who desire to be involved in aquatic sports and other physical activities. They are most useful for patients with malignancies, coagulopathy, haemolytic syndromes, and renal failure, all of which require continuous vascular access. Low-profile ports with 5- or 6-Fr catheters are available for use in infants. Larger ports are available with dual lumens. High-flow ports are available (Power Port Bard Access Systems, Salt Lake City, UT) that allow high-pressure injection of intravenous contrast for radiologic imaging. Ports require special noncoring needles to keep the septum from leaking. The reservoir should be implanted in a subcutaneous pocket, over a firm base such as the chest wall. Preferred sites for port placement include the pectoral area, parasternal area, (above and medial to the areola), and the subclavicular area (medial to the anterior auxiliary fold). In females with a concern for cosmoses, the low presternum area and the lateral chest wall (Fig. **1.7**) are locations that hide the scar when the port is eventually removed. Ports have been shown to be associated with lower complications in children undergoing outpatient cancer treatment when compared with PICCs and CVCs [26].

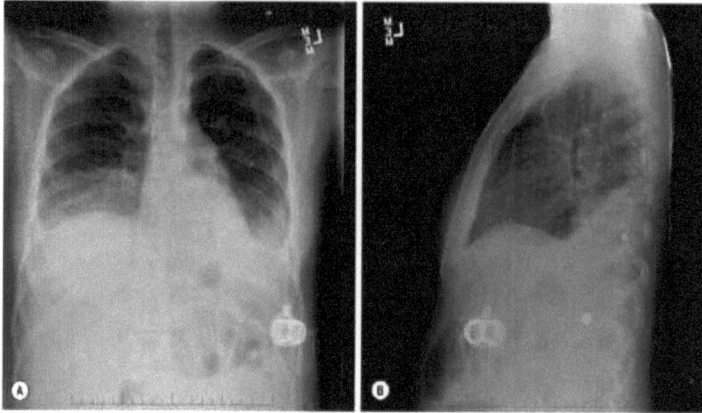

Fig. (1.7). This 17-year-old girl is being treated with chemotherapy. On the anteroposterior (A) and lateral (B) chest films, note the portacath has been placed on the lateral aspect of the left thoracic cage, and below her left breast.

Intraosseous Access

Several studies have been published over the past 60 years establishing the safety and electiveness of IO access for infusion of fluids and medications in children, including neonates [27, 28]. IO access has also been shown to be faster than access with a PIV3 and safer than an emergency CVC. Bone marrow consists of rich lattice network of vessels. Whereas the peripheral veins collapse in patients in shock, the vascular spaces in the bone marrow do not [60]. The bioavailability of resuscitative drugs administered through IO access has been well established and shown to be better than that of those administered through an Endotracheal tube [30, 31]. The current Paediatric Advanced Life Support (PALS) recommendation is to establish IO access promptly if PIV access cannot be attained rapidly in neonates and children of all ages who need intravenous drugs or fluids urgently.32In children, the long bones of the lower extremities are used preferentially for IO placement. The proximal tibia is the most common site, followed by the distal femur. With full sterile precautions, a needle designed for bone marrow aspiration is advanced through the cortical bone to access the bone marrow. In an infant, a spinal needle may be used, but in an older child, a generic bone marrow needle or a purpose-designed IO needle such as the widely used Jamshidi needle (Cardinal Health, McGraw Park, IL) is used [30 - 34]. The anteromedial flat surface of the tibia, 1–3 cm caudal to the tibial tuberosity, is the best site. A small skin incision is made using the tip of a pointed scalpel or a large-bore hypodermic needle. The IO needle is positioned pointing posteriorly and angled slightly caudad. It is then advanced through the cortical bone using ascrewing and unscrewing motion with constant pressure. Once the needle penetrates the outer cortex, a sudden "give" is felt. The needle is held in this position, and the obdurate is removed. A syringe is attached, and bone marrow is aspirated to confirm correct placement. The IO needle is stabilized with a dressing. The distal femur location is accessed by placing the needle 1–3 cm cephalad to the patella, and angled slightly cranial to avoid the growth plate. Contraindications to IO placement include injury or suspected injury to the bone or soft tissue overlying the placement site.

Venous Cutdown

Paediatric surgeons should maintain the knowledge and skills required to perform this procedure [9]. The vessel of choice is the long saphenous vein near the medial malleolus. The vein is superficial, it is of satisfactory size, and there is minimal subcutaneous fat in this location. A transverse incision is made anterior and cephalad to the medial malleolus. The vein is readily identified by dissecting through the thin subcutaneous tissue and is stabilized by placing proximal and distal stay ligatures. The vein is then directly cannulated using a venous catheter of appropriate size relative to the vein, and the catheter is anchored to the adjacent skin.

Arterial Catheter

Intra-arterial catheters allow continuous hemodynamic monitoring and blood sampling. The radial artery at the wrist is most commonly used for intra-arterial access due to the excellent collateral circulation. The dorsalis pedis and posterior tibial arteries are other peripheral sites that may sometimes be used. Femoral arteries are frequently used by cardiologists for catheter-based cardiac interventions and occasionally for monitoring. However, in general, it is advisable not to use the main artery of an extremity for chronic arterial catheter placement to avoid thromboembolic and ischemic complications [5]. Adequacy of collateral arterial supply through the ulnar artery should be confirmed before placement of a radial arterial line by using the Allen test [34]. The right radial artery allows predictable monitoring and sampling.

Hemodialysis Catheters

The current recommendation is to use an autologous arteriovenous fistula (AVF) as the route of choice for hemodialysis. AVFs permit high-flow rates that facilitate effective dialysis [35, 36]. They also are reliable, durable, and, once established, have low complication rates. Because patients are often referred late, and AVFs take time to mature, there is frequently a need for CVCs for immediate dialysis. Temporary and tunnelled long-term, double-lumen hemodialysis catheters are placed preferentially through the right IJV, either percutaneous or by cut down (Fig. **1.8**). The larger size of the vein and the straight internal path of the catheter allow a larger catheter to be placed safely through the right IJV.

Additionally, use of the IJV avoids possible injury or thrombosis to the SCV, which must be patent to develop a functioning AVF at the wrist. The long- term, cuffed hemodialysis catheters are precurved to allow right IJV placement with tunnelling to the pectoral area. Flow rates achieved through hemodialysis catheters tend to be lower, and they last a relatively short time. AVF is also an option for management of young children with severe haemophilia [37].

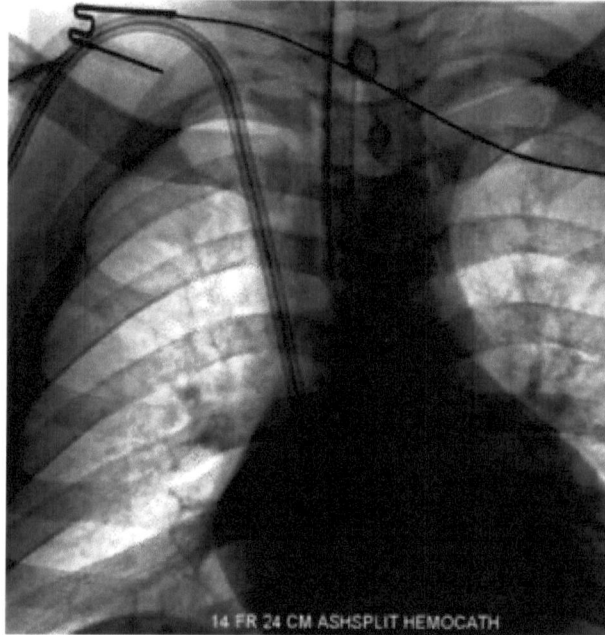

14 FR 24 CM ASHSPLIT HEMOCATH

Infection continues to be a significant source of mortality and morbidity for children despite improvements in antimicrobial therapy, aseptic surgical technique, and postoperative intensive care. Widespread unchecked antibiotic use has led to the development of more resistant organisms, leading to a rather complex and arduous process of selecting the appropriate antibiotic, especially as newer antibiotics is continually developed [1, 2]. In addition, infections with uncommon organisms are becoming more frequent with diminished host resistance from immunosuppressive states such as immaturity, cancer, systemic diseases, and transplant procedures. Surgical infections, by definition, often require some operative intervention, such as incision and drainage (I&D) of an abscess or removal of necrotic tissue, and often do not respond to antibiotics alone.

Pathogenesis of Infection

The evolution of infection involves a complex interaction between the host and the infectious agent. Four components are important: virulence of the organism, size of the inoculums, presence of a nutrient source for the organism, and a breakdown in the host's defence.

Virulence

The virulence of any microorganism depends on its ability to cause damage to the host. Exotoxin, such as streptococcal hyaluronidase, is digestive enzymes released locally by some organisms that allow the spread of infection by breaking down host extracellular matrix proteins. End toxins, such as lipopolysaccharide, are components of gram-negative cell walls that are released only after bacterial cell death. Once systemically absorbed, end toxins trigger a severe and rapid systemic inflammatory response by releasing various endogenous mediators such as cytokines, bradykinine, and prostaglandins.3Surgical infections occasionally may be polymicrobial, involving various interactions among the microorganisms and toxins.

Inoculum

The size of the inoculums is the second important component of an infection. The number of colonies of microorganisms per gram of tissue is the key determinant. Predictably, any decrease in host resistance decreases the absolute number of colonies necessary to cause clinical disease. In general, if the bacterial population in a wound exceeds 100,000 organisms per gram of tissue, an invasive infection is present [4].

Nutrients

For any inoculums, the environment determines the viability and survival. Therefore, the presence of suitable nutrients for the organism is essential and comprises the third component of any clinical infection. Accumulation of necrotic tissue, hematoma, and foreign matter is an excellent nutrient medium for continued organism growth and spread. Of special importance to the surgeon is the concept of necrotic tissue and infection [5] when present at an infected site, this tissue often needs to be debrided to restore the host–bacterial balance and lead to effective wound healing [6].

Host Defence

Finally, for a clinical infection to arise, the body's defences must be overwhelmed. Even highly virulent organisms can be eradicated before clinical infection occurs if the host resistance is intact.

DEFENCE AGAINST INFECTION

Anatomic Barrier

Intact skin and mucous membranes provide an effective surface barrier to infection [7]. These tissues barriers are not merely a mechanical obstacle, but rather possess physiologic characteristics that provide an extra layer of protection. In the skin, thermoregulation, the constant turnover of keratinocytes, and acid secretion from sebaceous glands inhibits bacterial cell growth. The mucosal surfaces like-wise have developed advanced defence mechanisms to prevent and combat microbial invasion, where specialized epithelial layers provide resistance to infection.

Immune Response

The immune system involves complex pathways and many specialized effector responses. The initial line of defence is the more primitive and nonspecific innate system, which consists primarily of phagocytic Neutrophils and the serum- based complement system. The Neutrophil is able to rapidly migrate to the source of the infection and engulf and destroy the infecting organisms by phagocytosis. In the complement system, cytokines, low molecular weight proteins including tumour necrosis factor (TNF), and many interleukins that attract and activate Neutrophils, play a significant role in mediating the inflammatory response.

Humoral and Cell-Mediated Immunity

The more specialized, adaptive immune system involves a highly specific response to antigens as well as the eventual production of a variety of humoral mediators [8] B-cell immunity is provided by antibodies. The first exposure of an antigen leads to the production of IgM antibodies, whereas subsequent exposure to the same antigen results in rapid production of IgG antibodies. Humoral antibodies may neutralize toxins, tag foreign matter to aid phagocytosis (opsonization), or lyse invading cellular pathogens, plasma cells and nonthymicdependent lymphocytes that reside in the bone marrow and in the germinal centres and medullary cords of lymph nodes produce the reactive components of this humoral system. These agents account for most of the human immunity against extracellular bacterial species. The T-cell component of immunity is based on sensitized lymphocytes located in the sub cortical regions of lymph nodes and in the arterial spaces of the spleen. T-cells are specifically responsible for immunity to viruses, most fungi, and intracellular bacteria. They produce a variety of lymphocytes, such as transfer factors, which further activate lymphocytes; chemotactic factors; leukotrienes; and interferon.

Immunodeficiencies

Susceptibility to infection is increased when one of the components of the host defence mechanism is absent, reduced in numbers, or dysfunctional. Some of these derangements may be congenital in nature, although the majority is acquired as a direct result of medications, radiation, endocrine disease, surgical ablation, tumours, or bacterial toxins. Immunodeficiencies from any cause significantly increases the risk of infection both in hospitalized and postoperative patients. Mycotic (fungal) infections are an increasing problem, especially in immunocompromised paediatric patients [8].

Antibiotics

Antibiotics are classified based on their molecular structure, mechanism, and site of action. The varying antibiotic classes can be divided into bacteriostatic (which inhibit bacterial growth) and bactericidal (which destroy bacteria). Monitoring drug dosages in infants and children is important when treating them with antibiotics. The efficacy and safety of many drugs have not been established in children, especially in the newborn. Dosages based on paediatric pharmacokinetic data over the most rational approach. Dosage requirements constantly change as a function of age and body weight. Furthermore, the volume of distribution and half-life of many medications are often increased in neonates and children compared with adults for a variety of reasons [9, 10].

Prevention of Infections

The most effective way to deal with infectious complications is to prevent their occurrence. The clinician must there- fore be cognizant of the variables that increase the risk of infection and attempt to mitigate them. The World Health Organization, American College of Surgeons, and Centre for Disease Control all has recently published guidelines for prevention of surgical site infection (SSI) [11 - 14].

Patient Characteristic

In adults, comorbdities often increase the risk of a SSI. However, these chronic diseases are infrequently encountered in children. Attempting to reduce SSI with preoperative patient optimization continues to be a topic of investigation for surgeons. Adults with positive nasal methicillin-resistant *Staphylococcus aureus* (MRSA) have been shown to have a higher chance of MRSA SSI; however, the rate of MRSA SSI was <2% in one study [15]. Recent paediatric evidence suggests there is no correlation between positive nasal swabs and wound infection for elective surgeries, and *Staphylococcus aureus* eradication may not be needed preoperatively [16].

Surgical Preparation

Preoperative preparation of the surgical site and the sterility of the surgical team are very important in reducing the risk of postoperative infection. Hand hygiene remains the most important proactive mechanism to reduce infection by reducing the number of microorganisms present on the skin during an operation. In the United States, the conventional method for surgical team scrubbing has been a 5-minute first scrub followed by subsequent 2- or 3-minute scrubs for subsequent cases with either 5% povidoneiodine or 4% chlorhexidine gluconate. These scrubbing protocols can achieve a 95% decrease in skin flora [17, 18]. However, newer alcohol-based antiseptic cleaners with shorter applications, usually 30 seconds, have been shown to be as effective as, or even more effective than, hand washing in decreasing bacterial contamination [19 - 21]. Normothermia has also been suggested as a means to decrease the incidence of wound infections [38]. Infants and children are at particular risk for experiencing hypothermia during surgery due to an increased area-to-body weight ratio leading to greater heat loss [23]. Intraoperative hypothermia can potentially lead to serious complications, including coagulopathy, SSIs, and cardiac complications. Finally, adequate control of glucose levels preoperatively has also been demonstrated to decrease morbidity and mortality in both adult and paediatric surgical patients, particularly in those patients undergoing cardiac surgery [24 - 27].

Wound Classification

The infection risk for operative cases can be stratified into one of four levels Table **1.6**, with the risk of SSI increasing with each higher classification level. Preoperative, wound classification has commonly been used for SSI risk stratification, which is now used as a quality measure by hospitals and third-party payers [28 - 30]. Classifying the operation has also been incorporated into the routine preoperative time-out sessions.

Table 1.6. Wound classification.

Class	Definition
Clean	An uninfected operative wound in which no inflammation is encountered and the respiratory, alimentary, genital, or infected urinary tract is not entered. In addition, clean wounds are closed primarily and, if necessary, drained with closed drainage
Clean-contaminated	An operative wound in which the respiratory, alimentary, genital, or urinary tract is entered under controlled conditions and without unusual contamination

Contaminated	Open, fresh, accidental wounds. This includes operations with major breaks in sterile technique or gross spillage from the gastrointestinal tract and incisions in which acute, no purulent inflammation is encountered
Dirty	Old traumatic wounds with retained devitalized tissue and those that involve existing clinical infection or perforated viscera

Antibiotic Prophylaxis

Important points for preoperative antibiotic prophylaxis include using agents that cover the most probable intraoperative contaminants for the operation, optimal timing for the initial dose of antibiotic so that bactericidal concentrations are reached at the time of incision, and maintaining the appropriate serum levels throughout the operation [31]. Timing of the Perioperative antibiotic coverage is crucial. The first dose is generally given 30 minutes to 1 hour before the start of the operation. In operations that take more than the half-life of the administered drug, a second dose of prophylactic antibiotics is needed to reachieve adequate serum levels [32]. In paediatric surgery, it is clear that antibiotic coverage is required during clean contaminated, contaminated, or dirty cases. Antibiotic prophylaxis in clean cases, such as inguinal hernias, orchidopexy, and laparoscopic pyloromyotomies, has not been shown to decrease SSI and is probably not warranted [33, 34].

Bowel Preparation

The current bowel prep recommendations for adults under- going an elective colorectal operation is combined isosmotic mechanical bowel prep along with oral antibiotics [35]. The bowel prep includes mechanical irrigation and flushing of the colon to remove stool, oral antibiotics against colonic aerobes and anaerobes, and preoperative intravenous antibiotics that cover both common skin and colonic flora [36]. A recent large retrospective database study found that mechanical bowel preparation along with oral antibiotics reduced SSI, anastigmatic leak, and ileums for adult elective colorectal cases in comparison to mechanical bowel preparation alone and no mechanical bowel prep [37].

TYPES OF INFECTION

Postoperative Surgical Site Infection

Despite meticulous technique and Perioperative antibiotics, infectious complications still occur. Postoperative wound infections can be divided into superficial or deep [38]. Early diagnosis and prompt intervention help to avoid morbidity and occasional mortality. Erythema, fever, leukocytosis, tenderness, crepitus, and suppuration are concerning diagnostic signs but are not always present. When confronted with one or more of these signs, clinical judgment is important. Treatment may include oral or intravenous antibiotics, I&D, or extensive surgical debridement with supportive wound care (Fig. **1.9**). An abscess is a localized collection of pus in a cavity formed by an expanding infectious process (Fig. **1.9 A**). Pus is a combination of leukocytes, necrotic material, bacteria, and extracellular fluid. The usual cause is the staphylococcal species, especially methicillin-susceptible *Staphylococcus aureus* and MRSA [39] The Infectious Diseases Society of America (IDSA) practice guidelines recommend I&D for purulent skin and soft tissues infections (Fig. **1.9 B**) [40]. A phlegm on is an area of diffuse inflammation with little pus and some necrotic tissue. A phlegmon can often be treated with antibiotics, although it can progress to an abscess, which may require I&D Streptococcal soft tissue infections are probably the most virulent and can arise within a few hours after a surgical procedure (Fig. **1.10**). High fever, delirium, leukocytosis, and severe pain are hallmarks of these infections. Bacillus infections are the next most virulent infection. Inspection of the wound will show dark, mottled areas, as opposed to the bright pink of streptococcal cellulites. Fewer than half of patients with Bacillus infections have detectable gas crepitation. Severe pain is the most telling clinical symptom of this type of infection. High doses of penicillin and operative debridement of the necrotic tissue are the hallmarks of treatment for these patients.

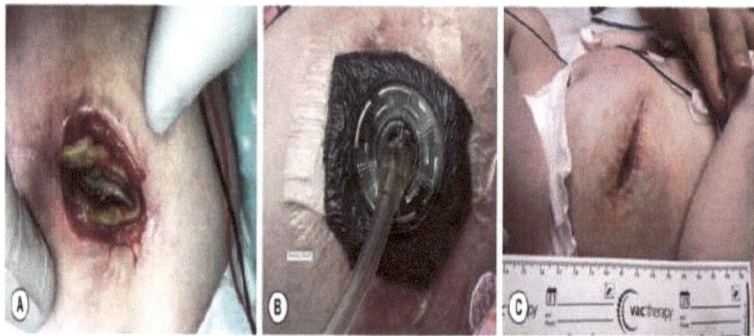

Fig. (1.9). This newborn underwent open left congenital diaphragmatic hernia repair using mesh for diaphragmatic replacement along with an abdominal wall mesh bridge. An infection developed in the left upper abdominal incision (A) that required removal of the mesh. After removing the mesh, the wound was left open and a Wound V.A.C.® was placed for wound healing (B). The wound healed nicely, and the Wound V.A.C.® was able to be removed. The photograph in C shows almost complete healing of the wound.

Nosocomial Infection

Nosocomial infections are defined as those infections that are hospital acquired [41]. As such, they are a potential threat to all hospitalized patients and significantly increase morbidity and mortality. Their incidence appears to be increasing as surgical care becomes more complicated and patients survive longer. The recent focus on patient safety has made prevention of nosocomial infections increasingly important. Pneumonia can be a lethal nosocomial infection, with mortality ranging from 20– 70%, and accounting for 10–15% of all paediatric hospital-acquired infections (HAIs) [42] The mortality rate is dependent on the causative organism.The risk factors for nosocomial pneumonia in the paediatric population include serious underlying illness, immunosuppressant, and length of time on a ventilator. Measures to prevent ventilator-associated pneumonia in children include elevating the head of the bed, daily assessment of readiness for extubation, and age-appropriate mouth care [43].

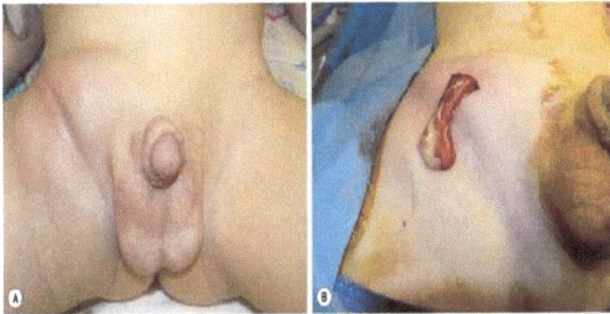

Fig. (1.10). This young boy developed a large expanding right inguino femoral abscess (A), (B) the abscess has been drained, and the purulent fluid is seen draining from the abscess.

Clostridium difficile is a well-recognized cause of infectious diarrhea that develops after antibiotic therapy in many patients, although it likely accounts for only 15–25% of antibiotic-associated diarrhea. It is a very common cause of HAI, and its incidence is increasing in frequency with associated increasing mortality [44 - 46]. The best method of prevention is the judicious and appropriate use of antibiotics.

Catheter Infections

Central venous catheters (CVCs) are essential for managing critically ill patients. CVCs include peripherally inserted CVC (PICC), no tunnelled/ tunnelled CVC, and venous access ports [47]. The use of CVCs in infants and children has increased as prolonged vascular access has become increasingly necessary to provide parenteral nutrition, chemotherapy, antimicrobial therapy, and hemodynamic monitoring.However, central-line associated blood stream infections (CLABSIs) are common, despite considerable effort to reduce their occurrence, and are associated with increased hospital costs, length of stay, and morbidity/mortality [48, 49]. CLABSIs are manifested as erythema at the site of insertion, tachycardia, and/or leukocytosis. Rates of infection are influenced by patient-related factors, by type and severity of illness, and by catheter-related parameters (catheter type, purpose, and conditions under which it was placed)

[50]. Coagulate-negative staphylococci, followed by *Staphylococcus aureus*, were the most frequently isolated causes of hospital-acquired blood stream infections in a report from the National Nosocomial Infections Surveillance System [51]. A number of factors are associated with the development of CLABSIs, including the sterility of the insertion technique, type of solution being administered through the line, care of the catheter once inserted, proximity of the catheter to another wound, and the presence of another infection elsewhere. Absolute sterile techniques should be maintained in all instances of line insertion whenever possible. Emergency situations may necessitate less-than-sterile technique. The use of maximal sterile barriers, including sterile gown, gloves, and a large sterile sheet, has been shown in adults to greatly reduce the risk of CLABSI [53]. The single most important factor in preventing CLABSI is hand hygiene. Standardized hand hygiene programs in neonatal care units have been found to decrease CLABSI rates [54, 55]. Studies suggest that chlorhexidine, compared with povidoneiodine, significantly reduces the incidence of CLABSI and microbial colonization, and 2% chlorhexidine preparations with alcohol are now recommended for skin antisepsis [52 - 57]. The skin and catheter hub are the most common sites/ sources of colonization and infection. Thus, various methods have been used to combat these risks. Chlorhexidine bathing has been shown to decrease CLABSI rates in the NICU, but its efficacy is unknown for children in the non- ICU setting [58]. Catheters have been coated with chlorhexidine/silver sulfadiazine as well as minocycline/Rifampin along with other agents [59, 60]. The use of these antibacterial-coated catheters has been approved by the U.S. Food and Drug Administration for use in patients weighing >3 kg. It is likely that the efficacy for reducing infection decreases after being in place for longer than 3 weeks because of a decrease in the antimicrobial activity [61].

OTHER INFECTIONS REQUIRING SURGICAL CARE AND TREATMENT

Necrotizing Soft Tissue Infection

Necrotizing soft tissue infection (NSTI) is a rapidly progressing infection of the facial tissues and overlying skin, with a hospital mortality of 7% [62]. Although these infections can occur as a postoperative complication or as a primary infection, necrotizing fasciitis is more likely in immunocompromised patients [63]. However, in the paediatric population, necrotizing fasciitis often effects previously healthy children and infants [64]. Because the diagnosis is often not obvious, the physician must look for clinical clues such as edema beyond the area of erythema, crepitus, skin vesicles, or cellulites refractory to intravenous antibiotics. Skin necrosis is generally a late sign and is indicative of thrombosis of vessels in the subcutaneous tissue. Necrotizing fasciitis often occurs in the truncal region in children as opposed to adults, in whom infection in the extremities is most common (Fig. **1.11**) [65]. Although infections with a single organism often occur in adults with necrotizing fasciitis, polymicrobial infections predominate in children [66]. Prompt surgical intervention, including wide excision of all necrotic and infected tissue, along with the institution of broad-spectrum antibiotics, is important to avoid progression and mortality. Necrotizing fasciitis can also occur as a complication of chickenpox [67]. In neonates, necrotizing fasciitis is seen secondary to omphalitis, balanitis, and fatal monitoring [68].

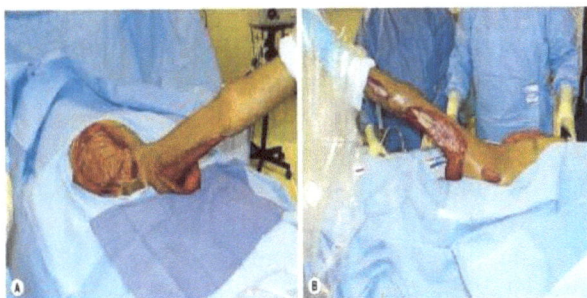

Fig. (1.11). This 15-year-old was ill for 2 weeks with perforated appendicitis and presented in shock. After a midline incision for exploration for a rigid abdomen, his appendix was removed.

Sepsis

Sepsis is defined as life-threatening organ dysfunction caused by a dysregulated host response to infection [69, 70]. The diagnostic criteria for sepsis differs for the paediatric population and is defined as: signs and symptoms of inflammation plus infection with hypo- or hyperthermia, tachycardia, and organ dysfunction (altered mental status, hypoxemia, increased serum lactate, or bounding pulses) [70]. Although there has been a decrease in the mortality rate among children with sepsis, the prevalence of severe sepsis in children has risen [71, 72]. Neonatal sepsis is defined as a generalized bacterial infection accompanied by a positive blood culture within the first month of life.Neonatal sepsis occurring during the first week of life is caused primarily by maternal organisms transferred during delivery. Maternal contamination can be transmitted through the placenta to the newborn *via* the birth canal or by direct contamination of the amniotic fluid. The mortality of this early onset sepsis approaches 50%. Late-onset neonatal sepsis is primarily nosocomial and is most often secondary to indwelling catheters or bacterial translocation from the gut.In the surgical neonate, three factors promote bacterial translocation and sepsis: (1) intestinal bacterial colonization and overgrowth, (2) com- promised host defences, and (3) disruption of the mucosal epithelial barrier [73]. The mortality associated with late- onset sepsis approaches 20%. The clinician must be alert for the subtle signs and symptoms of neonatal sepsis, which include lethargy, irritability, temperature instability, and a change in respiratory or feeding pattern. Neonates may not demonstrate leukocytosis. Empirical broad-spectrum coverage may be started, pending the results of blood and other cultures.

Peritonitis

Peritonitis is defined as inflammation of the peritoneum [74], it is divided into primary, secondary, and tertiary. Spontaneous primary peritonitis is a bacterial infection without enteric perforation. Primary peritonitis is usually caused by a single organism. An infant with primary peritonitis usually does not exhibit profound signs of peritonitis but may have poor feeding, lethargy, dissention, vomiting, and mild to severe abdominal tenderness. Definitive treatment may only require a course of broad-spectrum antibiotics.Secondary peritonitis is associated with gastrointestinal tract disruption. This can be caused by intestinal perforation, bowel wall necrosis, trauma, or postoperatively as a result of iatrogenic injury or an anastigmatic leak. In addition, secondary peritonitis also may result from an indwelling dialysis catheter or ventriculoperitoneal shunt [75]. These infections are generally polymicrobial. Treatment of secondary peritonitis is a combination of operative intervention, removal of any prosthetic device, and antibiotics. Tertiary peritonitis, also called recurrent peritonitis, is characterized by organ dysfunction and systemic inflammation in association with recurrent infection. The mortality rate is high, and management is difficult [76]. Treatment consists of broad-spectrum antibiotics because the infection often includes nosocomial organisms and multidrug-resistant bacteria.

The peritoneal cavity was extensively and copiously irrigated, and the abdominal incision was left open. He returned to the operating room 2 days later for evaluation and was found to have necrotizing fasciitis of the rectus abdominal muscles bilaterally. Eventually, despite aggressive surgical debridement, this process spread to the retro peritoneum and down the left inguinal canal through a patent process esvaginitis. One week postoperatively, he was found to have edema and erythema of the left leg that prompted exploration. The necrotizing fasciitis had progressed down all compartments of the left thigh and the lateral compartment of the left lower leg. In the upper thigh, the semimembranosus and semitendinosus muscles had to be excised due to necrotic musculature. These photographs were taken on his ninth postoperative day. (A) The abdomen is seen to be open, and the medial aspect of the left thigh is visualized. (B) The incisions in the left buttock area, the left lateral thigh, and the left lateral lower leg are seen.

CONSENT FOR PUBLICATION

Not applicable.

CONFLICT OF INTEREST

The author declares no conflict of interest, financial or otherwise.

ACKNOWLEDGEMENTS

Declared none.

REFERENCES
PHYSIOLOGY OF NEW BORN & ANESTHETIC CONSIDERATIONS FOR PAEDIATRIC SURGICAL CONDITIONS

[1]   Guillen U, Weiss E, Munson D, *et al.* Guidelines for the management of extremely premature deliveries: a systematic review. Pediatrics 2015; 136: 342-50.

[2]   Simmons R. Abnormalities of fetal growth.Avery's Diseases of the Newborn. Philadelphia: Saunders 2012.

[3]   Sarafoglou K, Hoffmann G, Roth K. Pediatric Endocrinology and Inborn Errors of Metabolism. China: The McGraw-Hill Companies, Inc 2009.

[4]   Dweck HS, Cassady G. Glucose intolerance in infants of very low birth weight. I: incidence of hyperglycemia in infants of birth weights1,110 grams or less. Pediatr 1974; 53: 189-95.

[5]   Hsu SC, Levine MA. Perinatal calcium metabolism: physiology and pathophysiology. Semin Neonatol 2004; 9: 23-6.

[6]   Thomas TC, Smith JM, White PC, *et al.* Transient neonatal hypocal-cemia: presentation and outcomes. Pediatrics 2012; 129: e1461-7.

[7]   Bauer C, Ludwig I, Ludwig M. Different effects of 2,3-diphosphoglyc- erate and adenosine triphosphate on the oxygen affinity of adult and fetal human hemoglobin. Life Sci 1968; 7: 1339.

[8]   Asch J, Wedgwood JF. Optimizing the approach to anemia in the preterm infant: is there a role for erythropoietin therapy? J Perinatol 1997; 17: 276-82.

[9]   Maisels MJ, Bhutani VK, Bogen D, *et al.* Hyperbilirubinemia in the newborn infant ≥35 weeks gestation: an update with clarifications. Pediatrics 2009; 124(4): 1193-8.

[10]   Fujiwara R, Maruo Y, Chen S, *et al.* Role of extrahepatic UDP- glucuronosyltransferase 1A1: advances in understanding breast milk-induced neonatal hyperbilirubinemia. Toxicol Appl Pharmacol. 2015; 289(1): 124–132.

[11]   Osborn LM, Lenarsky C, Oakes RC, *et al.* Phototherapy in full-term infants with hemolytic disease secondary to ABO incompatibility. Pediatrics 1984; 73: 520-6.

[12]   Saugstad O. Optimal oxygenation at birth and in the neonatal period. Neonatology 2007; 91: 319-22.

[13]   Jordan CO. Retinopathy of prematurity. Pediatr Clin North Am 2014; 61: 567-77.

[14]   Cryotherapy for retinopathy of prematurity cooperative group. Multicenter trial of cryotherapy for retinopathy of prematurity. Arch Ophthalmol 1988; 106: 471-9.

[15]   Ng E, Connolly B, McNamara J, *et al.* A comparison of laser photocoagulation with cryotherapy for threshold retinopathy of prematurity at 10 years: part 1. Visual function and structural outcome. Ophthalmology 2002; 202: 928-35.

[16]   Shalev B, Farr A, Repka M. Randomized comparison of diode laser photocoagulation versus cryotherapy for threshold retinopathy of prematurity: seven-year outcome. Am J Ophthalmol 2002; 132: 76-80.

[17]   Connolly B, McNamara J, Sharma S, *et al.* A comparison of laser phototherapy with trans-scleral cryotherapy for the treatment of threshold retinopathy. Ophthalmology 1998; 105: 1628-31.

[18]   Section on Ophthalmology, AAo Ophth, AAo Ophth/Strabismus. Screening examination of premature infants for retinopathy of prematurity. Pediatrics 2006; 117: 572-6.

[19]   Lorenz JM, Kleinman LI, Kotagal UR, *et al.* Water balance in very low birth weight infants: relationship to water and sodium intake and effect on outcome. J Pediatr 1982; 101: 423-32.

[20]   Parrillo JE. Septic shock in humans. Advances in the understanding of pathogenesis, cardiovascular dysfunction, and therapy. Ann Intern Med 1990; 113: 227-42.

[21]   McCloskey RV, Straube KC, Sanders C, *et al.* Treatment of septic shock with human monoclonal antibody HA-1A. A randomized, double-blind, placebo-controlled trial. CHESS Trial Study Group. Ann Intern Med 1994; 121: 1-5.

[22]   Rogy MA, Moldawer LL, Oldenburg HS, *et al.* Anti-endotoxin therapy in primate bacteremia with HA-1A and BPI. Ann Surg 1994; 220: 77-85.

[23]   Ziegler EJ, Fisher CJ Jr, Sprung CL, *et al.* Treatment of gram-negative bacteremia and septic shock with HA-1A human monoclonal antibody against endotoxin. A randomized, double-blind, placebocontrolled trial. The HA-1A Sepsis Study Group. N Engl J Med 1991; 324: 429-36.

[24]   Cates KL, Rowe JC, Ballow M. The premature infant as a compromised host. Curr Probl Pediatr 1983; 13: 1-63.

[25]   Zuckerberg AL. A hot mnemonic for the treatment of malignant hyperthermia. Anesth Analg 1993; 77: 1077.

[26]   Shete MM, Stocks RM, Sebelik ME, *et al.* Effects of adeno-tonsillectomy on polysomnography patterns in Down syndrome children with obstructive sleep apnea: a comparative study with children without Down syndrome. Int J Pediatr Otorhinolaryngol 2010; 74: 241-4.

[27]   Cook-Sather SD, Harris KA, Chiavacci R, *et al.* A liberalized fasting guideline for formula-fed infants does not increase average gastric fluid volume before elective surgery. Anesth Analg 2003; 96: 965-9.

[28]   Cook-Sather SD, Harris KA, Chiavacci R, *et al.* A liberalized fasting guideline for formula-fed infants does not increase average gastric fluid volume before elective surgery. Anesth Analg 2003; 96: 965-9.

[29]   Yamashita M, Chin I, Horigome H. Sudden fatal cardiac arrest in a child with an unrecognized anterior mediastinal mass. Resuscitation 1990; 19: 175-7.

[30]   Viswanathan S, Campbell CE, Crok RC. Asymptomatic undetected mediastinal mass: a death during ambulatory anesthesia. J Clin Anesth 1995; 7: 151-5.

[31]   Stricker PA, Gurnaney HG, Litman RS. Anesthetic management of children with an anterior mediastinal mass. J Clin Anesth 2010; 22: 159-63.

[32]   Hack HA, Wright NB, Wynn RF. The anaesthetic management of children with anterior mediastinal masses. Anaesthesia 2008; 63: 837-46.

[33]   Rushani D, Kaufman JS, Ionescu-Ittu R, *et al.* Infective endocarditis in children with congenital heart disease: cumulative incidence and predictors. Circulation 2013; 128: 1412-9.

[34]   Hakim TS, Michel RP, Chang HK. Effect of lung inflation on pulmonary vascular resistance by arterial and venous occlusion. J Appl Physiol 1982; 53: 1110-5.

[35]   Jardin F, Vieillard-Baron A. Right ventricular function and positive pressure ventilation in clinical practice: from hemodynamic subsets to respiratory settings. Intensive Care Med 2003; 29: 1426-34.

[36]   Murat I, Constant I, Maud'huy H. Perioperative anaesthetic morbidity in children: a database of 24,165 anaesthetics over a 30-month period. Paediatr Anaesth 2004; 14: 158-66.

[37]   Patel RI, Hannallah RS. Anesthetic complications following pediatric ambulatory surgery: a 3-year study. Anesthesiology 1988; 69: 1009-12.

[38]   Watcha MF, White PF. Postoperative nausea and vomiting: its etiology, treatment, and prevention. Anesthesiology 1992; 77: 162-84.

[39]   Weir PM, Munro HM, Reynolds PI, *et al*. Propofol infusion and the incidence of emesis in pediatric outpatient strabismus surgery. Anesth Analg 1993; 76: 760-4.

[40]   Schreiner MS. Preoperative and postoperative fasting in children. Pediatr Clin North Am 1994; 41: 111-20.

[41]   Schreiner MS, Nicolson SC, Martin T, *et al*. Should children drink before discharge from day surgery? Anesthesiology 1992; 76: 528-33.

[42]   Koka BV, Jeon IS, Andre JM, *et al*. Postintubation croup in children. Anesth Analg 1977; 56: 501-5.

[43]   Schreiner MS, O'Hara I, Markakis DA, *et al*. Do children who experience laryngospasm have an increased risk of upper respiratory tract infection? Anesthesiology 1996; 85: 475-80.

[44]   von Ungern-Sternberg BS, Boda K, Chambers NA, *et al*. Risk assessment for respiratory complications in paediatric anaesthesia: a prospective cohort study. Lancet 2010; 376: 773-83.

[45]   Malviya S, Polaner DM, Berde C. Acute pain.A Practice of Anesthesia for Infants and Children. 4th ed. Philadelphia: Saunders Elsevier 2009; pp. 939-78.

[46]   Merkel SI, Voepel-Lewis T, Shayevitz JR, *et al*. The FLACC: a behavioral scale for scoring postoperative pain in young children. Pediatr Nurs 1997; 23: 293-7.

[47]   Nelson KL, Yaster M, Kost-Byerly S, *et al*. A national survey of American Pediatric Anesthesiologists: patient-controlled analgesia and other intravenous opioid therapies in pediatric acute pain management. Anesth Analg 2010; 110: 754-60.

[48]   Birmingham PK, Tobin MJ, Henthorn TK, *et al*. Twenty-four hour pharmacokinetics of rectal acetaminophen in children. Anesthesiology 1997; 87: 244-52.

[49]   Montgomery CJ, McCormack JP, Reichert CC, *et al*. Plasma concentrations after high-dose (45 mg•kg-1) rectal acetaminophen in children. Can J Anaesth 1995; 42: 982-6.

VASCULAR ACCESS

[1]   Rauch D, Dowd D, Eldridge D, *et al*. Peripheral difficult venous access in children. Clin Pediatr (Phila) 2009; 48: 895-901.

[2]   de Caen A. Venous access in the critically ill child: when the peripheral intravenous fails! Pediatr Emerg Care 2007; 23.

[3]   Keir A, Giesinger R, Dunn M. How long should umbilical venous catheters remain in place in neonates who require long-term (>5-7 days) central venous access? J Paediatr Child Health 2014; 50: 649-52.

[4]   O'Grady NP, Alexander M, Burns LA, *et al*. Guidelines for the prevention of intravascular catheter-related infections. Clin Infect Dis 2011; 52: e162-93.

[5]   Holzmann-Pazgal G, Kubanda A, Davis K, *et al*. Utilizing a line maintenance team to reduce central-line-associated bloodstream infections in a neonatal intensive care unit. J Perinatol 2012; 32: 281-6.

[6]   Legemaat MM, Jongerden IP, van Rens RM, *et al*. Effect of a vascular access team on central line-associated bloodstream infections in infants admitted to a neonatal intensive care unit: a systematic review. Int J Nurs Stud 2015; 52: 1003-10.

[7]   Stevens TP, Schulman J. Evidence-based approach to preventing central line-associated bloodstream infection in the NICU. Acta Paediatr 2012; 101: 11-6.

[8]   Heinrichs J, Fritze Z, Klassen T, *et al*. A systematic review and metaanalysis of new interventions for peripheral intravenous cannulation of children. Pediatr Emerg Care 2013; 29: 858-66.

[9]   Haas NA. Clinical review: vascular access for fluid infusion in children. Crit Care 2004; 8: 478.

[10]   Keyes LE, Frazee BW, Snoey ER, *et al.* Ultrasound-guided brachial and basilic vein cannulation in emergency department patients with difficult intravenous access. Ann Emerg Med 1999; 34: 711-4.

[11]   Schindler E, Schears GJ, Hall SR, *et al.* Ultrasound for vascular access in pediatric patients. Paediatr Anaesth 2012; 22: 1002-7.

[12]   Miyake RK, Zeman HD, Duarte FH, *et al.* Vein imaging: a new method of near infrared imaging, Where a processed image is projected onto the skin for the enhancement of vein treatment. Dermatol Surg 2006; 32: 1031-8.

[13]   Butler-O'Hara M, Buzzard CJ, Reubens L, *et al.* A randomized trial comparing long-term and short-term use of umbilical venous catheters in premature infants with birth weights of less than 1251 grams. Pediatrics 2006; 118e25

[14]   Ramasethu J. Complications of vascular catheters in the neonatal intensive care unit. Iatrog Dis 2008; 35: 199-222.

[15]   Kim JH, Lee YS, Kim SH, *et al.* Does umbilical vein catheterization lead to portal venous thrombosis? Prospective US evaluation in 100 neonates 1. Radiology 2001; 219: 645-50.

[16]   Linck DA, Donze A, Hamvas A. Neonatal peripherally inserted central catheter team: evolution and outcomes of a bedside-nurse–designed program. Adv Neonatal Care 2007; 7: 22-9.

[17]   Racadio JM, Doellman DA, Johnson ND, *et al.* Pediatric peripherally inserted central catheters: complication rates related to catheter tip location. Pediatrics 2001; 107E28

[18]   Earhart A, Jorgensen C, Kaminski D. Assessing pediatric patients for vascular access and sedation. J Infus Nurs 2007; 30: 226-31.

[19]   Pettit J. Assessment of infants with peripherally inserted central catheters: part 1. Detecting the most frequently occurring complications. Adv Neonatal Care 2002; 2: 304-15.

[20]   Abboud P-AC, Kendall JL. Ultrasound guidance for vascular access. Emerg Med Clin North Am 2004; 22: 749-73.

[21]   Hind D, Calvert N, McWilliams R, *et al.* Ultrasonic locating devices for central venous cannulation: meta-analysis. BMJ 2003; 327.

[22]   Hosokawa K, Shime N, Kato Y, *et al.* A randomized trial of ultrasound image–based skin surface marking versus real-time ultrasoundguided internal jugular vein catheterization in infants. Anesthesiology 2007; 107: 720-4.

[23]   Maecken T, Grau T. Ultrasound imaging in vascular access. Crit Care Med 2007; 35: S178-85.

[24]   Pirotte T. Ultrasound-guided vascular access in adults and children: beyond the internal jugular vein puncture. Acta Anaesthesiol Belg 2007; 59: 157-66.

[25]   Wigmore T, Smythe J, Hacking M, *et al.* Effect of the implementation of NICE guidelines for ultrasound guidance on the complication rates associated with central venous catheter placement in patients presenting for routine surgery in a tertiary referral centre. Br J Anaesth 2007; 99: 662-5.

[26]   Bratton J, Johnstone PA, McMullen KP. Outpatient management of vascular access devices in children receiving radiotherapy: complications and morbidity. Pediatr Blood Cancer 2014; 61: 499-501.

[27]   DeBoer S, Russell T, Seaver M, *et al.* Infant intraosseous infusion. Neonatal Netw 2008; 27: 25-32.

[28]   Engle WA. Intraosseous access for administration of medications in neonates. Clin Perinatol 2006; 33: 161-8.

[29]   Calkins MD, Fitzgerald G, Bentley TB, *et al.* Intraosseous infusion devices: a comparison for potential use in special operations. J Trauma 2000; 48.

[30]   Blumberg SM, Gorn M, Crain EF. Intraosseous infusion: a review of methods and novel devices. Pediatr Emerg Care 2008; 24: 50-6.

[31] Buck ML, Wiggins BS, Sesler JM. Intraosseous drug administration in children and adults during cardiopulmonary resuscitation. Ann Pharmacother 2007; 41: 1679-86.

[32] de Caen AR, Kleinman ME, Chameides L, *et al.* Part 10: paediatric basic and advanced life support: 2010 international consensus on cardiopulmonary resuscitation and emergency cardiovascular care science with treatment recommendations. Resuscitation 2010; 81: e213-59.

[34] Boon J, Gorry D, Meiring J. Finding an ideal site for intraosseous infusion of the tibia: an anatomical study. Clin Anat 2003; 16: 15-8.

[35] Kohonen M, Teerenhovi O, Terho T, *et al.* Is the Allen test reliable enough? Eur J Cardiothorac Surg 2007; 32: 902-5.

[36] Matoussevitch V, Taylan C, Konner K, *et al.* AV fistula creation in paediatric patients: outcome is independent of demographics and fistula type reducing usage of venous catheters. J Vasc Access. 2014;16:382–387. 77. T D'Cunha P, Besarab A. Vascular access for hemodialysis: 2004 and beyond. Curr Opin Nephrol Hypertens 2004; 13: 623-9.

[37] Mancuso M, Berardinelli L. Arteriovenous fistula as stable venous access in children with severe haemophilia. Haemophilia 2010; 16: 25-8.

SURGICAL INFECTION

[1] Brueggemann AB. Antibiotic resistance mechanisms among pediatric respiratory and enteric pathogens: a current update. Pediatr Infect Dis J 2006; 25: 969-73.

[2] Liu HH. Antibiotics and infectious diseases. Prim Care 1990; 17: 745-74.

[3] DeLa Cadena RA, Majluf-Cruz A, Stadnicki A, *et al.* Activation of the contact and fibrinolytic systems after intravenous administration of endotoxin to normal human volunteers: correlation with the cytokine profile. Immunopharmacology 1996; 33: 231-7.

[4] Robson MC, Stenberg BD, Heggers JP. Wound healing alterations caused by infection. Clin Plast Surg 1990; 17: 485-92.

[5] Baxter CR. Immunologic reactions in chronic wounds. Am J Surg 1994; 167: 12S-4S.

[6] Bowler PG. Wound pathophysiology, infection and therapeutic options. Ann Med 2002; 34: 419-27.

[7] Forslind B, Lindberg M, Roomans GM, *et al.* Aspects on the physiology of human skin: studies using particle probe analysis. Microsc Res Tech 1997; 38: 373-86.

[8] Fleisher TA. Back to basics: Primary immune deficiencies: windows into the immune system. Pediatr Rev 2006; 27: 363-72.

[9] Hall P, Kaye CM, McIntosh N, *et al.* Intravenous metronidazole in the newborn. Arch Dis Child 1983; 58: 529-31.

[10] Routledge PA. Pharmacokinetics in children. J Antimicrob Chemother 1994; 34 (Suppl. A): 19-24.

[11] Berrios-Torres SI, Umscheid CA, Bratzler DW, *et al.* Centers for disease control and prevention guideline for the prevention of surgical site infection. JAMA Sur 2017.

[12] Ban KA, Minei JP, Laronga C, *et al.* American College of Surgeons and Surgical Infection Society: surgical site infection guidelines, 2016 update. J Am Coll Surg 2017; 224: 59-74.

[13] Allegranzi B, Zayed B, Bischoff P, *et al.* New WHO recommendations on intraoperative and postoperative measures for surgical site infection prevention: an evidence-based global perspective. Lancet Infect Dis 2016; 16: e288-303.

[14] Allegranzi B, Bischoff P, de Jonge S, *et al.* New WHO recommendations on preoperative measures for surgical site infection prevention: an evidence-based global perspective. Lancet Infect Dis 2016; 16: e276-87.

[15] Kalra L, Camacho F, Whitener CJ, *et al.* Risk of methicillin-resistant *Staphylococcus aureus* surgical site infection in patients with nasal MRSA colonization. Am J Infect Control 2013; 41: 1253-7.

[16]   Steiner Z, Natan OB, Sukhotnik I, *et al.* Does *Staphylococcus aureus* nasal carriage require eradication prior to elective ambulatory surgery in children? Pediatr Surg Int 2014; 30: 521-5.

[17]   Pereira LJ. LeeGM,WadeKJ. The effect of surgical handwashing routines on the microbial counts of operating room nurses. Am J Infect Control 1990; 18: 354-64.

[18]   Wheelock SM, Lookinland S. Effect of surgical hand scrub time on subsequent bacterial growth 1997.

[19]   Tanner J, Swarbrook S, Stuart J. Surgical hand antisepsis to reduce surgical site infection. Cochrane Database Syst Rev 2008.CD004288

[20]   Parienti JJ, Thibon P, Heller R, *et al.* Hand-rubbing with an aqueous alcoholic solution vs traditional surgical hand-scrubbing and 30-day surgical site infection rates: a randomized equivalence study. JAMA 2002; 288: 722-7.

[21]   Girou E, Loyeau S, Legrand P, *et al.* Efficacy of handrubbing with alcohol based solution versus standard handwashing with antiseptic soap: randomised clinical trial. BMJ 2002; 325: 362.

[22]   Madrid E, Urrutia G, Roque i Figuls M, *et al.* Active body surface warming systems for preventing complications caused by inadvertent perioperative hypothermia in adults. Cochrane Database Syst Rev 2016; 4Cd009016

[23]   Serour F, Weissenberg M, Boaz M, *et al.* Intravenous fluids warming by mattress is simple and efficient during pediatric surgery. Acta Anaesthesiol Scand 2002; 46: 80-4.

[24]   Wu Y, Pei J, Yang XD, *et al.* Hyperglycemia and its association with clinical outcomes for patients in the pediatric intensive care unit after abdominal surgery. J Pediatr Surg 2013; 48: 801-5.

[25]   Wu Y, Lai W, Pei J, *et al.* Hyperglycemia and its association with clinical outcomes in postsurgical neonates and small infants in the intensive care unit. J Pediatr Surg 2016; 51: 1142-5.

[26]   Krinsley J. Perioperative glucose control. Curr Opin Anaesthesiol 2006; 19: 111-6.

[27]   Yates AR, Dyke PC, Taeed R, *et al.* Hyperglycemia is a marker for poor outcome in the postoperative pediatric cardiac patient. Pediatr Crit Care Med 2006; 7: 351-5.

[28]   Gibbons C, Bruce J, Carpenter J, *et al.* Identification of risk factors by systematic review and development of risk-adjusted models for surgical site infection. Health Technol Assess 2011; 15: 1-156. [iii-iv.].

[29]   Mu Y, Edwards JR, Horan TC, *et al.* Improving risk-adjusted measures of surgical site infection for the national healthcare safety network. Infect Control Hosp Epidemiol 2011; 32: 970-86.

[30]   Kao LS, Ghaferi AA, Ko CY, *et al.* Reliability of superficial surgical site infections as a hospital quality measure. J Am Coll Surg 2011; 213: 231-5.

[31]   Mangram AJ, Horan TC, Pearson ML, *et al.* Guideline for prevention of surgical site infection, 1999. Centers for Disease Control and Prevention (CDC) Hospital Infection Control Practices Advisory Committee. Am J Infect Control 1999; 27: 96-134.

[32]   Nichols RL. Preventing surgical site infections. Clin Med Res 2004; 2: 115-8.

[33]   Katz MS, Schwartz MZ, Moront ML, *et al.* Prophylactic antibiotics do not decrease the incidence of wound infections after laparoscopic pyloromyotomy. J Pediatr Surg 2011; 46: 1086-8.

[34]   Vaze D, Samujh R, Narasimha Rao KL. Risk of surgical site infection in paediatric herniotomies without any prophylactic antibiotics: a preliminary experience. Afr J Paediatr Surg 2014; 11: 158-61.

[35]   Holubar SD, Hedrick T, Gupta R, *et al.* American Society for Enhanced Recovery (ASER) and Perioperative Quality Initiative (POQI) joint consensus statement on prevention of postoperative infection within an enhanced recovery pathway for elective colorectal surgery. Perioper Med (Lond) 2017; 6: 4.

[36]   Le TH, Timmcke AE, Gathright JB, *et al.* Outpatient bowel preparation for elective colon resection. South Med J 1997; 90: 526-30.

[37]   Shah M, Ellis CT, Phillips MR, *et al.* Preoperative bowel preparation before elective bowel resection or ostomy closure in the pediatric patient population has no impact on outcomes: a prospective randomized study. Am Surg 2016; 82: 801-6.

[38]   Upperman JS, Sheridan RL, Marshall J. Pediatric surgical site and soft tissue infections. Pediatr Crit Care Med 2005; 6: S36-41.

[39]   Frei CR, Makos BR, Daniels KR, *et al.* Emergence of communityacquired methicillin-resistant *Staphylococcus aureus* skin and soft tissue infections as a common cause of hospitalization in United States children. J Pediatr Surg 2010; 45: 1967-74.

[40]   Stevens DL, Bisno AL, Chambers HF, *et al.* Practice guidelines for the diagnosis and 999management of skin and soft tissue infections: 2014 update by the infectious diseases society of America. Clin Infect Dis 2014; 59: e10-52.

[41]   Allen U, Ford-Jones EL. Nosocomial infections in the pediatric patient: an update. Am J Infect Control 1990; 18: 176-93.

[42]   Stein F, Trevino R. Nosocomial infections in the pediatric intensive care unit. Pediatr Clin North Am 1994; 41: 1245-57.

[43]   Sandora TJ. Prevention of healthcare-associated infections in children: new strategies and success stories. Curr Opin Infect Dis 2010; 23: 300-5.

[44]   Ananthakrishnan AN. Clostridium difficile infection: epidemiology, risk factors and management. Nat Rev Gastroenterol Hepatol 2011; 8: 17-26.

[45]   Benson L, Song X, Campos J, *et al.* Changing epidemiology of *Clostridium difficile*-associated disease in children. Infect Control Hosp Epidemiol 2007; 28: 1233-5.

[46]   Nylund CM, Goudie A, Garza JM, *et al. Clostridium difficile* infection in hospitalized children in the United States. Arch Pediatr Adolesc Med 2011; 165: 451-7.

[47]   Chesshyre E, Goff Z, Bowen A, *et al.* The prevention, diagnosis and management of central venous line infections in children. J Infect 2015; 71 (Suppl. 1): S59-75.

[48]   Goudie A, Dynan L, Brady PW, *et al.* Attributable cost and length of stay for central line-associated bloodstream infections. Pediatrics 2014; 133: e1525-32.

[49]   Niedner MF, Huskins WC, Colantuoni E, *et al.* Epidemiology of central line-associated bloodstream infections in the pediatric intensive care unit. Infect Control Hosp Epidemiol 2011; 32: 1200-8.

[50]   O'Grady NP, Alexander M, Dellinger EP, *et al.* Guidelines for the prevention of intravascular catheter-related infections. The Hospital Infection Control Practices Advisory Committee, Center for Disease Control and Prevention. US Pediatrics 2002; 110e51

[51]   Weiner LM, Webb AK, Limbago B, *et al.* Antimicrobial-resistant pathogens associated with healthcare-associated infections: summary of data reported to the National Healthcare Safety Network at the Centers for Disease Control and Prevention, 2011-2014. Infect Control Hosp Epidemiol 2016; 37: 1288-301.

[52]   Loveday HP, Wilson JA, Pratt RJ, *et al.* Epic3: national evidencebased guidelines for preventing healthcare-associated infections in NHS hospitals in England. J Hosp Infect 2014; 86 (Suppl. 1): S1-S70.

[53]   Raad II, Hohn DC, Gilbreath BJ, *et al.* Prevention of central venous catheter-related infections by using maximal sterile barrier precautions during insertion. Infect Control Hosp Epidemiol 1994; 15: 231-8.

[54]   Boyce JM, Pittet D. Guideline for Hand Hygiene in Health-Care Settings. Recommendations of the Healthcare Infection Control Practices Advisory Committee and the HIPAC/SHEA/APIC/IDSA Hand Hygiene Task Force. Am J Infect Control 2002; 30: S1-S46.

[55]   Capretti MG, Sandri F, Tridapalli E, *et al.* Impact of a standardized hand hygiene program on the

incidence of nosocomial infection in very low birth weight infants. Am J Infect Control 2008; 36: 430-5.

[56]   Lai NM, Lai NA, O'Riordan E, *et al.* Skin antisepsis for reducing central venous catheter-related infections. Cochrane Database Syst Rev 2016; 7Cd010140

[57]   Maki DG, Ringer M, Alvarado CJ. Prospective randomised trial of povidone-iodine, alcohol, and chlorhexidine for prevention of infection associated with central venous and arterial catheters. Lancet 1991; 338: 339-43.

[58]   Quach C, Milstone AM, Perpete C, Bonenfant M, Moore DL, Perreault T. Chlorhexidine bathing in a tertiary care neonatal intensive care unit: impact on central line-associated bloodstream infections. Infect Control Hosp Epidemiol 2014; 35: 158-63.

[59]   Weber JM, Sheridan RL, Fagan S, *et al.* Incidence of catheterassociated bloodstream infection after introduction of minocycline and rifampin antimicrobial-coated catheters in a pediatric burn population. J Burn Care Res 2012; 33: 539-43.

[60]   Bertini G, Elia S, Ceciarini F, *et al.* Reduction of catheter-related bloodstream infections in preterm infants by the use of catheters with the AgION antimicrobial system. Early Hum Dev 2013; 89: 21-5.

[61]   Veenstra DL, Saint S, Saha S, *et al.* Efficacy of antiseptic-impregnated central venous catheters in preventing catheter-related bloodstream infection: a meta-analysis.

[62]   Endorf FW, Garrison MM, Klein MB, *et al.* Characteristics, therapies, and outcome of children with necrotizing soft tissue infections. Pediatr Infect Dis J 2012; 31: 221-3.

[63]   Farrell LD, Karl SR, Davis PK, *et al.* Postoperative necrotizing fasciitis in children. Pediatrics 1988; 82: 874-9.

[64]   Bingöl-Koloğlu M, Yildiz RV, Alper B, *et al.* Necrotizing fasciitis in children: diagnostic and therapeutic aspects. J Pediatr Surg 2007; 42: 1892-7.

[65]   Murphy JJ, Granger R, Blair GK, *et al.* Necrotizing fasciitis in childhood. J Pediatr Surg 1995; 30: 1131-4.

[66]   Moss RL, Musemeche CA, Kosloske AM. Necrotizing fasciitis in children: prompt recognition and aggressive therapy improve survival. J Pediatr Surg 1996; 31: 1142-6.

[67]   Waldhausen JH, Holterman MJ, Sawin RS. Surgical implications of necrotizing fasciitis in children with chickenpox. J Pediatr Surg 1996; 31: 1138-41.

[68]   Hsieh WS, Yang PH, Chao HC, *et al.* Neonatal necrotizing fasciitis: a report of three cases and review of the literature. Pediatrics 1999; 103e53

[69]   Singer M, Deutschman CS, Seymour CW, *et al.* The Third International consensus definitions for sepsis and septic shock (Sepsis-3). JAMA 2016; 315: 801-10.

[70]   Dellinger RP, Levy MM, Rhodes A, *et al.* Surviving sepsis campaign: international guidelines for management of severe sepsis and septic shock: 2012. Crit Care Med 2013; 41: 580-637.

[71]   Hartman ME, Linde-Zwirble WT, Angus DC, *et al.* Trends in the epidemiology of pediatric severe sepsis*. Pediatr Crit Care Med 2013; 14: 686-93.

[72]   Balamuth F, Weiss SL, Neuman MI, *et al.* Pediatric severe sepsis in U.S. children's hospitals. Pediatr Crit Care Med 2014; 15: 798-805.

[73]   Jackson RJ, Smith SD, Wadowsky RM, *et al.* The effect of *E coli* virulence on bacterial translocation and systemic sepsis in the neonatal rabbit model. J Pediatr Surg 1991; 26: 483-6.

[74]   Heemken R, Gandawidjaja L, Hau T. Peritonitis: pathophysiology and local defense mechanisms. Hepatogastroenterology 1997; 44: 927-36.

[75]   Levy M, Balfe JW, Geary D, *et al.* Exit-site infection during continuous and cycling peritoneal dialysis in children. Perit Dial Int 1990; 10: 31-5.

[76]   Nathens AB, Rotstein OD, Marshall JC. Tertiary peritonitis: clinical features of a complex nosocomial infection. World J Surg 1998; 22: 158-63.

Essentials of Pediatric Surgery, 2021, 49-61

CHAPTER 2

Head and Neck Surgery

Karrar K. Abdulsahib[1] and **Sultan M. Ghanim[2,*]**

[1] *6th Grade Medical College, Faculty of Medicine, University of Kufa, Iraq*

[2] *ME Unit, Medical College, Faculty of Medicine, University of Kufa, Iraq*

Abstract: Based on the investigation or attribution of the cause in children, lesions of the head and neck can be divided into different categories. Infection, Trauma, neoplasm, or congenital origin are some of the cause of lesions. The hemangioma, Lymphangiomas and cystic hygroma in children, are the widespread benign neoplasm. In children, the malignant neoplasms may include neuroblastoma, lymphoma, and rhabdomyosarcoma. The abnormal growth of cells like primary or metastatic masses in the head and neck, thyroid and parathyroid lesions, or the traumatic injuries of the head and neck represents malignant neoplasm. This chapter discusses the common congenital head and neck malformations as well as inflammatory lesions.

Keyword: Neck, Pediatric, Surgery.

THYROGLOSSAL DUCT CYST

Thyroglossal duct cyst is considered as one of the most common lesions in the midline of the neck, found in 7% of the population and most are asymptomatic [1, 2]. These lesions are rarely manifested in infants and usually appear in pre-school children [3] at age 2-4 years. Thyroglossal duct cyst affects both males and females children equally (Fig. **2.1**).

Classically is located in the midline or appear just below the hyoid bone. Most cases present as painless, nontender and soft mass. The complaint of bad taste in the mouth by the patient could be the early symptom and soon there appears a spontaneous decompression of a cyst [4].

The reliable sign to diagnose Thyroglossal cyst is the movement of the cyst with swallowing or protrusion of tongue, still it is difficult to assess in pediatric age group. Unusual presentation in pediatric age group with severs respiratory distress

* **Corresponding author Sultan M. Ghanim:** ME Unit, Medical College, Faculty of Medicine, University of Kufa, Iraq; Tel: +9647816669997; E-mail: sultanmalsaadi@uokufa.edu.iq

Sultan M. Ghanim, Najah R. Hadi and Nada Al-Haris (Eds.)

or sudden infant death [4, 5]. Work up should be done as neck examination and preoperative US, CT, MRI [9] and fine needle aspiration in some cases.

Submental lymphadenopathy and midline dermoid cysts [8], Hodgkin's disease [6] and coexistence of thyroglossal and branchial cleft cyst [7] can be confused with a Thyroglossal duct cyst. Rarely, midline ectopic thyroid tissue sometimes appear similar to that of a Thyroglossal duct cyst and may represent the patient's only thyroid tissue [10 - 14]. So if there is a suspicion of ectopic thyroid, should obtain nuclear thyroid scan to confirm the diagnosis which can be treated without need to surgery.

Treatment, if abscess present then should start with drainage and antibiotics therapy, definitive treatment sistrunk operation [15 - 17] which is curative in >90% of patients. The risk of recurrence is low, 2–5% [18 - 21].

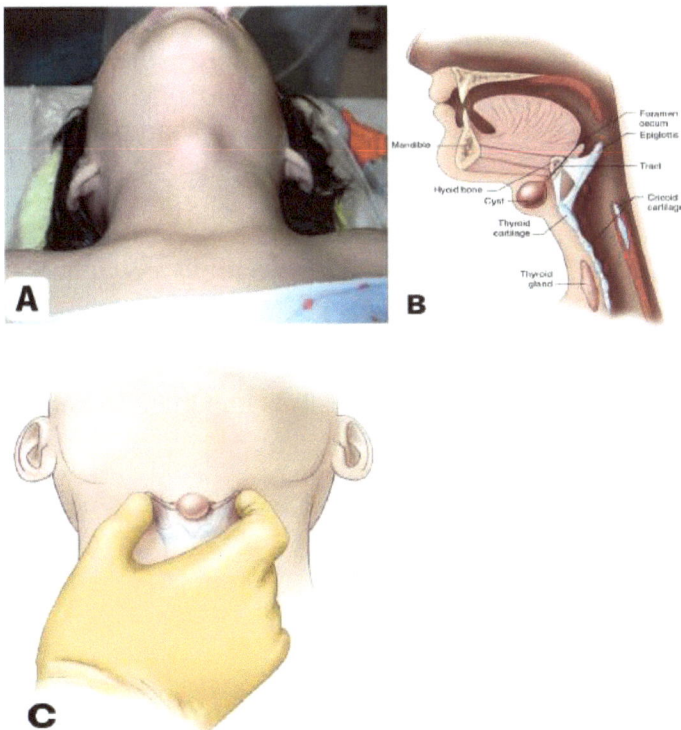

Fig. (2.1). A. Thyroglossal duct cyst traditionally manifests as a painless midline anterior cervical mass that often moves with swallowing B. The cyst occasionally communicates with the skin as a draining sinus, and its tract always extends through the center of the hyoid bone to terminate at the tongue base. C. The greater horns of the hyoid bone may be palpated bilaterally and moved side to side, which will result in cyst movement.

Cystic Hygroma

Lymphangiomas are benign masses with multinodular cysts of different sizes and content, microcysts (<1cm) more likely to contain blood and macrocysts (>1cm) more likely to contain lymph, so called cystic hygroma (Fig. **2.2**) [22 - 26].

Cystic hygroma occurs as a result of sequestration or obstruction of developing lymph vessels in about 1:12000 birth [27]. The most common sites are posterior triangle of neck, axilla, groin and mediastinum [27]. It presents as swelling usually occurs in the neck and may involve the parotid, submandibular, tongue and floor of mouth areas. Visibly increasing in size when the child coughs or cries, the characteristic that distinguishes it from all other neck swellings is that it is brilliantly translucent. It may be apparent at birth or appear and enlarge rapidly in early weeks or months of life as lymph accumulates, most present by age of 2 years. Extension of lesion into axilla or mediastinum occurs in about 10% [27].

Bleeding of its vessels or infection (by streptococcus or staphylococcus) lead to rapid growth and blockage of the airway passage. In this case it may need percutaneous aspiration to relive the respiratory distress, diagnosis made by prenatal U/S, before 30 weeks' gestation. The associated abnormalities like abnormal karyotyping and hydrops fetalis, and very large lesions may be present that may block the airway in the fetus resulting in polyhydraminous by the inability of the fetus to swallow the amniotic fluid, so need to secure the airway at delivery by EXIT procedure; an orotracheal intubation or emergency tracheostomy [27].

Treatment by surgical excision, image-guided sclerotherapy or combination of both and post operative wound drainage is important. It is important to know that recurrence occur with incomplete removal.

Cosmetic deformity and/or nerve injury can result when extensive surgical dissection is preformed for large lesions.

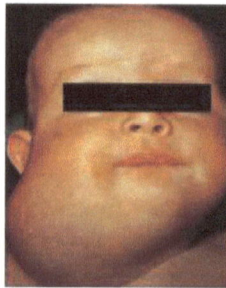

Fig. (2.2). Cystic hygroma.

Lymphadenopathy

The enlargement of lymph nodes is reported in 28% to 55% of the infants and children that may have no other symptoms, and this enlargement may be the cause of a neck mass (Fig. **2.3**) [28, 29]. A bacterial infection (Staphylococcus or Streptococcus) could be the possible reason for this enlargement. This infection appears in in infants of ages 1 to 5. Usually the infants of age less than 1 show no signs of this condition [30]. The entry of the infectious organism takes place through mucous membranes of the pharynx. Another infection called *M. tuberculosis* is usually a kind of pulmonary infection that may spread in supraclavicular nodes. Atypical strains sometimes may also cause infections spreading to higher cervical nodes, the submandibular or sub maxillary (Fig. **2.4**). Treatment of the primary cause (*e.g.*, otitis media or pharyngitis) with antibiotics often is all that is necessary. It has no evidence that the disease spread from one person to another. Another infection with atypical mycobacterium is also limited to lymph nodes, but fluctuance and spontaneous drainage occur in up to 50% of cases, with sinus tracts forming in up to 10%. In some cases there is regression of atypical nodal infection, but it usually breaks the nodes, sinus or fistula formation

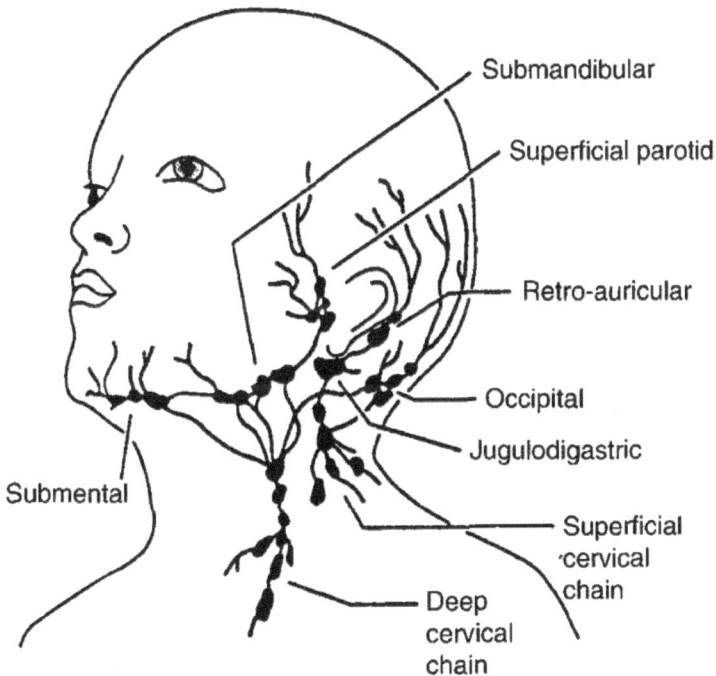

Fig. (2.3). Regional lymph node present in the head and neck.

Even after antibiotic therapy, there is a risk of malignancy of some lesions that become chronic or persist and surgical intervention indicated in conditions such as atypical mycobacterium adenitis as well as cat-scratch fever [31]. If there is persistent lymphadenopathy, for more than 6-8 weeks, even after two weeks of antibiotic therapy, an excisional biopsy is required to get rid of malignancy suspicions. The biopsy done for the adenopathy with no clear diagnosis, unilateral adenopathy involving supraclavicular or posterior triangle of the neck. The excisional biopsy is also suggested if there is firm and fix neck nodes and other nodes present in axilla or groin and there is a history that suggests lymphoma. To help distinguishing if the lesion is solid, cystic or mixed by using the diagnostic imaging [32].

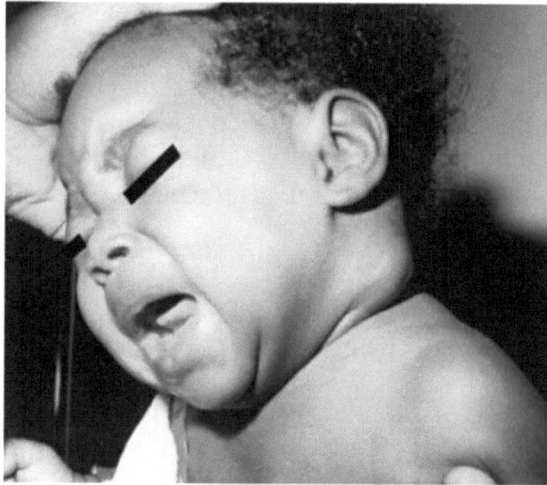

Fig. (2.4). Acute suppurative cervical adenitis is marked by the shiny and taut skin over the centralized abscess cavity.

Cat-Scratch Disease

Non-bacterial chronic lymphadenopathy [33] may cause cat-scratch disease. This disease is prevalent in developed countries of the world. *Bartonella henselae*, a gram-negative, rickettsial bacteria that considered as causative organisms [34]. The scratch caused by the cat, dog or monkey may result in a wound on the superficial skin of the body, and the disease is transmitted by this scratch, the most common carrier of the causative organism is kitten. A superficial infection on the site of scratch may result in pustule forming in initial 3-5 days. The resulting regional adenopathy in 1 to 2 weeks. Usually the axilla is the most common location of this infection, tender lymphadenopathy and few other systemic symptoms may also be included.

Diagnosis for the detection of antibody or PCR [34], Or even sometimes complete removal of the node involved is recommended to ensure the diagnosis. The other complications may include encephalitis, retinitis, and osteomyelitis, but these are rare to some extent. The treatment of the disease is symptomatic. It could resolve in weeks or months with only occasional suppuration. Antibiotics that are commonly prescribed include Azithromycin, Rifampin, ciprofloxacin, and trimethoprim- sulfamethoxazole [35, 36].

Branchial Cleft Anomalies

More than 90% of Branchial cleft anomalies are estimated to arise from the second branchial system [37], and about 10% of second branchial remnants being bilateral [38].

During embryonic development, the penetration of second cleft tract into the platysma and cervical fascia takes place. The carotid sheath is raised above the level of hyoid bone. Remnants may be present along the course of this embryonic path. Although the internal opening can be anywhere in the nasopharynx or pharynx, it is most commonly found in the tonsillar fossa. When a sinus is present, most Branchial anomalies can be diagnosed in the first 10 years of life of the child. But in the absence of external sinus, it becomes difficult to diagnose this until the age of puberty (Fig. **2.5**).

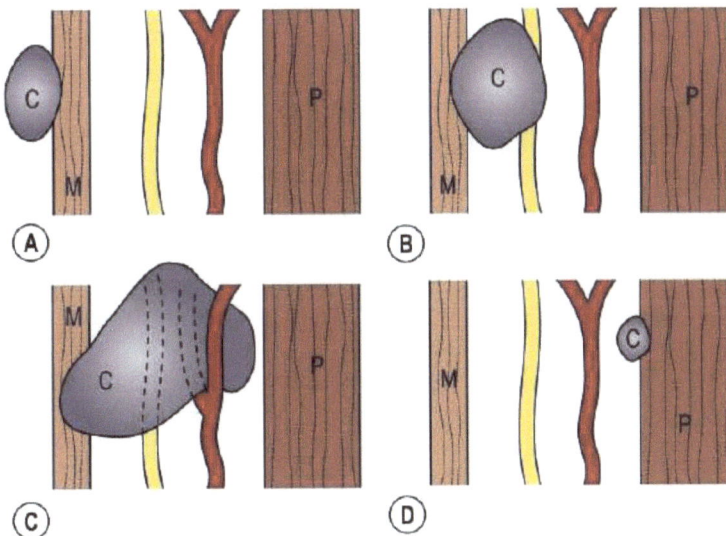

Fig. (2.5). Second Branchial cleft anomalies. Figure (A) shows a cyst (C) that is superficial to the sternocleidomastoid muscle (M). Figure(B) the cyst is no more superficial and lies near the carotid sheath. Figure (C) the passing of cyst between the internal and external carotid arteries to the lateral wall of the pharynx (P). Figure (D) shows the cyst penetrated in the carotid sheath abutting the pharynx.

The presence of a drainage from tiny pit in the skin anterior to the lower third of the sternocleidomastoid muscle, indicates the presence of a second Branchial cleft sinus or fistula. All of a sudden a painful mass in this location, gives the first indication of any of the lesions. The associated features may include the presence of a stridor, pharyngeal cyst resulting in sore throat or feeling of fullness in the throat, hyponasal speech, dysphagia or odynophagia *etc*. The other features may include a cold nodule, a hot nodule on thyroid scan [39], an isolated hypoglossal nerve palsy [40]or multiple cranial nerve palsies [41].

Surgery is required as it may cause the risk of developing of infection. When operating on a fistula, dissection of the tract is made with great care while undergoing resection to protect the spinal accessory, hypoglossal, and vagus nerves. Infant wait until 3 to 6 month of age to do the surgery. An alternative to open resection of the fistula is a stripping technique utilizing a guide wire passed between the opening in the neck and the internal opening in the tonsillar fossa (But the long-term recurrence risk is unknown) [42]. Two thirds of the patients may have recurrence.

Neonatal or Infantile Primary Hyperparathyroidism

It is considered as a rare disorder that is often fatal [44]. Solitary hyper functioning adenoma results in this disorder. The diffuse hyperplasia of all four glands could be the possible cause of this disorder sometime but this one is a very rare cause. The hyperplasia in all four glands gives rise to the Hyperparathyroidism which is a common feature of MEN1. This one is a familial component in 50% of the cases. Pathologically, there is usually diffuse parathyroid gland hyperplasia, developed in first three months after the birth. The possible symptoms may be hypotonicity, respiratory distress, and failure to thrive, elevated serum PTH level, lethargy and polyuria. If not diagnosed at an early stage, this may lead to abnormal growth and development in neonates.

In children, the primary hyperparathyroidism is not managed medically. The resection of parathyroid tissue is advised as soon its diagnosis is established. Total parathyroidectomy with heterotopic auto-transplantation ensures more chances of survival in neonates showing the symptoms of severe hyperkalemia. A dosage of vitamin D and calcium is advised for the patients with total parathyroidectomy and autotransplantation. This dosage is essential and supplemented till the heterotopic tissue start functioning [45].

Torticollis

The presence of a lateral neck mass in infancy in association with rotation of the head toward the opposite side of the mass.

It could be congenital, and the most common type [46 - 48]. The fibrosis of the sternocleidomastoid muscle may give rise to this mass (Fig. **2.6**). The possible reasons could be the collagen and fibroblast deposition around the atrophied muscle cells, breech presentation and other abnormal obstetric positions. This acquired torticollis is attributed due to the cervical hemivertebrae and imbalance of the ocular muscles. The acquired torticollis may have some other associated problems as well, including otolaryngologic infection, gastroesophageal reflux (Sandifer syndrome), or the possibility of a neoplastic condition [49, 50]. Acquired type may develop at any age. In two third of the cases, this mass is big enough to be palpated around the area of muscle that is affected. With the passage of time, other associated features like facial and cranial asymmetry may be caused. The facial structures may undergo flattening on the side of the lesion. In some cases, these features may be reversed around the age of 12, although reports have described good results when the operative correction is performed after age 10 [51, 52]. In 90% of the cases, the therapy based on the passive and regular stretching of the affected muscle proved beneficial. The key is early recognition and action. Parents should regular conduct an exercise session based on the exercises suggested by the doctor as a treatment.

1-Diagnosis in children having age more than a year [53].
2- The head rotation is limited by Persistent sternomastoid in children having age between 12 to 15 months (Fig. **2.7**) [54].
3-Persistent sternomastoid tightness accompanied with progressive facial hemihypoplasia.

Surgical transaction of the sternocleidomastoid is rarely indicated.

The need for potential surgical intervention is associated with the severity of the rotational deficit, an older age at presentation, and the presence of 'tumor' rather than fibrosis without tumor [55]. Ultrasound helps in both leading to a diagnosis as well as indicating the children which require operative therapy. The need for surgery is also indicated by the longitudinal extent of fibrosis in the sternocleidomastoid muscle [56]. The development of facial hemihypoplasia also points out towards the need for a surgery [57].

While conducting the surgery, a muscle can be incised anywhere. But a lateral collar incision conducting in the middle third is the simplest approach. The scar by this incision is the most aesthetically acceptable one. This incision also leads to the division of fascia colli of the neck, which is often tight. This may need to be divided anteriorly up to the midline and posteriorly up to the anterior border of the trapezius. No postoperative restriction of movement is necessary. Intensive physiotherapy is instituted as soon as possible. For optimal results, application of a soft cervical collar for at least 3 months following fibrous band release is recommended [59]. Some authors advise delaying operative intervention until the patient is at least five years of age (Better outcomes and improved compliance) [58]. Complications of the operation includes Hematoma and Persistent torticollis if not well divided and the recurrent is rare, less than 3% [60].

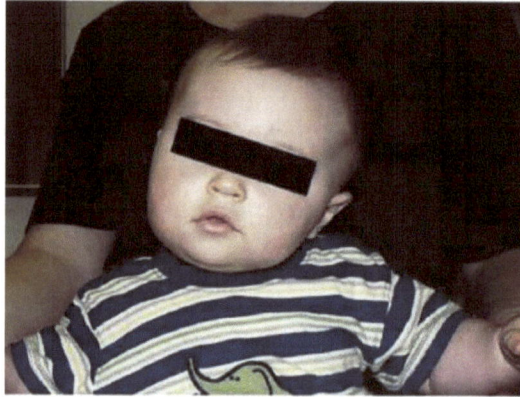

Fig. (2.6). Restriction of rotation of the stern mastoid muscle. The right stern mastoid muscle is shown by the black bars and its rotation is limited when it is unable to lengthen itself.

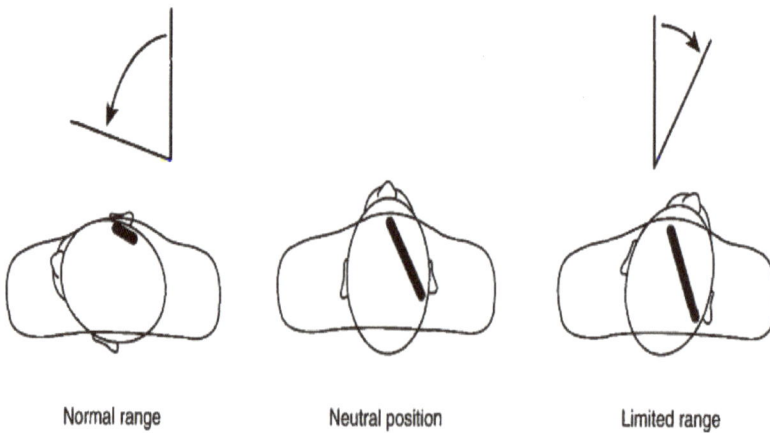

Normal range   Neutral position   Limited range

Fig. (2.7). This young child has left torticollis. He is sitting on his mother's lap. The face and chin are tilted away from the involved side, and the head is tilted toward the ipsilateral shoulder.

CONSENT FOR PUBLICATION

Not Applicable.

CONFLICT OF INTEREST

The author declares no conflict of interest, financial or otherwise.

ACKNOWLEDGEMENTS

Declared none.

REFERENCES

[1]   Telander RL, Deane SA. Thyroglossal and branchial cleft cysts and sinuses. Surg Clin North Am 1977; 57(4): 779-91.
        [http://dx.doi.org/10.1016/S0039-6109(16)41288-0] [PMID: 897966]

[2]   Enepekides DJ. Management of congenital anomalies of the neck. Facial Plast Surg Clin North Am 2001; 9(1): 131-45.
        [PMID: 11465000]

[3]   Filston HC. Head and neck-sinuses and masses. In: Holder TM, Ashcraft KW, Eds. Pediatric Surgery. Philadelphia: WB Saunders 1980; pp. 1062-79.

[4]   Samuel M, Freeman NV, Sajwany MJ. Lingual thyroglossal duct cyst presenting in infancy. J Pediatr Surg 1993; 28(7): 891-3.
        [http://dx.doi.org/10.1016/0022-3468(93)90689-I] [PMID: 8229561]

[5]   Byard RW, Bourne AJ, Silver MM. The association of lingual thyroglossal duct remnants with sudden death in infancy. Int J Pediatr Otorhinolaryngol 1990; 20(2): 107-12.
        [http://dx.doi.org/10.1016/0165-5876(90)90075-3] [PMID: 2286503]

[6]   Good GM, Isaacson G. Hodgkin's disease simulating a pediatric thyroglossal duct cyst. Am J Otolaryngol 2000; 21(4): 277-80.
        [http://dx.doi.org/10.1053/ajot.2000.8384] [PMID: 10937915]

[7]   LaRiviere CA, Waldhausen JH. Congenital cervical cysts, sinuses, and fistulae in pediatric surgery. Surg Clin North Am 2012; 92(3): 583-97.

[8]   Drucker C, Gerson CR. Sublingual contiguous thyroglossal and dermiod cyst in a neonate. Int J Pediatr otorhinolaryngol 23: 181.

[9]   Faerber EN, Swartz JD. Imaging of neck masses in infants and children. Crit Rev Diagn Imaging 1991; 31(3-4): 283-314.
        [PMID: 2036174]

[10]   Strickland AL, Macfie JA, Van Wyk JJ, French FS. Ectopic thyroid glands simulating thyroglossal duct cysts. Hypothyroidism following surgical excision. JAMA 1969; 208(2): 307-10.
        [http://dx.doi.org/10.1001/jama.1969.03160020075007] [PMID: 5818483]

[11]   Nanson EM. Salivary gland drainage into the thyroglossal duct. Surg Gynecol Obstet 1979; 149(2): 203-5.
        [PMID: 462351]

[12]   Radkowski D, Arnold J, Healy GB, *et al.* Thyroglossal duct remnants. Preoperative evaluation and management. Arch Otolaryngol Head Neck Surg 1991; 117(12): 1378-81.
        [http://dx.doi.org/10.1001/archotol.1991.01870240070011] [PMID: 1845265]

[13]   Gupta P, Maddalozzo J. Preoperative sonography in presumed thyroglossal duct cysts. Arch Otolaryngol Head Neck Surg 2001; 127(2): 200-2.
        [http://dx.doi.org/10.1001/archotol.127.2.200] [PMID: 11177039]

[14]   Kessler A, Eviatar E, Lapinsky J, Horne T, Shlamkovitch N, Segal S. Thyroglossal duct cyst: is thyroid scanning necessary in the preoperative evaluation? Isr Med Assoc J 2001; 3(6): 409-10.

[PMID: 11433631]

[15]   Sistrunk WE. Technique of removal of cyst and sinuses of the thyroglossal duct. Surg Gynecol Obstet 1928; 46: 109-12.

[16]   Bennett KG, Organ CH Jr, Williams GR. Is the treatment for thyroglossal duct cysts too extensive? Am J Surg 1986; 152(6): 602-5.
        [http://dx.doi.org/10.1016/0002-9610(86)90434-4] [PMID: 3789282]

[17]   Obiako MN. The Sistrunk operation for treatment of thyroglossal cysts and sinuses. Ear Nose Throat J 1985; 64(4): 196-201.
        [PMID: 3996268]

[18]   Foley DS, Fallat ME. Thyroglossal duct and other congenital midline cervical anomalies. Semin Pediatr Surg 2006; 15(2): 70-5.
        [http://dx.doi.org/10.1053/j.sempedsurg.2006.02.003]

[19]   Foley DS, Fallat ME. Thyroglossal duct and other congenital midline cervical anomalies. Semin Pediatr Surg 2006; 15(2): 70-5.
        [http://dx.doi.org/10.1053/j.sempedsurg.2006.02.003] [PMID: 16616309]

[20]   Ein SH, Shandling B, Stephens CA, Mancer K. The problem of recurrent thyroglossal duct remnants. J Pediatr Surg 1984; 19(4): 437-9.
        [http://dx.doi.org/10.1016/S0022-3468(84)80270-5] [PMID: 6481589]

[21]   Mickel RA, Calcaterra TC. Management of recurrent thyroglossal duct cysts. Arch Otolaryngol 1983; 109(1): 34-6.
        [http://dx.doi.org/10.1001/archotol.1983.00800150038007] [PMID: 6848104]

[22]   Banieghbal B, Davies MR. Guidelines for the successful treatment of lymphangioma with OK-432. Eur J Pediatr Surg 2003; 13(2): 103-7.
        [http://dx.doi.org/10.1055/s-2003-39581] [PMID: 12776241]

[23]   Bouchard S, Johnson MP, Flake AW, *et al.* The EXIT procedure: experience and outcome in 31 cases. J Pediatr Surg 2002; 37(3): 418-26.
        [http://dx.doi.org/10.1053/jpsu.2002.30839] [PMID: 11877660]

[24]   Charabi B, Bretlau P, Bille M, Holmelund M. Cystic hygroma of the head and neck--a long-term follow-up of 44 cases. Acta Otolaryngol Suppl 2000; 543: 248-50.
        [http://dx.doi.org/10.1080/000164800454530] [PMID: 10909034]

[25]   Hirose S, Farmer DL, Lee H, Nobuhara KK, Harrison MR. The ex utero intrapartum treatment procedure: Looking back at the EXIT. J Pediatr Surg 2004; 39(3): 375-80.
        [http://dx.doi.org/10.1016/j.jpedsurg.2003.11.011] [PMID: 15017555]

[26]   Schuster T, Grantzow R, Nicolai T. Lymphangioma colli--a new classification contributing to prognosis. Eur J Pediatr Surg 2003; 13(2): 97-102.
        [http://dx.doi.org/10.1055/s-2003-39583] [PMID: 12776240]

[27]   Samuel M, McCarthy L, Boddy SA. Efficacy and safety of OK-432 sclerotherapy for giant cystic hygroma in a newborn. Fetal Diagn Ther 2000; 15(2): 93-6.
        [http://dx.doi.org/10.1159/000020983] [PMID: 10720873]

[28]   Hartzog LW: Prevalence of lymphadenopathy of the head and neck in infants and children. Clin Pediatr 1983; 22: 485.
        [http://dx.doi.org/10.1177/000992288302200703]

[29]   Larsson LO, Bentzon MW. BergKelly K, Mellander L:Palpable lymph nodes of the neck in Swedish school children. Acta Paediatr 1994; 83: 1091.
        [http://dx.doi.org/10.1111/j.1651-2227.1994.tb12992.x] [PMID: 7841711]

[30]   Bodenstein L, Altman RP. Cervical lymphadenitis in infants and children. Semin Pediatr Surg 1994; 3(3): 134-41.

[PMID: 7987628]

[31]   Filston HC. Common lumps and bumps of the head and neck in infants and children. Pediatr Ann 1989; 18(3): 180-182, 184, 186.
[http://dx.doi.org/10.3928/0090-4481-19890301-07] [PMID: 2664678]

[32]   Elden LM, Grundfast KM, Vezina G. Accuracy and usefulness of radiographic assessment of cervical neck infections in children. J Otolaryngol 2001; 30(2): 82-9.
[http://dx.doi.org/10.2310/7070.2001.20808] [PMID: 11770961]

[33]   Carithers HA. Cat-scratch skin test antigen: purification by heating. Pediatrics 1977; 60(6): 928-9.
[PMID: 600610]

[34]   Scott MA, McCurley TL, Vnencak-Jones CL, *et al.* Cat scratch disease: detection of Bartonella henselae DNA in archival biopsies from patients with clinically, serologically, and histologically defined disease. Am J Pathol 1996; 149(6): 2161-7.
[PMID: 8952548]

[35]   Chia JKS, Nakata MM, Lami JLM, Park SS, Ding JC. Azithromycin for the treatment of cat-scratch disease. Clin Infect Dis 1998; 26(1): 193-4.
[http://dx.doi.org/10.1086/517061] [PMID: 9455538]

[36]   Margileth AM. Antibiotic therapy for cat-scratch disease: clinical study of therapeutic outcome in 268 patients and a review of the literature. Pediatr Infect Dis J 1992; 11(6): 474-8.
[http://dx.doi.org/10.1097/00006454-199206000-00010] [PMID: 1608685]

[37]   Gatti WM, Zimm J. Bilateral branchial cleft fistulas: diagnosis and management of two cases. Ear Nose Throat J 1988; 67(4): 256-61.
[PMID: 3383763]

[38]   Soper RT, Pringle KC. Cysts and sinuses of the neck. In: Welch K, Ed. Pediatric Surgery. 4th ed. Chicago: Year Book Medical 1986; pp. 539-51.

[39]   Sonnino RE, Spigland N, Laberge JM, Desjardins J, Guttman FM. Unusual patterns of congenital neck masses in children. J Pediatr Surg 1989; 24(10): 966-9.
[http://dx.doi.org/10.1016/S0022-3468(89)80192-7] [PMID: 2809966]

[40]   Gatot A, Tovi F, Fliss DM, Yanai-Inbar I. Branchial cleft cyst manifesting as hypoglossal nerve palsy. Head Neck 1991; 13(3): 249-50.
[http://dx.doi.org/10.1002/hed.2880130317] [PMID: 2037480]

[41]   Durrant TJ, Sevick RJ, Lauryssen C, MacRae ME. Parapharyngeal branchial cleft cyst presenting with cranial nerve palsies. Can Assoc Radiol J 1994; 45(2): 134-6.
[PMID: 8149269]

[42]   Van Zele T, Katrien B, Philippe D, Hubert V. Stripping of a fistula for complete second branchial cleft. J Plast Reconstr Aesthet Surg 2010; 63(6): 1052-4.
[http://dx.doi.org/10.1016/j.bjps.2009.11.013] [PMID: 20005791]

[43]   Ross AJ III. Parathyroid surgery in children. Prog Pediatr Surg 1991; 26: 48-59.
[http://dx.doi.org/10.1007/978-3-642-88324-8_7] [PMID: 1904598]

[44]   Kulczycka H, Kamiński W, Woźniewicz B, Pronicka E. Primary hyperparathyroidism in infants. Diagnostic and therapeutic difficulties. Klin Padiatr 1991; 203(2): 116-8.
[http://dx.doi.org/10.1055/s-2007-1025412] [PMID: 2033903]

[45]   Wells SA Jr, Farndon JR, Dale JK, Leight GS, Dilley WG. Long-term evaluation of patients with primary parathyroid hyperplasia managed by total parathyroidectomy and heterotopic autotransplantation. Ann Surg 1980; 192(4): 451-8.
[http://dx.doi.org/10.1097/00000658-198010000-00003] [PMID: 7425691]

[46]   Jones PG. Torticollis. In: Welch KJ, Ed. Pediatric Surgery. 4th ed. Chicago: Year Book Medical 1986; pp. 552-6.

[47] Mickelson MR, Cooper RR, Ponseti IV. Ultrastructure of the sternocleidomastoid muscle in muscular torticollis. Clin Orthop Relat Res 1975; (110): 11-8.
[http://dx.doi.org/10.1097/00003086-197507000-00003] [PMID: 1157372]

[48] Dunn PM. Congenital postural deformities: perinatal associations. Proc R Soc Med 1972; 65(8): 735-8.
[http://dx.doi.org/10.1177/003591577206500836] [PMID: 4673597]

[49] Kahn ML, Davidson R, Drummond DS. Acquired torticollis in children. Orthop Rev 1991; 20(8): 667-74.
[PMID: 1923581]

[50] Bredenkamp JK, Maceri DR. Inflammatory torticollis in children. Arch Otolaryngol Head Neck Surg 1990; 116(3): 310-3.
[http://dx.doi.org/10.1001/archotol.1990.01870030074012] [PMID: 2306349]

[51] Yu SW, Wand NH, Chin LS, *et al.* Surgical correction of muscular torticollis in older children. Chung Hua I HsuehTsaChih Taipei 1995; 5: 168-71.

[52] Cheng JCY, Tang SP. Outcome of surgical treatment of congenital muscular torticollis. Clin Orthop Relat Res 1999; (362): 190-200.
[http://dx.doi.org/10.1097/00003086-199905000-00028] [PMID: 10335298]

[53] Demirbilek S, Atayurt HF. Congenital muscular torticollis and sternomastoid tumor: results of nonoperative treatment. J Pediatr Surg 1999; 34(4): 549-51.
[http://dx.doi.org/10.1016/S0022-3468(99)90070-2] [PMID: 10235319]

[54] Wei JL, Schwartz KM, Weaver AL, Orvidas LJ. Pseudotumor of infancy and congenital muscular torticollis: 170 cases. Laryngoscope 2001; 111(4 Pt 1): 688-95.
[http://dx.doi.org/10.1097/00005537-200104000-00023] [PMID: 11359141]

[55] Cheng JC, Tang SP, Chen TM, Wong MW, Wong EM. The clinical presentation and outcome of treatment of congenital muscular torticollis in infants--a study of 1,086 cases. J Pediatr Surg 2000; 35(7): 1091-6.
[http://dx.doi.org/10.1053/jpsu.2000.7833] [PMID: 10917303]

[56] Lin JN, Chou ML. Ultrasonographic study of the sternocleidomastoid muscle in the management of congenital muscular torticollis. J Pediatr Surg 1997; 32(11): 1648-51.
[http://dx.doi.org/10.1016/S0022-3468(97)90475-9] [PMID: 9396548]

[57] Soeur R. Treatment of congenital torticollis. J Bone Joint Surg 1940; 38: 35-40.

[58] Shim JS, Jang HP. Operative treatment of congenital torticollis. J Bone Joint Surg Br 2008; 90(7): 934-9.
[http://dx.doi.org/10.1302/0301-620X.90B7.20339] [PMID: 18591606]

[59] Lee IJ, Lim SY, Song HS, Park MC. Complete tight fibrous band release and resection in congenital muscular torticollis. J Plast Reconstr Aesthet Surg 2010; 63(6): 947-53.
[http://dx.doi.org/10.1016/j.bjps.2009.05.017] [PMID: 19539550]

[60] Wirth CJ, Hagena FW, Wuelker N, Siebert WE. Biterminal tenotomy for the treatment of congenital muscular torticollis. Long-term results. J Bone Joint Surg Am 1992; 74(3): 427-34.
[http://dx.doi.org/10.2106/00004623-199274030-00015] [PMID: 1548271]

CHAPTER 3

Thoracic Surgery

Houreleen H. Salman[1], **Noor Al-Huda I. Khalaf**[1] and **Sultan M. Ghanim**[2,*]

¹ 6ᵗʰ Grade Medical College, Faculty of Medicine, University of Kufa, Iraq

² ME Unit, Medical College, Faculty of Medicine, University of Kufa, Iraq

Abstract: This chapter will include the most common cases of thoracic surgery in the pediatric age group, it ranges from congenital such as diaphragmatic hernia, lung emphysema to acquired conditions such as corrosive injury.Usually two types of deformities considered as Congenital are found to be associated with the chest wall. One may cause depression or protuberance due to overgrowth of the cartilages and the other one causing aplasia or dysplasia. Pectus carinatum (PC), is a protuberance of chest all which makes up to 10% of the chest wall abnormalities while combined PE/PC makes up 5%, while Pectus excavatum (PE) cause a depression in the chest, thus may be called as sunken, or funnel chest. Jeune syndrome is another syndrome that may exhibit mixed features of PE/PC but is rarely found.

Keywords: Chest, Diaphragm, Pulmonary.

CHEST WALL DEFORMITIES

Pectus Excavatum

Pectus excavatum is the most common chest wall deformity in children.There is a depression in the chest wall and its severity may vary (Fig. **3.1**). Depression may show different shapes like cup or saucer-shaped (Fig. **3.2**). The depth of the depression is related to the seriousness of the deformity. More depth may be associated with more cardiac and pulmonary compression. It is noted in infancy in many patients. With the growth and development in the children this may progress until puberty, but only one third of such patients may require surgery. Pectus excavatum occurs in approximately 1 in 1000 children, and it has a male-to-female ratio of 3-4:1 [1]. A genetic predisposition of this deformity reveals that associated scoliosis is more prevalent in female patients, thus linking it to the chromosomal make-up [2, 3]. The disease may sometime be associated with the disorder of connective tissue. 17% of such patients showed the symptoms of Mar-

* **Corresponding author Sultan M. Ghanim:** ME Unit, Medical College, Faculty of Medicine, University of Kufa, Iraq; Tel: +9647816669997; E-mail: sultanmalsaadi@uokufa.edu.iq

fan syndrome and 0.7% showed the indication of Ehlers–Danlos. 20% of patients showed the signs of Mild scoliosis. In many cases, an early treatment of the Pectus excavatum resulted in the improvement of mild scoliosis.

CLINICAL FEATURES

No symptoms are prevalent in most of the patients, however the rigidity of the chest wall becomes obvious with the passage of time and age. Such children may face difficulty while taking part in aerobic games. This leads to vicious cycle and further deterioration in the physical condition as the children stop taking part in games. Such children are shy of showing their chest by removing shirts while playing games, thus affecting their physical capabilities to further extent. "Pectus" posture, thoracic hypnosis, forward sloping shoulders, and a protuberant abdomen are some of the features associated with this deformity (Fig. **3.3**). The sternum is depressed even further due to change in posture. The treatment may include some exercising based on the breathing pattern, before and after the surgery. In some cases the deformity is not serious, but obviously this is not going to be resolved without any treatment. During puberty, the condition may become serious in such patients within a period of less than half a year, seeking an examination and advice from the doctor. The symptoms in such patients are more complex. The may show shortness of breath, exhausted by even little exercises, including chest pain. Complains of long term infections in the respiratory tract associated with features of asthma may also be present (Table **3.1**) [4].

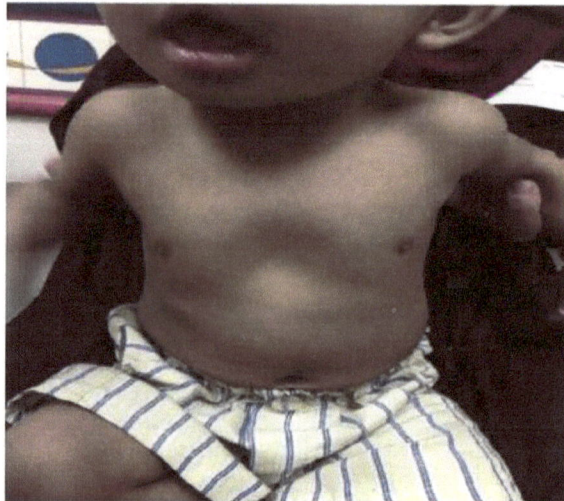

Fig. (3.1). Pectus excavatum is often seen in infants. This 11-month-old child was evaluated for a Pectus excavatum. Observation was recommended.

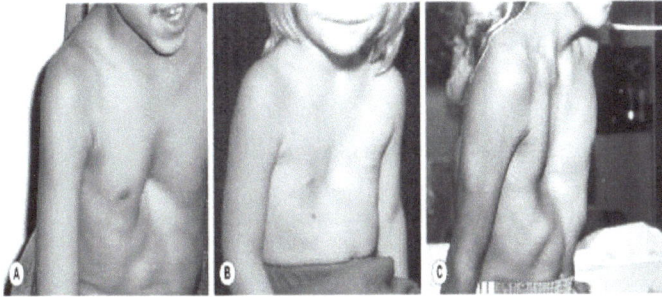

Fig. (3.2). Figure (A) shows Localized or 'cup-shaped' Pectus excavatum. Figure (B) shows Diffuse or 'saucer-shaped deformity. Figure (C) shows Eccentric deformity.

An inferiority complex related to self-worth may be associated with such patients due to poor shape of the body. If left untreated, this may have far reaching consequences on the physiologic and psychological health of the adolescent [5].

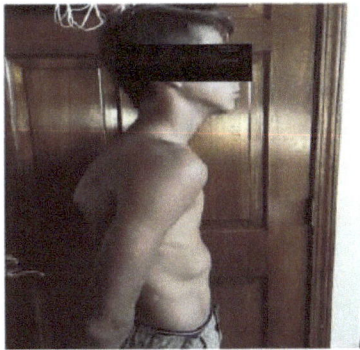

Fig. (3.3). This boy has the classic Pectus posture with thoracic hypnosis, forward-sloping shoulders, and lumbar lordosis.

Evaluation and Indications for Operation

The treatment may start with the evaluation or assessment of the history of the patients. Photographs of the body are also taken during the examination. An exercise program is advised to stop the further progression of the deformity in patients which don't show serious condition. Many follow-up checkups may be required. Serious pateints may also be treated by exercise and posture program, before making the decision regarding the surgery. A wide range of test like PFTs, CT, MRI and ECG may be conducted in order to make a clear assessment. The extent of depression leading to the compression of various vital organs in the chest is shown by CT scan. Asymmetry of the chest, sterna torsion, compensatory development of a barrel-chest deformity are the features that are also evaluated before making any decision. The calculation of CT index is important to get a comparison of severity among similar patients (Fig. **3.4**).

Table 3.1. List of Symptoms in patients undergone correction of Pectus excavatum.

Symptoms	Percent %
Shortness of breath, lack of endurance, exercise intolerance	80
Chest pain, with or without exercise.	70
Frequent respiratory infections	20
Cardiology indicators	
Cardiac compression	85
Cardiac displacement by computed tomography	75
Murmurs	25
Mitral valve prolapsed	13
Pulmonary indicators	
FVC <80%	24
FEV1% <80%	29
FEF25-75% <80%	43

Despite the fears of radiation exposure, CT scan is preferred over MRI. The surgery may be required if two or more of the following results are obtained during the physical examination:

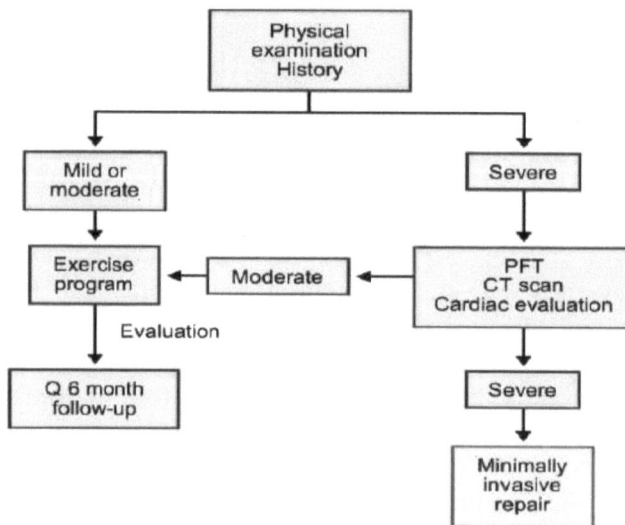

Fig. (3.4). An Algorithm used to evaluate and treat the patients with Pectus deformities.

1. If CT Index is more than 3.2 or correction index greater than 24%
2. PFTs revealing restrictive airway disease
3. If cardiac evaluation reveals cardiac compression resulting in murmurs, mitral valve prolepses, cardiac displacement, or conduction abnormalities
4. Evidences of progression of the condition
5. A failed Ravitch procedure
6. A failed MIRPE indicating towards a condition or deformity that may require surgery [6, 7].

Treatment

In the last few years, newer options for treatment of PE have been developed. An option that is being used internationally is the vacuum bell device as a sterna lifter (Fig. **3.5**). Whether this technique is effective for all patients with PE is not yet known but is unlikely but was most effective in patients with low body weight and smaller chest depth. Another innovation has been the development the Magnetic Mini-Mover, which is currently envisioned for treatment of prepubertal patients with PE [7, 8].

OPERATIVE APPROACHES

Minimally Invasive Pectus Repair (The MIRPE); involves making incisions on each side of the chest and creating a subcutaneous tunnel from the lateral thoracic incision to the top of the Pectus ridge on each side. Sterna elevation, by use of a crane (Rultract, Inc., Cleveland, OH, or other device), vacuum bell, or sturdy assistant, can be used to help lift the sternum away from the heart. At the top of the ridge, bilateral thoracotomy incisions are created and a large introducer is inserted into the chest cavity under thoracoscopic visualization. The patient is discharged within 3-4 days after surgery and advised not to take part in games for a period of two months. The posture and exercise program is advised by the healthcare team to improve and maintain the posture. A variety of measures have been used for pain management in the postoperative period. Many surgeons use a combination of intravenous narcotics, benzodiazepines, and nonsteroidal anti-inflammatory agents. Transition to oral medications is usually attempted on either the second or third postoperative day in preparation for discharge on day 4 or 5 [9, 10].

Open Technique

The preoperative measures required are same as that for MIRPE. Since this surgery may interfere with growth plates and development of asphyxiating chondrodystrophy, the surgery is conducted patients undergoing puberty. The surgery is suitable for patients with asymmetric or eccentric deformities or showing mixed PE/PC deformities. It is the only approach we have found effective for chondromanubrial deformities (also called Currarino–Silverman syndrome or Pectus arcuatum) [11, 12].

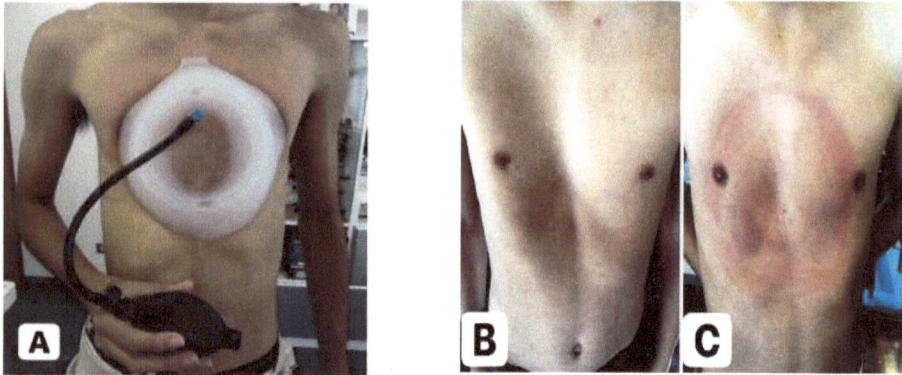

Fig. (3.5). A-The vacuum bell corrects Pectus excavatum by suction of anterior sternum. (Photograph courtesy Dr. Carlos Segura.). B- Chest wall before using the vacuum bell. C-the Pectus excavatum following after several months' usage of the vacuum bell.

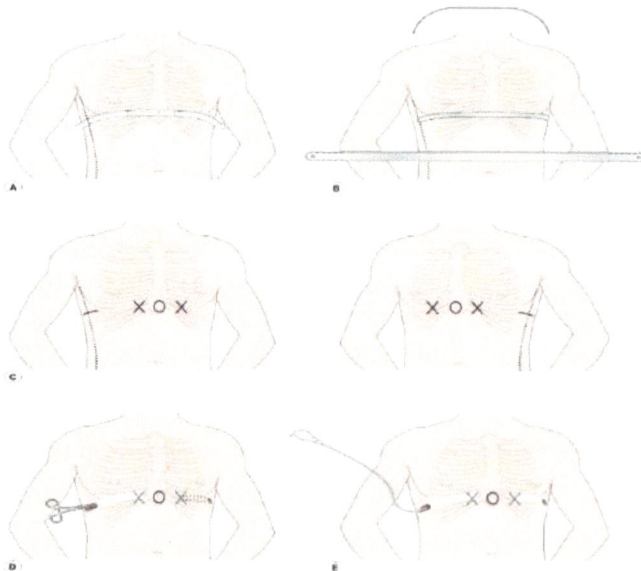

Fig. (3.6). (A) The procedure of calculation of the length of the Pectus bar (measure the distance from right to left midaxillary line and subtract 1–2 cm (1 inch) (B) The conformation of Lorenz Pectus support to the desired chest wall level requires its bending (C) A marking pen is used to Mark the deepest point of the Pectus excavatum. This point sets the horizontal plane bar for insertion (D) making of lateral thoracic skin incisions and raising of skin flaps anteriorly toward the X marked on the external skin at the top of the Pectus ridge (E) Retraction of the skin incision anteriorly allows visualization of the intercostals space.

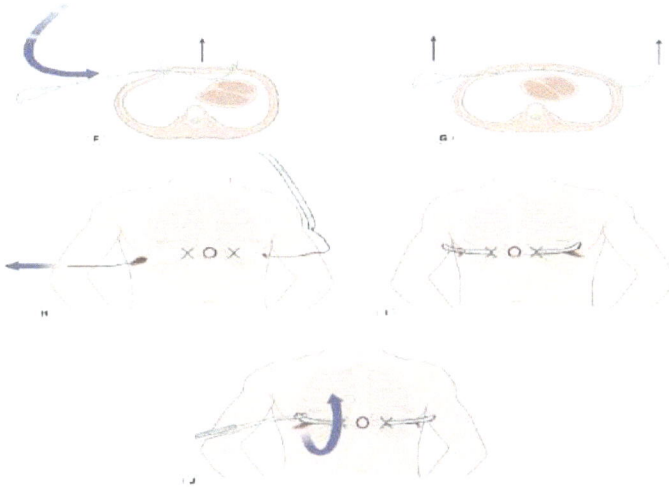

Fig. (3.7). (F) After completion of substernal tunnel, gentle pushing of the tip of the introducer through the contra lateral intercostals space at the previously marked 'X' (G) Elevation of sternum using introducer takes place.H) The Pectus bar is attached to the umbilical tape and guides through the tunnel with the use of umbilical tape for traction (I) The bar is inserted with the convexity facing posteriorly (J) When the bar is in position, use the specially designed Lorenz bar rotational instrument (bar flipper) to turn the bar over.

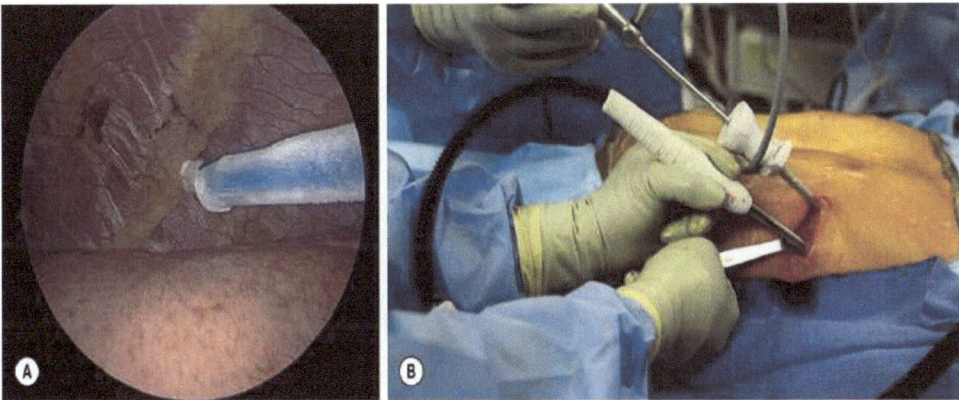

Fig. (3.8). The use of cryoablation is a new technique to reduce/eliminate pain in the postoperative period. On the left (A) thecryoablation probe is being applied to the intercostals nervebundle below the third rib on the right side. It takes approximately 2 minutes to cryoablate each intercostal bundle. Note the ice forming along the cryoablation probe. On the right (B) the probe has been inserted into the right chest through the lateral chest wall incision. Note the cannula and telescope that have been introduced into the right thoracic cavity through the same lateral chest wall incision. It is important to retract the inferior aspect of the incision so as not to cryoablation the skin as well.

The MIRPE is widely acceptable as it does not involve rib resection or sterna osteotomy. There is less blood loss and operating time. The patient is also discharged within a week.

COMPLICATIONS

Early and the most feared complication is injury to the heart during insertion of the substernal bar. This appears to be more common with the MIRPE approach than with the open operation. Other complications include pneumothorax, haemothorax, and plural effusion, and pericarditis, metal allergy, bar displacement, wound infection, overcorrection, and failure of the repair. Bar displacement and Metal allergy remains a challenging issue as a Late Complications.

LONG-TERM FOLLOW-UP

The follow-up checkups are usually advised after 6 to 12 months until the deformaity is treated completely. The postoperative results are classified into various scales depending upon the success of the repair. If the Pectus deformity is resolved without any recurring symptoms, the result is considered as excellent. A good repair is synonymous with improved condition but the shape of the chest wall is not normal so far and some signs of the deformity are also there. If the PE remains there to some extent, the results are marked as fair. If the deformity still recurs with symptoms, this may be called as failed repair and the surgery is advised again. The Pectus bar is advised to be left in place for 2–3 years. There is strict monitoring of the patients after surgery with regard to their growth and activity, pulmonary and cardiac functioning and activity levels. The bar wall remains there in the patients having ages between 3 to 6 years as they show limited growth while it has to remove in 2 years in teenagers since they show massive growth and development of the chest wall. The exercise program advised has the significance equal to that of surgery. The passive lifestyle in children and adults don't result in expansion of the lungs more than 10% of total lung capacity or the resting tidal volumes. Exercises and games like running (*e.g.*, soccer, basketball) and swimming are important for the expansion of the lungs. Breath holding for 10–15 seconds is also an important exercise. Most bar removals are uneventful and managed as outpatient procedures. However, complications can develop, including significant hemorrhage, wound infection, hematoma, and even cardiac arrest and death (Table **3.2**).

Table (3.2). Complications observed after initial Pectus excavatum repair.

Complication	Percentage (number)
Pneumothorax w\spontaneous resolution	55.7% (815)
Pneumothorax w\chest tube	3.8% (56)
Bar displacement requiring revision	3.7% (54)
Overcorrection	3.15 (47)
Bar allergy	2.9%(39)
Suture site infection	1.2%(18)
Pneumonia	0.9% (13)
Haemothorax	0.36% (6)
Haemothorax (post-traumatic)	0.1% (2)
Pericarditis	0.6%(9)
Pleural effusion(requiring drainage)	0.9%(13)
Temporary paralysis	<0.1%(2)
Death	0%
Cardiac perforation	0%
Recurrence	0.9% (13)

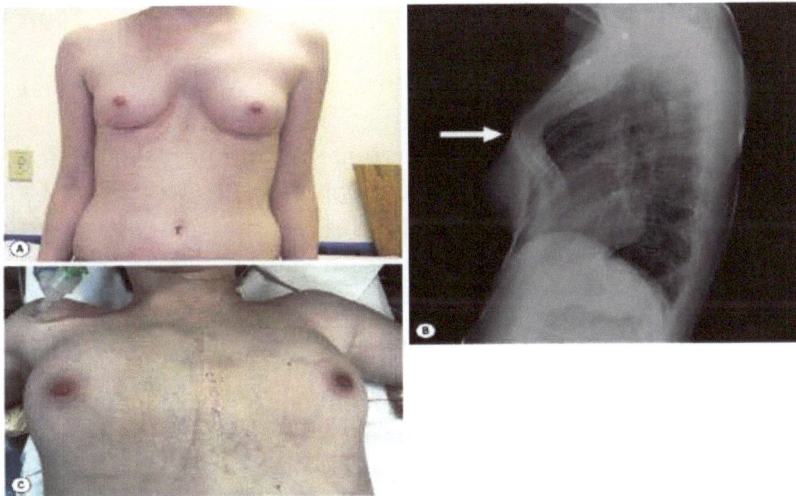

Fig. (3.9). This girl has the typical features of Currarino–Silverman syndrome (A). It looks like she has a Pectus excavatum, but she really has a variant of Pectus carinatum. The sternum is short, and there is marked posterior angulations (arrow) at the site of the normal chondromanubrial junction (B). The photograph in (C) was taken 18 months postoperatively at the time of removal of the substernal bar that was placed at the time of her initial operation (Ravitch-type repair).

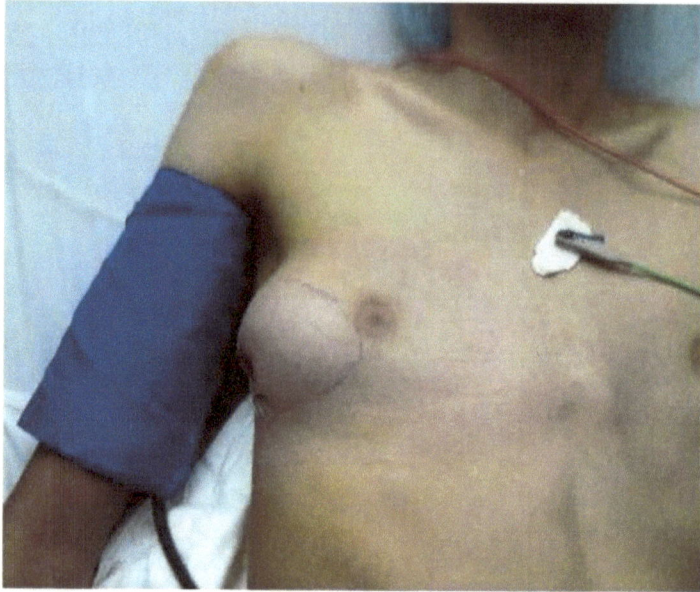

Fig. (3.10). This patient has undergone removal of the bar, but a hematoma developed around the right lateral chest wall incision after bar removal. The hematoma resolved by wrapping the chest wall with an elastic bandage (Photo courtesy Dr Michele Ugazzi).

Pectus Carinatum: is protrusion deformity of the chest, and it comprises about 5% of patients with chest wall deformities, although PC is the second most frequent chest wall malformation. Its occurance is less than that of Pectus excavatum in most countries. It is traditionally referred to as the "undertreated chest wall deformity" due to lack of referrals from primary care practitioners and an underestimation of its incidence and prevalence [13]. The protrusion or prominence if found in upper manubrium of the sternum is known as a chondromanubrial deformity, while in lower part of the sternum is known as chondrogladiolar, the later one being more common. It have a genetic predisposition as 80% of the patients are boys with a ratio with a ratio of 3:1 or 4:1. The age of adolescence is the time while this disease start developing, because the deformity usually is not appreciated until after 11 years of age and then worsens with puberty [15 - 17]. The etiology is unknown, a genetic component of causation is suggested by the approximately 25% of patients with a family history of a chest wall defect, and has also been reported to occur after treatment for Pectus excavatum, and following surgically corrected congenital diseases (*e.g.*, diaphragmatic hernia) or sternotomy, mostly performed for cardiac surgical procedures [18]. PC is far from being a cosmetic condition, and patients often manifest psychological problems and disorders (discomfort, shame, shyness, anxiety, anguish, depression, and impairment in sports, partner, and social activities). In addition, they also exhibit signs/symptoms such as chondrosternal and/or chondrocostal pain, backache, inability to sleep in the prone position, posterior asymmetry, impaired shoulders, sterna rotation, scoliosis, and hypnosis. Cardio respiratory disorders are very rare in PC patients, yet dyspnea, reduced endurance, tachypnea with exertion, asthma, associated mitral valve disease are widely attributed with PC [19 - 21]. Other associations include Marfan, Noonan, and von Recklinghausen syndromes (in 15%) (Fig. **3.11**). Progressive thoracic cage deformation becomes evident with age in all cases.

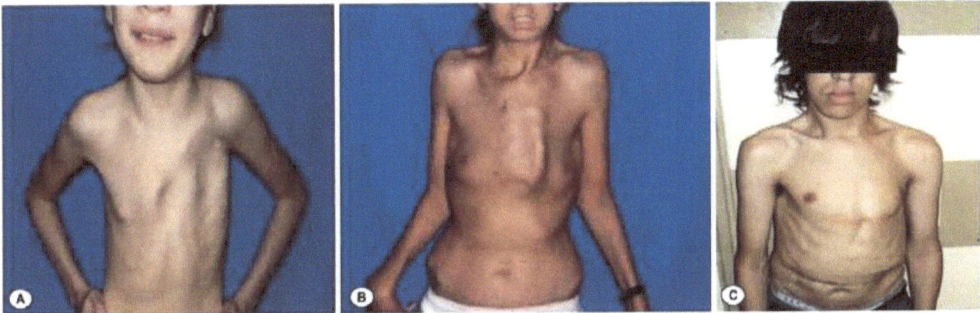

Fig. (3.11). These three children exhibit features of Poland (A), Marfan (B), and von Recklinghausen (C) syndromes in association with their Pectus carinatum. In A, note the absence of the left pectorals major and minor muscles along with the serratus anterior and latissimus dorsi muscles.

For the patient diagnosed with a PC, the position of the protruion, symmetry/asymmetry of the deformity, degree of sterna rotation, chest wall compliance, and presence of a concomitant PE should be assessed in addition to any clinical signs and symptoms or psychological problems and disorders. A physical evaluation for scoliosis is mandatory because the association with this condition is seen in about 20% of cases. Follow-up with photographs and different measurement methods is important to evaluate the evolution of the deformity. Imaging studies such as chest radiographs or CT scans should only be reserved for the most severe cases or when concomitant skeletal deformities are suspected. When PC represents a significant deviation from normal, operative or nonoperative corrective therapy is indicated. A classification of the available treatments for PC is seen in Table **3.3**. The use of Orthotic bracing is widespread in patients of PC. The deformity has been reported to be treated by the use of brace similar to that utilized in the treatment of scoliosis [22, 23]. About 85% of our brace patients have been successfully treated without operation. In the remainder, minimally invasive or open operation is performed. Patients must be operated by an experienced surgeon associated with big medical centers to reduce the chances of recurrence [24]. An unusual atypical form of Pectus carinatum occurs with a short, thick, and wide nondemented sternum and marked posterior angulations at the site of the normal chondromanubrial junction (Currarino–Silverman syndrome). Also, congenital heart disease is often present. Although its etiology is unclear, early fusion of the sterna plates is postulated as the cause of this deformity [25, 26]. Repair is best performed with an open Ravitch-type repair using an open technique with subparachondral resection of the second to seventh costal cartilages and a broad wedge-shaped osteotomy through the anterior cortex of the sternum at the point of maximal angularization. The lower sternum is then displaced anteriorly with sutures while the costal cartilages regenerate. The confusing part about this anomaly is that it may appear to be a Pectus excavatum deformity when, in fact, it is an uncommon variant of Pectus carinatum (Fig. **3.9**) [27].

Table (3.3). Classification of treatment of pectus carinatum.

Open. Ravitch
Robiseck
Willlital
Welch
Resective
intrathoracic Kim
Thoracoscopic. Varela
Extrathoracic. Schaarschmidt
Surgical
Abramson
Extrathoracic. Yuksel
Zip-Back
Non Resective
Kalman
Combined
intrathoracia and extrathoracic. Perez
thoracic. Park (sandwich technique)
Nonsurgical. classic bracing
Pressure controlled bracing

*We define a respective surgery as a surgical procedure in which the cartilages are either transected or partially or totally resected [28].

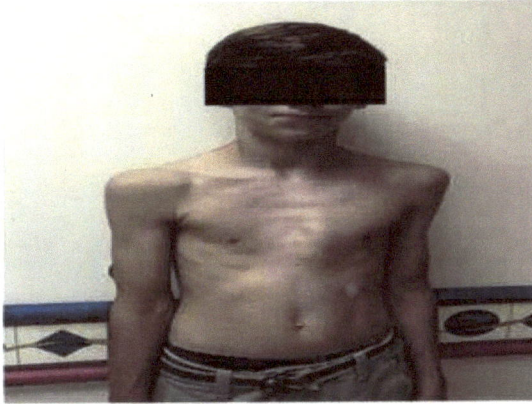

Fig. (3.12). This child has a mixed pectus excavatum and carinatum. The left costal margin is involved with the carinatum, and he has a mild pectus excavatum on the right side of his anterior chest wall.

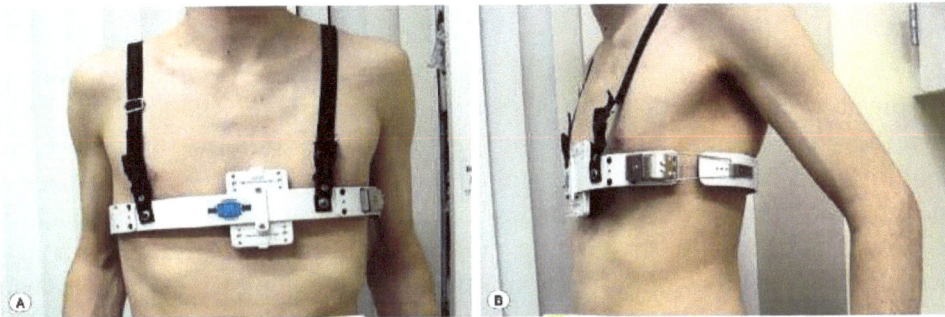

Fig. (3.13). A patient being treated with dynamic compression bracing for a prominent pectus carinatum, (A) front view, (B) lateral view. The advantage of this brace is that it allows a preset pressure to be used to compress the carinatum.

POLAND SYNDROME

Poland syndrome had been The description of Poland syndrome dates back to 1826 and 1839 in the French and German literature [30].The cause of the disease is not quite obvious so far but it is associated with the embryonic tissues forming the pectorals muscles, hyperplasia of the subclavian artery, or in utero trauma. Out of 30000 birth, usually one infant is affected by this disease, thus the disease has an irregular occurrence pattern, showing no signs of genetic disorder so far although having a history in the same families [29 - 32]. Sometimes it may be associated with a group of abnormalities in different ways. The right side of the body is more affected in 70% of the cases [33]. Another correlation is with breast hypoplasia/aplasia, as 15% of such patients may have Poland syndrome [34].

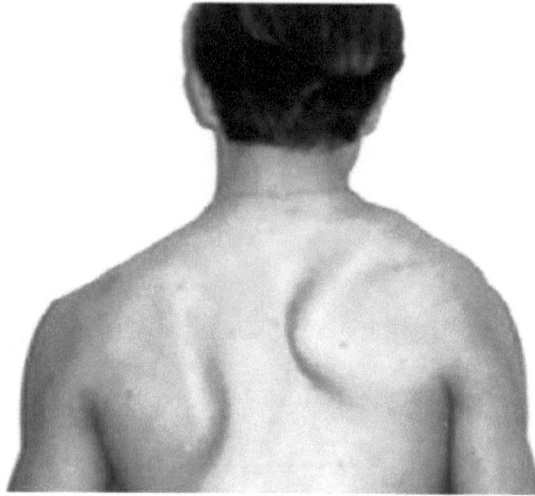

Fig. (3.14). A 12 yearold boy with Poland syndrome showing winged scapula on the right.

The extent of anomaly of the hand and chest wall may also vary from mild hyperplasia to total aplasia of muscles, ribs, and cartilage. The total aplasia may affect the chest wall depression and paradoxical respiratory motion. Clinical symptoms may include all or any of the following: absence of the pectoralis major, pectorals minor, serratus anterior, rectus abdominis, and latissimus dorsi muscles. Athelia or amastia, nipple deformities, limb deformities (syndactyly, brachydactyly), absent axillaries hair, and limited subcutaneous fat can also be found (Fig. **3.14**). Patients showing symtoms of aplasia of the ribs or a major depression deformity may require repair otherwise chest wall reconstruction with correction of contra lateral carinatum-type protrusions is the viable remedy. Autologous rib grafts, or a variety of bioprosthetic agents, with or without a latissimus dorsi flap can also be used. The usage of custom-made chest wall prostheses may sometimes be associated with some problems like migration, erosion of local tissues, and optimal cosmesis. In female patients having hyperplasia or aplasia of the breast, Chest wall reconstruction is done prior to the breast reconstruction.

STERNAL DEFECTS

Sterna defects starting from midline of the upper torso up to benign sterna cleft may be found in children and neonates. The benign sterna cleft does not show displacement of the heart while thoracic ectopic cordis being the rare and fatal one pushes the heart out of chest having no covering of the skin (Fig. **3.15**). Cleft sternum is also a rare form of chest malformations and indicates towards the partial or total failure of sterna fusion at an early stage of embryonic development.

The sternal clefts may be divided into complete, superior or inferior forms [35].

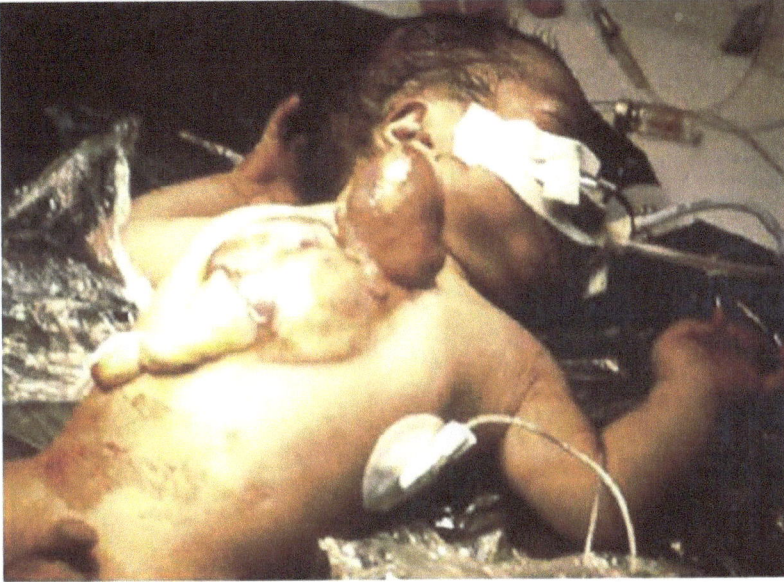

Fig. (3.15). This older photograph shows a thoracic ectopic cordis. The heart does not have any overlying somatic structures, and there is an associated upper abdominal wall defect. Note the apex of the heart in a vertical direction rather than oriented inferiorly.

Superior clefts are usually isolated, U-shaped or V-shaped, and exhibit minor lesions. The location and position of the heart is normal without cardiac malfunctioning. After the successful diagnosis, the operation is suggested which is usually very successful. If operation is conducted in neonatal period, the chances of the success are bright due to flexible and minimal compression of meditational structures, it is much easier to approximate the sterna edges. The repair after one year may involve complex procedures like the use of use of autologous structures (costal cartilage, ribs) or prosthetic materials [36, 37]. Thoracic ectopic cordis is a rare lesion in which heart is deprived of overlying somatic structures, very often resulting in mortality. Its incidence is 5.5 to 7.9 per million births and usually occurs with some form of an abdominal wall defect, with the heart sitting on the chest and the apex pointed toward the chin [38]. Intrinsic cardiac anomalies like tetralogy of Fallout, pulmonary artery stenosis, transposition of the great arteries, and ventricular septal defects (VSD) are frequently associated with it. During repair, torsion of the great vessels and compression of the heart may result in the death of the patient. Thus it is difficult to reduce the heart back into the chest. The therapy is conducted to ensure spontaneous ventilation. The therapy may include covering the heart, prevent kinking of vessels, repairing the associated abdominal wall defect, and stabilizing the thoracic cavity [39, 40]. The lesion in which the heart is covered by an omphalocele-like membrane [41] is known as Thoracoabdominal ectopic cordis. It also shows Intrinsic cardiac anomalies, with tetralogy of Fallout and VSDs. Cantrell's pentalogy consists of an inferior sterna cleft, ectopic cordis, midline abdominal wall defects or omphalocele, pericardial defects, and one or more cardiac defects. The surgery conducted to repair in these patients have better chances of success. Initially the issues like lack of skin overlying the heart and abdominal cavity is addressed and later repair is conducted to provide coverage of the midline defects, separate the abdominal and pericardial compartments, and the diaphragm. The procedure involved may include Various techniques for closure include flap mobilization, skin closure only, and the use of some bioprosthetic agents, then the congenital heart defect is taken care of.

Thoracic Insufficiency Syndrome Associated with Diffuse Skeletal Disorders

The disease in which thorax is unable to support the normal respiration or lung growth is known as Thoracic insufficiency syndrome [42]. Various disorders are associated with this, that include: (Jeune syndrome), acquired asphyxiating thoracic dystrophy (after open pectus excavatum repair), spondylothoracic dysplasia (Jarcho–Levin syndrome) Fig. (**3.16**), congenital scoliosis with multiple vertebral anomalies and fused or absent ribs (jumbled spine), unilateral thoracic hyperplasia seen with the VACTERL (vertebral defects, anal atresia, cardiac defects, trachea-esophageal fistula, renal anomalies, and limb abnormalities) syndrome and severe kyphoscoliosis. Each and every disorder is taken care of separately. Also may arise secondary to over-extensive Ravitch-type Pectus excavation repairs or repairs performed too early in life.

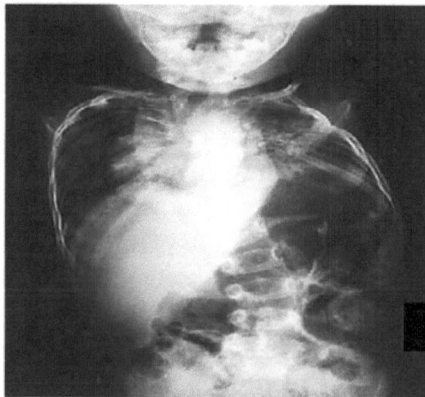

Fig. (3.16). Chest radiograph of a patient with Jarcho–Levin syndrome. The shortened thoracic spine gives a crab-like appearance.

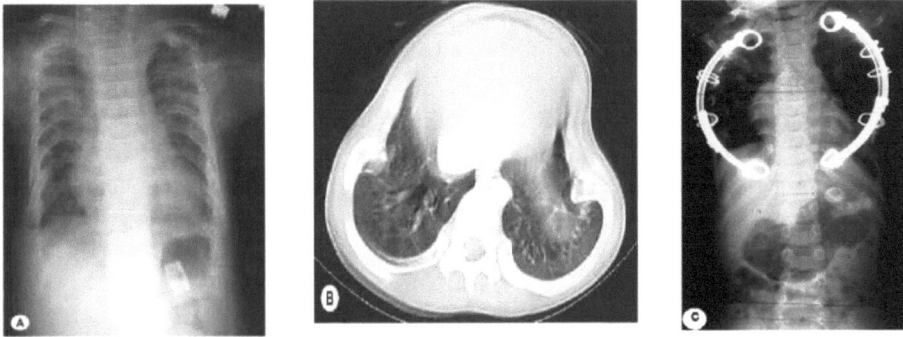

Fig. (3.17). (A) Chest radiograph of a patient with Jeune syndrome (asphyxiating thoracic dystrophy) showing narrowed thorax is narrow, with short and wide ribs (B) CT scans of Jeune syndrome (asphyxiating thoracic dystrophy) (C) Fixation of Bilateral vertical expandable prosthetic titanium ribs (VEPTR) with titanium in Jeune asphyxiating thoracic dystrophy seen in Figure 20.29 A.

The mild form of Jeune syndrome may support respiration while in severe cases the narrowing of chest transversely and vertically results in failure of respiration leading to death (Fig. **3.17**). The chest become rigid due to wide horizontal ribs and irregular costochondral junctions, with very little intercostal excursion, leading to ventilator dependence [44, 45]. This disease is an autosomal recessive inherited osteochondrodystrophy which express itself in various froms. The abnormalities associated with this also varies, despite normal bronchial development. The alveolar density is also variable [46, 47]. Extrinsic chest has a strong influence in underlying hyperplasia. The abnormalities of the muscles may include short stubby extremities, fixed elevated clavicles, hypo plastic iliac wings, and a high incidence of C1 spinal stenosis [48, 49]. The patients may also have renal dysplasia [50]. Spondylothoracic dysplasia (Jarcho–Levin) expresses itself in two inherited forms. Type I which is an autosomal recessive deformity expresses in multiple vertebral hemi vertebrae and posterior rib [51]. Thoracic spine shortens, and chest radiograph gives a crab-like chest image [52]. 30% of patients express anomalies involving cardiac and renal problems. This form is fatal and leads to death after 15 months. Type II which is spondylothoracic dysplasia and an autosomal dominant inheritance characterize near-normal longevity, which is widespread in white neonates. The operative repair in these diseases is associated with the correction of thoracic volume by different techniques. Anterior longitudinal sterna split with widening of the sternum is one such techniques acquired with methylmethacrylate. Another staged approach with a methylmethacrylate plate is also adopted that leads to secondary removal of the plate and latissimus dorsi flaps to cover the created sterna cleft. In patients of acquired thoracic dystrophy, elevation of the sternum is done by adopting open and the minimally invasive techniques that are commonly used for Pectus repair.

A lateral staged approach has also been useful. All approaches described above give variable success in enough growth of the chest wall that may lead to lung expansion.The lateral thoracic expansion may affect normal functioning of intercostal muscle. A promising technique to address this problem developed by Campbell and Smith is expansion thoracoplasty and the use of a vertically expandable prosthetic titanium rib (VEPTR) that addresses many of the problems found in the above mentioned disorders. These results in expansion of the chest wall allowing un-hindered growth of the thorax and spine. This technique is accompanied with anterior rib osteotomy adjacent to the costochondral junction and posterior osteotomy in the 3rd to 9th ribs of the spine. A segment of the chest wall is distracted with this techniques that is anchored to the VEPTR with 2 mm titanium rings, stabilizing the segment, and allowing re-ossification of the multiple osteotomies. The second phase of this stage is performed after 3 month and devices involved in the technique are expanded every six months. This technique is useful for patients with fused or absent ribs and scoliosis, and allows expansion of the chest, correction of the scoliosis and the rotational spinal deformity. The resulting increased spinal height in both congenital scoliosis and Jarcho Levin syndrome may involve the placement of bilateral devices [53 - 55].

Congenital Diaphragmatic Hernia

CDH is a defect in the posterolateral diaphragm, also called as foramen of Bochdalek. The abdominal viscera translocate through this defect into the chest during fetal development. The overall incidence of CDH is likely underestimated, as around 25–35% of fetuses that are prenatally diagnosed with CDH result in pregnancy termination, in utero demise, or death shortly after birth [56]. Thus, many infants with prenatally diagnosed CDH may never be seen or accounted for in a tertiary referral center [57]. CDH affects male infants more commonly, and the majority of posterlateral CDH are left sided (80%), with right sided (19%) and bilateral (1%) accounting for the rest [58 - 60]. Ninety percent of all CDH cases are located at the posterolateral or "**Bochdalek**" location, and the remainder is located anteriorly, termed "**Morgagni**" hernias, along with defects of the central septum transversum. Bilateral diaphragmatic hernias are more commonly associated with other congenital anomalies, and portend a much worse prognosis [60].

Associated Anomalies

Although approximately 60% of CDH cases are isolated, the others are associated with anomalies of the cardiovascular (27.5%), urogenital (17.7%), musculoskeletal (15.7%), and central nervous (9.8%) (CNS) systems [61], the impact of associated anomalies on prognosis and outcome cannot be overstated.

Although defect, size and the degree of CDH-PH are important contributors to overall survival, infants with isolated CDH demonstrate a significant survival advantage when compared with those with major concomitant cardiac, chromosomal, or associated structural anomalies (70–85% *vs* as low as 20%, depending on specific anomaly or anomalies) [62, 63].

Diaphragm Development and CDH Pathogenesis

Precursors to the development of human diaphragm begin to form during the fourth week of gestation. Historically, the diaphragm was thought to develop from the fusion of four embryonic components: anteriorly by the septum transversum, dorsolaterally by the pleuroperitoneal folds (PPFs), dorsally by the crura from the esophageal mesentery, and posteriorly by the body wall mesoderm [64, 65], the extension of the septum transversum divides the pleural and coelomic cavities during fetal development. This precursor of the diaphragm results in the separation of two cavities at the posterolateral aspects of this mesenchymally derived structure. Inadequate closure of the pleuroperitoneal canal allows the abdominal viscera to enter the thoracic cavity when they return from the extraembryonic coelom to herniate into the chest with the liver. As a result of the limited intrathoracic space, due to the visceral herniation, pulmonary hypoplasia develops.

Prenatal Diagnosis

Accurate prenatal diagnosis and prognostication of disease severity is an important adjunct to prenatal counseling, patient triage, and identification of high-risk infants with CDH. In obtaining an accurate diagnosis, it is important to differentiate CDH from other intrathoracic anomalies in which normal anatomy is otherwise undisturbed. These include CPAMs, bronchogenic cysts, bronchial atresia, or bronchopulmonary sequestrations, as well as meditational lesions, including enteric, neuronteric, or thymic cysts. Diaphragm eventration must also be included in the differential diagnoses [66], approximately 50–70% of infants with CDH are identified during pregnancy, and the frequency of prenatal detection has substantially improved in the past two decades [67 - 69]. The diagnosis of CDH is most often first made between the 18th and 22nd weeks of pregnancy on ultrasound (US) screening exams (Fig. **3.18**) [66]. Fetal US features include Polyhydramnios, intrathoracic fluid-filled bowel loops, an echogenic chest mass, meditational shift, and/or an intrathoracic stomach. Left-sided CDHs are more frequently detected prenatally [70] and feature meditational/cardiac shift to the right as well as herniation of the stomach, intestines, and/or spleen [67]. US of the fetal chest is best performed in the axial plane. The lung-to-head ratio (LHR) is a prenatal US assessment ratio, utilizing the contralateral lung area to the head circumference, which predicts CDH severity [71, 72]. If diaphragm pathology is suspected on fetal US, fetal magnetic resonance imaging (MRI) may add additional prognostic value [66], the percentage of liver herniation on fetal MRI correlates with pulmonary morbidity, with >20% liver herniation predicting more profound morbidity [73]. In addition, fetal MRI is an excellent modality for morphologic and volumetric measurements of the fetal lung (total fetal lung volume [TFLV]). It is especially advantageous in patients with oligohydramnios and maternal obesity.

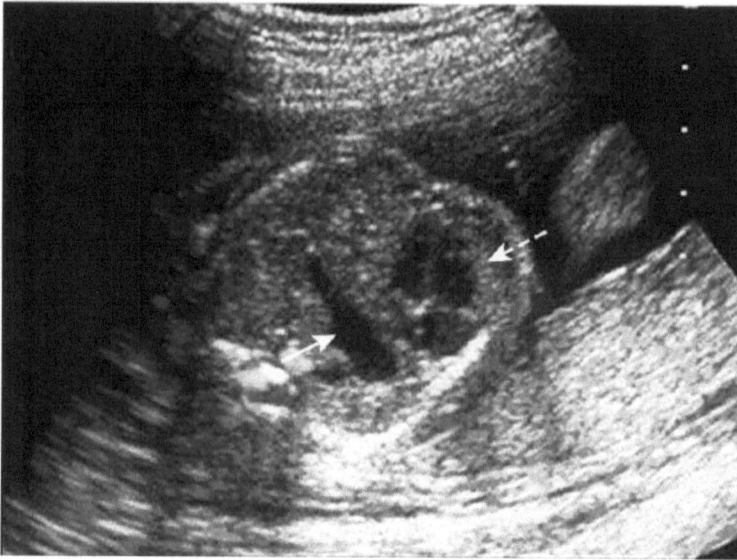

Fig. (3.18). Fetal ultrasound image at the level of the four-chamber heart (dotted arrow). Gastric bubble (solid arrow) at the level of the four chamber heart suggests CDH. This is the level used to calculate the lung-to-head ratio.

Clinical Presentation

Newborns with CDH typically present with respiratory distress. Clinical scenarios at birth range from immediate, profound respiratory distress with concomitant respiratory acidosis and hemodynamic instability, to an initial stable period with delayed respiratory distress, to an asymptomatic newborn. Initial signs associated with respiratory distress include tachypnea, chest wall retractions, grunting, cyanosis, and/or pallor. On physical examination, infants will often have a scaphoid abdomen and may have a subtle increase in thoracic diameter. The point of maximal cardiac impulse is often displaced, a physical finding with meditational shift. Bowel sounds may be auscultated within the thoracic cavity with a decrease in breath sounds bilaterally. Chest excursion may be reduced, suggesting a lower tidal volume. The diagnosis of CDH is typically confirmed by a chest radiograph demonstrating intestinal loops within the hemithorax, cephalad displacement of the stomach/Orogastric tube, and a meditational shift toward the contralateral hemithorax (Fig. **3.19**). The abdominal cavity may have minimal to no gas, particularly initially. Right-sided CDH can be challenging to diagnose (Fig. **3.20**). Salient features, such as intestinal and gastric herniation, may not be prominent, and the herniated right lobe of the liver can be mistaken for a right diaphragmatic elevation or eventration. Occasionally, features of lung compression may be the only radiographic sign, which can cause confusion with CPAMs, pulmonary sequestrations, bronchopulmonary cysts, neurogenic cysts, or cystic teratomas. Patients who present later in life have an excellent prognosis due to milder or absent associated complications, such as pulmonary hypoplasia and CDH-PH.

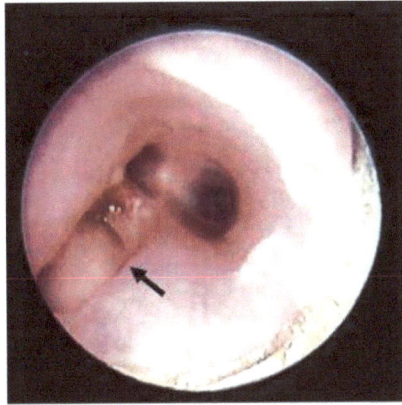

Fig. (3.19). (A) Anteroposterior chest radiograph in a neonate with a CDH demonstrating air-filled loops of bowel within the left chest. The heart and mediastinum are shifted to the right, and the hypoplastic left lung can be seen medially (B) Postoperative radiograph demonstrating hyperexpansion of the right lung with shift of the mediastinum to the left. The edge of the severely hypoplastic left lung is again easily visualized (arrow).

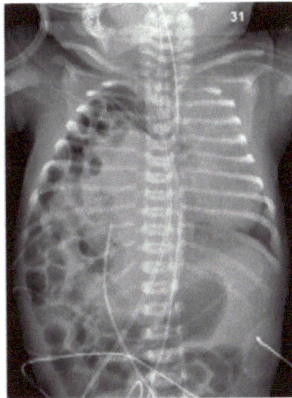

Fig. (3.20). This infant presented with respiratory distress and a right-sided CDH.

Treatment

The prenatal diagnosis of CDH continues to improve with the increased use and refinement of fetal US examination and advanced fetal MRI [74]. After initial screening, an advanced US helps to determine discordant size and dates, associated anomalies (cardiovascular, neurologic, other), as well as signs of fetal compromise (*i.e.*, hydrops fetalis). Further, an accurate LHR can estimate the probable severity, allowing informed counseling and consideration for appropriate prenatal monitoring and/or intervention. Once diagnosed, chromosomal screening *via* amniocentesis for karyotyping and chromosome microarray analysis is recommended [75]. Optimally, the mother and fetus should be referred to a tertiary perinatal center with protocolized fetal MRI and advanced maternal fetal medicine (a fetal center), neonatal, surgical, and critical care capabilities, including HFOV, ECMO, and pulmonary hypertension therapeutic expertise [75, 76]. A prenatal diagnosis enables informed counseling for the mother and family including treatment options and prognosis. After confirming the diagnosis, initial postnatal therapy is targeted at resuscitation and stabilization of the infant in cardiopulmonary distress. A rapid overall assessment is important to determine hemodynamic stability and the severity of disease. In most cases, prompt endotracheal intubation (without bag mask ventilation) and initiation of conventional mechanical ventilatory support is required. A nasogastric tube should be inserted to avoid gastric and intestinal distention. Arterial and venous access is necessary for resuscitative maneuvers. Acid–base balance and oxygenation–ventilation status should be carefully monitored. Invasive monitoring is important in accurately assessing the infant's overall perfusion and the severity of pulmonary hypertension and hypoplasia. Umbilical venous catheters may be helpful and, if possible, may be positioned in the right atrium to measure central venous pressures. In addition, an approximation of cerebral oxygenation and perfusion should be available using predictable oxygen content and/or saturation *via* either a right radial arterial catheter or a transcutaneous saturation probe. Targets for initial resuscitation include predictable arterial saturation (SaO2) between 80% and 90% with strictly limited positive airway pressures almost all infants with CDH and severe pulmonary hypertension exhibit some left ventricular dysfunction and emerging evidence continues to suggest cardiac dysfunction plays a prominent role in the outcomes of patients with CDH. Vasopressor agents such as dopamine, dobutamine, epinephrine, and Milrinone may be needed in hemodynamically unstable patients. These Inotropic agents can augment left ventricular output and increase systemic pressures in order to ameliorate right-to-left ductal shunting.

Operative Repair

With an improved understanding of its pathophysiology, repair of CDH is no longer considered an emergency procedure. However, the optimal timing for repair remains unclear. While delayed repair in most patients with CDH has become standard, in higher risk infants with CDH who require ECMO support, timing of repair as it relates to initiation of ECMO therapy remains controversial. Recently, there have been data suggesting that earlier repair when supported on ECMO results in improved survival [77]. There are two general approaches to the surgical repair of the diaphragmatic defect in CDH, open or minimally invasive. Open repair of CDH can be performed using a thoracic or abdominal approach. Advantages to laparotomy include easier reduction of intrathoracic viscera, the ability to mobilize the posterior rim of diaphragm, easier management of intestinal rotational anomalies (if necessary), and avoidance of thoracotomy-associated musculoskeletal sequelae. The vast majority of open neonatal repairs for CDH are through a subcostal incision (>90%). With advancing surgical techniques and optimization of Perioperative respiratory care, many surgeons have adopted minimally invasive surgical (MIS) approaches to CDH repair in efforts to avoid the respiratory sequelae and other morbidity seen after open repair [78, 79].

Outcomes

Clinical outcomes of infants with CDH have traditionally been difficult to generalize due to the low incidence of disease, varying patient characteristics and clinical practices, and single institution reports [80].

Risk Stratification in CDH

Defect size, associated anomalies, concomitant major congenital heart disease, and prematurity impose the greatest influence on patient survival in CDH. Thus, any comparative study on morbidity or mortality must risk-stratify across these known risk factors. Stratification by defect size correlates with disease severity [81, 82], and this association has prompted development of a universal grading system to define CDH defect size [80],based on intraoperative findings, the four classifications range from small defects that could be repaired primarily to total diaphragmatic agenesis. Congenital heart defects occur in 6–18% of CDH infants [80, 83]. However, when categorized into major (hemodynamically significant) and minor lesions (such asymptomatic ASD, VSD, or PDA), survival varies from 36% (major) to 67% (minor) [83]. When compared with infants without structural cardiac anomalies, the risk of hospital mortality was 2.2-fold higher in infants with major cardiac disease [83]. Defined as delivery <38 weeks of gestation, preterm birth occurs in approximately 23–30% of infants with CDH and the overall survival is approximately 50% for those born prematurely [84, 85]. Survival inversely correlates with prematurity. Infants born at <28 weeks of gestational age have been found to have a 32% chance of survival compared with 73.1% for those born at 37 weeks [84]. After adjusting for comorbdities and disease severity, prematurity had an increased odds ratio of 1.68 for death.

Bronchopulmonary Sequestration

BPS comprises approximately 10% of prenatally diagnosed BPMs and is defined as a portion of lung parenchyma that does not communicate with the normal tracheobronchial tree. These lesions have a systemic arterial blood supply, usually aorta and may have systemic and/or pulmonary venous return. Two different types of sequestrations are described: intralobar (iBPS) and extra lobar (eBPS), which differ in their prenatal and postnatal characteristics [86]. IBPS share the visceral pleural investment with the normal adjacent lung and have their venous return to the pulmonary vein, more commonly occurs within the parenchyma of the left lower lobe. In contrast, eBPS have a separate pleural investment and may have systemic and/or pulmonary venous drainage, located almost above the left diaphragm, it is commonly found in cases of CDH. The cause of sequestration is unknown but most probably involves an abnormal budding of the developing lung that picks up a systemic blood supply and never becomes connected with the bronchus or pulmonary vessels. Sequestrations may, in some cases, exhibit mixed pathology with components consistent with CCAMs. Extralobar sequestration is asymptomatic and is usually discovered incidentally on chest X-ray. If the diagnosis can be confirmed, *e.g.*, by CT scan, resection is not necessary. Diagnosis of intralobar sequestration may be made prenatally by Doppler US and confirmed on postnatal CT scan. Alternatively, the diagnosis of intralobar sequestration may be established after repeated infections manifested by cough, fever, and consolidation in the posterior basal segment of the left lower lobe.

Removal of the entire left lower lobe is usually necessary since the diagnosis often is made late after multiple infections. Occasionally segmental resection of the sequestered part of the lung can be performed using an open, or ideally, a thoracoscopic approach. If an open approach is used, it is important to open the chest through a low intercostal space (sixth or seventh) to gain access to the vascular attachments to the aorta. These attachments may insert into the aorta below the diaphragm; in these cases, division of the vessels as they traverse the thoracic cavity is essential.

Prognosis is generally excellent. However, failure to obtain adequate control of these vessels may result in their retraction into the abdomen and result in uncontrollable hemorrhage. It is also possible to perform a combined thoracoscopic and open approach, where the vessels are clipped and divided thoracoscopically and then the lesion safely removed through a limited thoracotomy.

Differential Diagnosis

The differential diagnosis of sub diaphragmatic BPS in the fetus or neonate includes neuroblastoma and adrenal hemorrhage, which can be differentiated on serial US imaging. BPS in close proximity to the esophagus can have an esophageal bronchus that needs to be identified and ligated during excision. There is debate regarding the postnatal management of a small intrathoracic or sub diaphragmatic BPS. Small BPSs with small feeding vessels have been reported to spontaneously regress [87], and carry a low risk of infection or malignancy. This has led some surgeons to avoid resection in such cases. Management of BPSs should be individualized, with the specific indications for resection shown in Box **3.1**. The surgical management of BPSs involves ligation and division of the systemic vasculature and removal of the mass. This must be done with care as systemic vessels arising from the abdominal aorta may cross the diaphragm and lead to difficult to control bleeding if not adequately ligated [88].

Box (3.1). Indications for Resection of Extralobar Bronchopulmonary Sequestrations.

Large systemic vascular supply.
Large lesions with compression of surrounding lung parenchyma or meditational shift.
Lesions with cystic components on prenatal ultrasound or postnatal CT scan.
Lesions that continue to grow postnatal.
Lesions within or under the diaphragm.

Congenital Lobar Emphysema

CLE is a condition characterized by overinflation and distension of one or more pulmonary lobes secondary to a one-way-valve mechanism, with variable degrees of compression of the adjacent lung. It occurs in 1; 20000-30000 live births. In half of cases, the cause is unknown. In the remaining half, the over distention results from dysplastic and weakened bronchial cartilage; end bronchial obstruction; extrinsic compression from vascular structures, cysts, tumors, *etc.*; or diffuse bronchial abnormalities related to infection. In the fetus, amniotic fluid trapping is analogous to postnatal air trapping, and can lead to lobar expansion [89]. The left upper lobe is the most frequently affected, followed by right middle and upper lobes, with rare bilateral or multifocal involvement. Most neonates/infants present with respiratory distress [90].

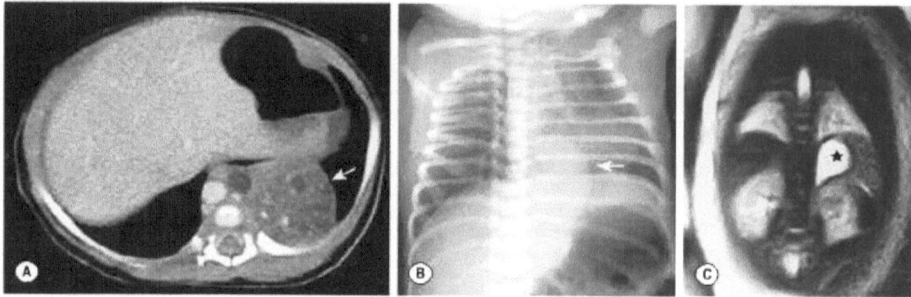

Fig. (3.21). (A) This CT scan shows an extralobar bronchopulmonary sequestration (eBPS) (arrow) in the typical basilar location in the left chest (B) In a different patient, the chest radiograph shows a large transdiaphragmatic eBPS (arrow) (C) This fetal MRI shows a left infradiaphragmatic eBPS (star).

Symptoms range from mild respiratory distress to full fledged respiratory failure with tachypnea, dyspnea, cough, and late cyanosis. The symptoms may be limited to this or may show progression resulting in recurrent pneumonia. Occasionally, infants with CLE present with failure to thrive, which likely reflects the increased work associated with the overexpanded lung. A hyperexpanded hemithorax in such infants on the ipsilateral side is pathogneumonic for CLE and is diagnosed by the chest X-ray. The mediastinum may be shifted resulting in the compression and atelectasis of the contralateral lung, (Fig. **3.22**). Barotraumas associated with Tx. of bronchopulmonary dysplasia in preterm infant can result in acquired emphysema in which multiple areas of hyperinflation may present most common in lower lobe, this help in differentiate congenital from acquired. Incidental Dx. need close monitoring due to rapid deterioration due to lesion regress. Long term pulmonary growth and function after lobectomy for CLE is excellent. Treatment is resection of the affected lobe, which can be safely, performed using either an open or thoracoscopic approach. Unless symptoms necessitate earlier surgery, resection can usually be performed after the infant is several months of age. The prognosis is excellent.

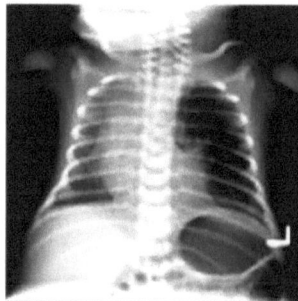

Fig. (3.22). Congenital lobar emphysema of the left upper lobe in a 2-week-old boy. Mediastinal shift is present.

Esophageal Atresia and Tracheo-esophageal Fistula

The esophagus and trachea share a common embryologic origin. At approximately 4 weeks' gestation, a diverticulum forms off the anterior aspect of the proximal foregut in the region of the primitive pharynx. This diverticulum extends caudally with progressive formation of the laryngotracheal groove, thus creating a separate trachea and esophagus. Successful development of these structures is the consequence of extremely intricate interplay of growth and transcription factors necessary for specification.. The birth incidence of this condition, EA/TEF is 1 in 2500–3000 live births [91 - 93], showing a slight male preponderance of 1.26:1. There is no evidence for a link between EA/ TEF and maternal age when chromosomal cases are excluded.. The risk of EA/TEF in second child increases from 0.5 to 2%. If parents already have more than one EA/TEF child, the risk may rise up to 20%. Certain environmental factors may be associated with EA/TEF that include use of methimazole in early pregnancy, contraceptive pills, progesterone and estrogen exposure, diabetes in mother, and thalidomide exposure [95 - 99]. Mothers suffering from fetal alcohol syndrome and phenylketonuria may also give rise to EA infants. Usually 6-10% of such infants also have Chromosomal anomalies [100, 101].

Anomalies Associated with EA

The factors that cause EA during organogenesis may also affect other organs as well during the embryonic development. Clinically, there are two types of EA. Isolated EA and syndromic EA, having the same rate of incidence [102]. The malformations associated with the syndromic EA are:

• Cardiac malformation (13–34%), the more significant one
• Vertebral malformation (6–21%)
• Limb malformation (5–19%)
• Anorectal malformation (10–16%)
• Renal malformation (5–14%)

There are numerous classifications for EA and TEF available in literature. Usually EA is considered as a spectrum of anomalies, (Fig. **3.23**) [103].

Gross Type A: Pure Esophageal Atresia without TEF

The incidence of EA is 7% . The proximal and distal esophagus end blindly in the posterior mediastinum. The proximal end is dilated and has a thickened wall as in the more common EA/TEF. If there is no concomitant proximal fistula, the upper esophagus ends at the level of the azygos vein. The distal esophagus is short and often suspended by a fibrotic band. The distance between the two segments is considerable, usually precluding immediate anastomosis.

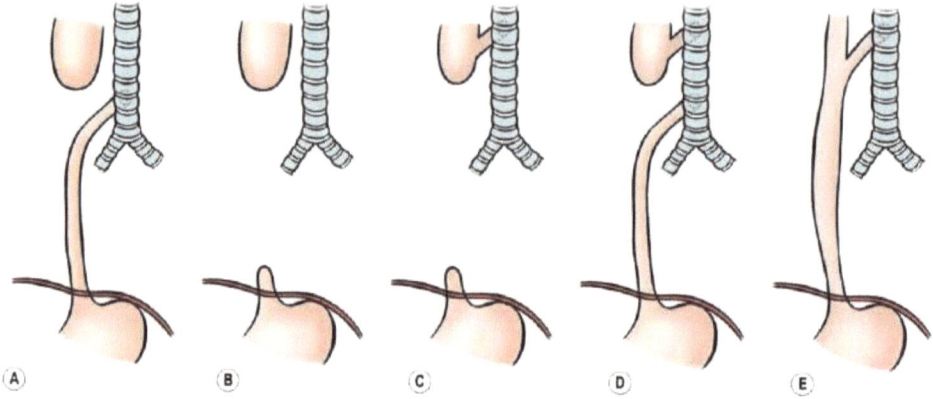

Fig. (3.23). Classification of EA and/or TEF (A) EA with distal TEF: Vogt IIIb, Ladd III, Gross C (B) EA without TEF: Vogt II, Ladd I, Gross A (C) EA with proximal TEF: Vogt IIIa, Ladd II, Gross B (D) EA with proximal and distal fistulas: Vogt IIIc, Ladd V, Gross D (E) TEF (H-type) without EA: Vogt IV, Gross E.

Gross Type B: Esophageal Atresia with Proximal Fistula

2% or more of the patient having EA may have a proximal fistula. This is not an upper esophageal fistula, as it is found proximally near the trachea and ends distally in the dilated proximal esophagus. It is somewhat similar to H-type. Sometime two or three fistulas may be found in some cases. The possible location of the fistula is thoracic aperture or higher in the neck. The length of the fistula is limited and the diameter is varying. In failure of diagnosis before operation, the bubbles seen on the opening the proximal esophagus may indicate its presence.

Gross Type C: Esophageal Atresia with Distal Fistula

Themost common type, thickened wall of the dilated proximal esophagus that descends into the superior mediastinum, is an indication of this anomaly that is found at a point between second to third and fourth thoracic vertebrae. At the level of carina, it posteriorly enters the trachea. The distance between both the esophageal ends may vary in this condition, from small to quite wide. The occlusion of the distal fistula may result into misdiagnosis of EA without distal fistula [105].

Gross Type D: Esophageal Atresia with Proximal and Distal Fistulas

In 1% of EA patinets, the EA is found to be associated with with proximal and distal fistulas. EA with one distal fistula and two proximal fistulas has also been described [106], also reported is a near-complete membranous obstruction of the esophagus in conjunction with a single TEF at the level of the membrane, communicating with both parts of the esophagus [107].

Gross Type E: H-type Fistula without Esophageal Atresia

H-type TEF without atresia is usually discussed together with EA because it may be part of the VACTERL association. It occurs with an incidence of about 4%. The fistula starts from the membranous trachea and runs caudad to enter the esophagus. Normally it is short, although the diameter may be variable. The fistula is usually situated at the thoracic aperture or higher in the neck [108].

Diagnosis

Polyhydraminous and an absent or small stomach bubble are the two possible non-specific signs of prenatal diagnosis of EA/TEF. Polyhydraminous is associated with anomalies that may have fetal origin. Ultrasonography (US) may indicate the absence of stomach bubble. In many patients, combination of a small stomach with a dilated cervical esophagus (the pouch sign) is the widely accepted diagnostic sign for EA [109 - 111].

Clinical Presentation of Infants with Esophageal Atresia and Tracheoesophageal Fistula

The anatomic variant of infants with EA-TEF predicts the clinical presentation. When the esophagus ends either as a blind pouch or as a fistula into the trachea (as in types A, B, C, or D), infants present with excessive drooling, followed by chocking or coughing immediately after feeding is initiated as a result of aspiration through the fistula tract. As the neonate coughs and cries, air is transmitted through the fistula into the stomach, resulting in abdominal distention. As the abdomen distends, it becomes increasingly more difficult for the infant to breathe. This leads to further atelectasis and respiratory compromise.In patients showing type C and D varieties, there are signs of pulmonary difficulties. The gastric juice passing from fistula, may be deposited in trachea and lungs, thus leading to a chemical pneumonitis. Very often this is diagnosed by a nursing staff when trying to feed the infant. The staff may witness the accumulation of oral secretions. Esophageal patency may be assessed in case of complicated pregnancy by the passage of a tube or catheter into the stomach. Similar is done when the infants exhibit anomalies that fit the VACTERL association. Due to blockage of lower esophagus the saliva accumulate in the mouth and oesophagus, and the process of feeding should be withheld until esophageal continuity is confirmed. This is best done by a stiff 10 French catheter inserted either through the oral or nasal cavity. The tip of the tube that is curled in the blind upper pouch around T2–T4, indicates towards atresia but also gives some information about length of the upper pouch. Air may be present in the stomach indicating the presence of a distal TEF. The tip of the catheter beyond the level of the carina may give rise to the questioning of the diagnosis of EA. Some conditions like esophageal stenosis, tracheal rings, and iatrogenic perforation of the esophagus may be regarded as EA which is wrong. Patients with type E TEFs (also called H-type) beyond newborn period may exhibit the symptoms like recurrent chest infections, bronchospasm, and failure to thrive.

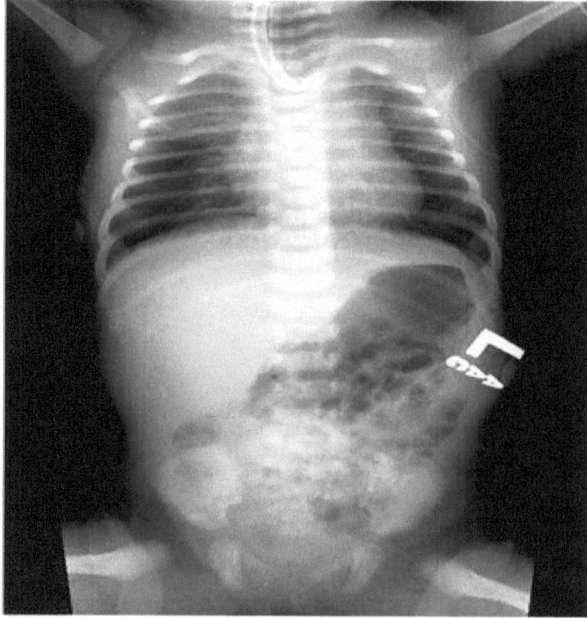

Fig. (3.24). This plain radiograph shows characteristics features present in infants with EA and TEF. A kinked nasoesophageal tube is seen in the upper pouch and an air in the stomach and bowel, represent a distal TEF.

PREOPERATIVE MANAGEMENT

As soon as the diagnosis of EA is made, the placement of a 10 French Replogle tube is advised in the upper esophagus, thus ensuring the continuous suction [112]. The head of the child is kept up. Intravenous access is essential, IV antibiotic therapy is initiated, vital signs are monitored and with the administration of warmed electrolyte solution. It is ensured that IV line is not placed on the right upper extremity, since this is going to hinder the surgical procedures. In cases of respiratory distress, endotracheal intubation and ventilation is required. Diaphragmatic splinting and even gastric rupture may result in case of forceful ventilation. To avoid this situation, low-pressure ventilation or high-frequency ventilation is maintained. In emergency conditions of the infants, emergency gastrostomy to decompress the stomach could be better.

Disadvantages like significant loss of tidal volume and respiratory issues are associated with this in some cases. The operative repair of EA/TEF is usually not required in emergency situation, thus healthcare staff has a lot of time in making diagnosis for associated anomalies. If the child is hemodynamically stable and is oxygenating well, definitive repair may be performed within 1 to 2 days after birth.

Operative Repair

In order to secure definitive repair, Primary Surgical Correction also called primary esophagoesophagostomy is conducted by two approaches, open thoracotomy or thoracoscopy.

COMPLICATIONS FROM OPERATIVE REPAIR

Anastomotic leaks

An overall leak rate of 3.5–17% has been reported by several authors [113-115]. These Anastomotic leaks may be seen immediately after the operation or several days after the repair. The reason for immediate leakage in first 24-48 hours could be pleural effusion, pneumothorax, and sepsis. The evaluation needs to be conducted immediately. Anastomosis is disrupted in such cases due to excessive tension, for this reason revision of anastomosis is required. If not, cervical esophagostomy and gastrostomy placement could be the possible option to ensure esophageal continuity. If these leakages are detected after some days of repair, immediate intervention may not be required. Administration of broad-spectrum antibiotics and pulmonary toilet are enough to treat this. A nutritional approach is also adopted in such cases. An esophagram that is conducted after a week or so may show the signs of resolution of the problem.

Strictures

Strictures may be there especially if the leakage has occurred. Its frequency could possibly be 10%–20%), and may become visible immediately after the surgery or many months or in some cases years later. Choking and gagging could be the possibly symptoms. These becomes visible as soon as the infants start eating solid food. A contrast swallow or esophagoscopy is often required to confirm the diagnosis, and simple dilatation is the possible corrective measure adopted widely [116].

Recurrent TEF

may represent a missed upper pouch fistula or a true recurrence. This may occur after an anastomotic disruption, during which the recurrent fistula may heal spontaneously. This may require the surgery again. The use of fibrin glue has widely been adopted in treating recurrent fistulas, currently.

Gastro Esophageal Reflux

During repair of EA/TEF, there may occur some alterations in esophageal motility and the anatomy of the gastroesophageal junction, giving rise to gastroesophageal reflux. The symptoms of this condition are same as that of primary gastroesophageal reflux disease. A loose antireflux technique, such as a Nissen fundoplication, may be adopted for the prevention of this condition, but this may lead to intrinsic dysmotility of the distal esophagus, creating feedig problems in the infants. An experienced healthcare may perform laproscopic fundoplication, but the care must be taken to ensure that the wrap is not excessively tight.

Corrosive Ingestion

Corrosive substances are chemical agents capable of injuring tissue on contact. Caustic ingestion in children, especially those <6 years old, is a global problem, especially in developing countries. In 20–40% of caustic ingestions some degree of esophageal injury will be produced [117], the extent of injury is dependent on several factors including the composition of the substance, volume, concentration, and duration of contact. Acidic injury results in immediate pain and liquefactive or coagulative necrosis with Escher formation, which likely limits tissue penetration and injury depth. Acidic ingestions most commonly cause gastric injury; more commonly result in esophageal injury. Alkalis combine with tissue proteins to cause liquefactive necrosis and saponification, and generally penetrate deeper into tissues, potentially leading to full thickness damage to the esophageal wall. Alkali absorption leads to vascular thrombosis, further impeding blood flow to the damaged tissue. Ingestion of granular products may result in more serious injuries due to prolonged contact time with the esophageal mucosa. Alkali ingestions have three phases of injury.

Liquefactive Necrosis, Reparative Phase, and Scar Retraction

In liquefactive necrosis, the injury rapidly penetrates the deep layers of the esophagus until the alkali is buffered by tissue fluids. Somewhere between 5 days and 2 weeks following injury is considered the reparative phase. Sloughing of the necrotic debris is followed by the development of granulation tissue and collagen deposition. The esophageal wall is thinnest during this sub acute phase and at highest risk for perforation. Scar formation begins after 2 weeks, during which there is deposition of collagen, potentially resulting in esophageal stricture formation. Subsequent strictures occur at the anatomic narrowed areas of the esophagus, cricopharyngeus, midesophagus, and gastroesophageal junction. The swallowing of an injurious substance may have no affects or symptoms but the child may not be able to swallow the saliva and drooling. The injury associated with this condition may be limited to pharynx and esophagus, or it may extend to include the stomach, may present with include nausea, vomiting, dysphagia, odynophagia, drooling, abdominal pain, chest pain, or stridor.

Management

Initial management of these patients should focus on airway management, volume resuscitation, and evaluation for esophageal or gastric perforation. Caregivers should be encouraged to bring in the ingested substance container if available. The oral cavity should be examined for signs of erythema or injury. Inducing emesis is discouraged because additional exposure to the substance can cause increased mucosal damage. There is no evidence to support dilution therapy with water or milk. Chest and abdominal radiographs should be obtained to look for signs of perforation. A chest CT can also be used in selected cases. In general, flexible upper endoscopy should be carried out in the first 24–48 hours after ingestion to characterize the degree of injury. Evidence of perforation is the only absolute contraindication to endoscopy. Because the burned esophagus is weakest between 7 and 21 days post ingestion, endoscopy generally should not be performed after 5 days to minimize the risks of perforation, fistula, and bleeding. Caustic injuries are classified similar to burns Table **3.4**.

Table (3.4). Incidence of morbidities in long term follow-up of patients with CDH.

Morbidity	Estimated frequency
Pulmonary Tracheostomy Decreased exercise intolerance Chronic recurrent pneumonia	4% 7-35% 7%
Neurodevelopmental Neuropathologic lesion Cognitive and motor dysfunction Emotional\behavioral problems	50% 20-73% 11-23%
Gastrointestinal GERD Long term carcinoma risk Failure to thrive	50-100% Unclear 50-60%
Musculoskeletal Pectus deformities Chest asymmetry Scoliosis	14-80% 48% 4-50%

Morbidity	Estimated frequency
Surgical complications Recurrence Small bowel obstruction	6-24% 1-8% (early)
Impact on family Caregiver impact Financial\time burden	20-40%

COMPLICATIONS

ESOPHAGEAL STRICTURE

Barret's Esophagus

Esophageal carcinoma is a late but serious complication of a severe caustic injury. The incidence is 1000 times the expected occurrence rate of patients of a similar age (Fig. **3.25**).

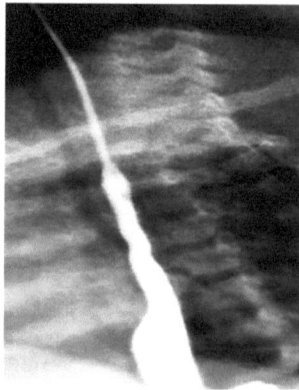

Fig. (3.25). This barium swallow was performed three weeks after lye ingestion. Note the significant narrowing in the proximal two-thirds of the esophagus.

Table (3.5). Classification of caustic esophageal injuries.

Grade	Endoscopic Findings
1	Mucosal edema and erythema
2a	Friability, hemorrhage, blisters, erosions, erythema, white exudates
2b	Findings of grade 2a plus deep or circumferential ulceration
3a	Small and scattered area of necrosis
3b	Extensive necrosis

Foreign Body

Foreign body ingestion is common in children. When a foreign body becomes impacted in the esophagus, it may erode into the airway, aorta, mediastinum, or pleural space, causing life-threatening complications (Table **3.5**) [118, 119]. Impaction is most likely to occur at one of the four sites of physiologic narrowing in the esophagus: the cricopharyngeus of the UES (the narrowest point in the GI tract), the aortic notch, the left main stem bronchus, and the LES. The epidemiology of swallowed foreign bodies depends on the cultural context. In Western countries, coins account for the majority of pediatric foreign body ingestions, while pieces of food account for 10–20%.

Clinical Presentation

Infants may present with excessive drooling, refusal to eat, and unexplained coughing or gagging. Older children can have dysphagia, vomiting, chest pain, or respiratory symptoms.

Diagnosis

The best initial diagnostic tests are anteroposterior and lateral chest radiographs. The flat surface of a coin is best seen on the anteroposterior view when it is lodged in the esophagus, whereas the lateral view will show the flat surface when it is lodged in the trachea (Fig. **3.26**). Radiographs will also differentiate coins from button batteries, which may have a halo sign, as well as the step-off between the positive and negative nodes the battery. If no radiopaque object is seen and suspicion is high, contrast esophagram or diagnostic endoscopy can be performed.

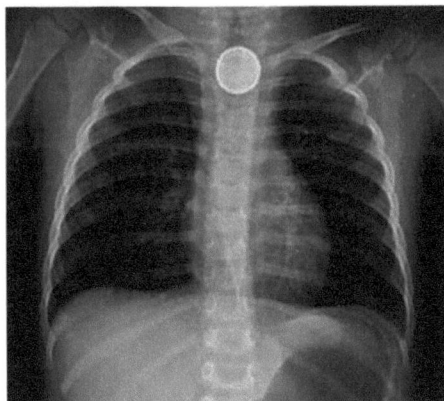

Fig. (3.26). This child presented within 12 hours of swallowing an unknown foreign body. However, the double contour rim raised suspicion of ingestion of a button battery. This was confirmed upon emergency removal of the battery *via* rigid esophagoscopy.

Management

Key principles of endoscopic management of esophageal foreign bodies are to protect the airway, maintain control of the object during extraction, and avoid causing additional damage. Many centers use flexible endoscopy to remove low-risk (smooth-surfaced) esophageal foreign bodies. Coins can be grasped with endoscopic (Magill) grasping forceps and extracted with the scope through the mouth, or pushed gently into the stomach to be retrieved with a basket (Fig. **3.27**). Other approaches have been described, including bougienage, Foley balloon extraction under fluoroscopy, and brief observation trials [123], around 40–50% of pediatric esophageal food impactions are associated with eosinophilic esophagitis. Current recommendations are to biopsy the proximal and distal esophagus at the time of endoscopic removal, treat with a proton pump inhibitor, and perform repeat endoscopy in 6–12 weeks [124, 125].

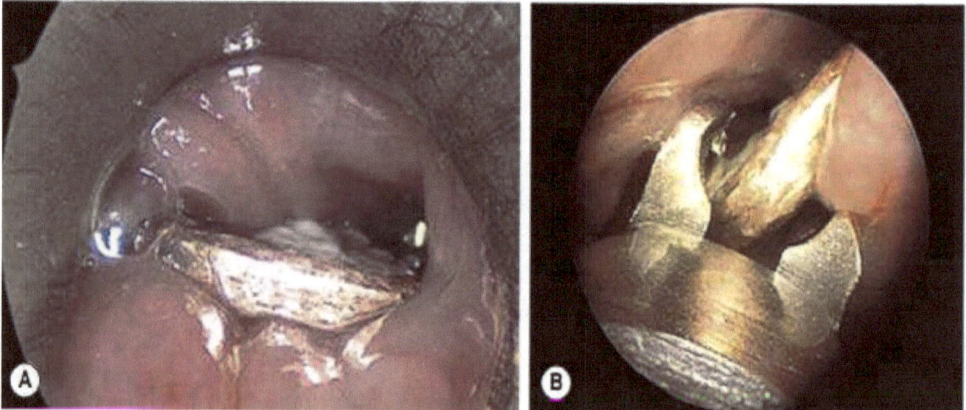

Fig. (**3.27**). This coin was lodged in the esophagus of a 2-year-old child. It was unclear how long the coin had been in the esophagus. Rigid esophagoscopy was performed (A) The coin is seen through the esophagoscope (B) The optical graspers are being used to grasp the coin and remove it. The safety and success rate for rigid esophagoscopy and coin removal approaches 100% with minimal complications. This is usually a safe and successful way to remove a coin in the esophagus of children in whom the Foley catheter technique is not appropriate.

For other objects or complicated presentations, removal with rigid esophagoscopy under general anesthesia is the gold standard. This procedure has been proven to be highly successful with low complication rates. Button batteries warrant special attention due to their potential for severe complications, including esophageal perforation, TEF, bilateral vocal cord paralysis, and death from aortoesophageal fistula (AEF) and uncontrollable hemorrhage (Fig. **3.28**). Most serious button battery injuries are caused by lithium batteries >20 mm AEF is the deadliest complication of impacted esophageal foreign bodies, with fatality rates of 40–70% (Fig. **3.29**). Delayed perforations or those involving other essential structures can be managed with positioning an endoscopic feeding tube past the injury, nil per os (NPO), and intravenous (IV) antibiotics for 4–6 weeks. If a contrast esophagram demonstrates resolution of the leak, oral feeds can be initiated. Otherwise, delayed repair can be performed.

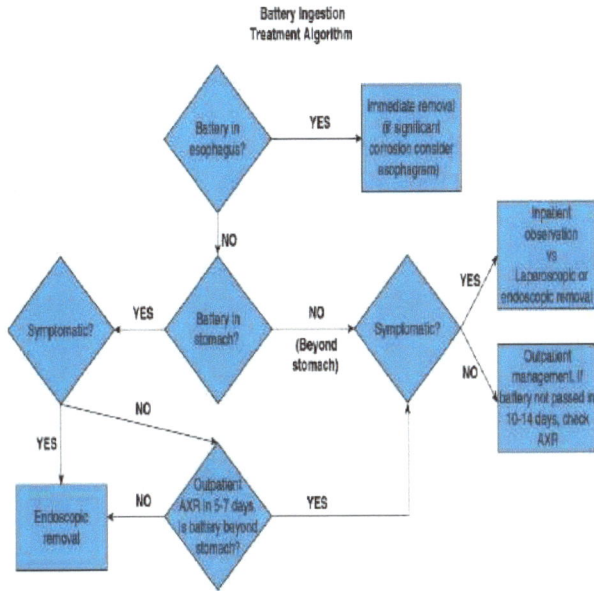

Fig. (3.28). Management algorithm for ingested batteries, AXR, abdominal radiograph (From Rosenfeld EH, Sola R, Yu YY, *et al.*, 53(8):1537–1541. Reprinted with permission).

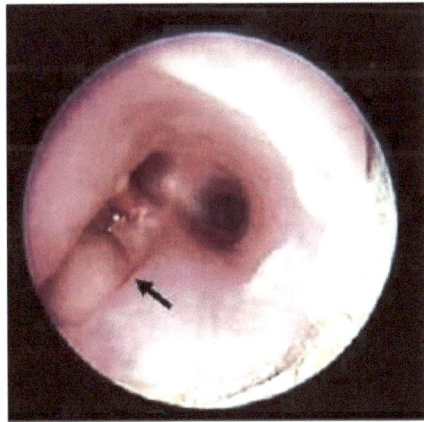

Fig. (3.29). This infant accidentally swallowed a lithium battery. The battery was removed within a few hours of its ingestion. However, 1 week later, the patient developed respiratory distress and bronchoscope revealed this tracheoesophageal fistula (arrow).

CONSENT FOR PUBLICATION

Not Applicable.

CONFLICT OF INTEREST

The author declares no conflict of interest, financial or otherwise.

ACKNOWLEDGEMENTS

Declared none.

REFERENCES

[1]   Shamberger RC. Congenital chest wall deformities. In: Grosfeld JL, O'Neill JA, Jr, Fonkalsrud EW, Coran AG, Eds. Pediatric Surgery. 5th ed. Philadelphia: Elsevier 1998; pp. 787-817.

[2]   Creswick HA, Stacey MW, Kelly RE Jr, *et al.* Family study of the inheritance of pectus excavatum. J Pediatr Surg 2006; 41(10): 1699-703.
[http://dx.doi.org/10.1016/j.jpedsurg.2006.05.071] [PMID: 17011272]

[3]   Horth L, Stacey MW, Proud VK, *et al.* Advancing our understanding of the inheritance and transmission of pectus excavatum. J Pediatr Genet 2012; 1(3): 161-73.
[PMID: 27625818]

[4]   Park JM, Farmer AR. Wolff-Parkinson-White syndrome in children with pectus excavatum. J Pediatr 1988; 112(6): 926-8.
[http://dx.doi.org/10.1016/S0022-3476(88)80219-1] [PMID: 3373400]

[5]   Lawson ML, Cash TF, Akers R, *et al.* A pilot study of the impact of surgical repair on disease-specific quality of life among patients with pectus excavatum. J Pediatr Surg 2003; 38(6): 916-8.
[http://dx.doi.org/10.1016/S0022-3468(03)00123-4] [PMID: 12778393]

[6]   Nuss D, Kelly RE Jr, Croitoru DP, Katz ME. A 10-year review of a minimally invasive technique for the correction of pectus excavatum. J Pediatr Surg 1998; 33(4): 545-52.
[http://dx.doi.org/10.1016/S0022-3468(98)90314-1] [PMID: 9574749]

[7]   Croitoru DP, Kelly RE Jr, Goretsky MJ, Lawson ML, Swoveland B, Nuss D. Experience and modification update for the minimally invasive Nuss technique for pectus excavatum repair in 303 patients. J Pediatr Surg 2002; 37(3): 437-45.
[http://dx.doi.org/10.1053/jpsu.2002.30851] [PMID: 11877663]

[8]   St Peter SD, Weesner KA, Weissend EE, *et al.* Epidural *vs* patient-controlled analgesia for postoperative pain after pectus excavatum repair: a prospective, randomized trial. J Pediatr Surg 2012; 47(1): 148-53.
[http://dx.doi.org/10.1016/j.jpedsurg.2011.10.040] [PMID: 22244408]

[9]   Martinez D, Juame J, Stein T, *et al.* The effect of costal cartilage resection on chest wall development. Pediatr Surg Int 1990; 5: 170-3.
[http://dx.doi.org/10.1007/BF00179655]

[10]   Haller JA Jr, Colombani PM, Humphries CT, Azizkhan RG, Loughlin GM. Chest wall constriction after too extensive and too early operations for pectus excavatum. Ann Thorac Surg 1996; 61(6): 1618-24.
[http://dx.doi.org/10.1016/0003-4975(96)00179-8] [PMID: 8651758]

[11]   Sauerbruch F. Operative BeseitigungderAngeborenenTrichterbrust. Dtsch Z Chir 1931; 234: 760.
[http://dx.doi.org/10.1007/BF02797645]

[12]   Gross RE. The Surgery of Infancy and Childhood. Philadelphia: WB Saunders 1953; pp. 753-61.

[13]   Shamberger RC, Welch KJ. Surgical correction of pectus carinatum. J Pediatr Surg 1987; 22(1): 48-53.
[http://dx.doi.org/10.1016/S0022-3468(87)80014-3] [PMID: 3819993]

[14]   Chin EF. Surgery of funnel chest and congenital sternal prominence. Br J Surg 1957; 44(186): 360-76.
[http://dx.doi.org/10.1002/bjs.18004418607] [PMID: 13510593]

[15]   Hosie S, Sitkiewicz T, Petersen C, *et al.* Minimally invasive repair of pectus excavatum-the Nuss procedure. A European multicentre experience. Eur J Pediatr Surg 2002; 12(4): 235-8.
[http://dx.doi.org/10.1055/s-2002-34486] [PMID: 12368999]

[16]   Robicsek F, Cook JW, Daugherty HK, Selle JG. Pectus carinatum. J Thorac Cardiovasc Surg 1979; 78(1): 52-61.
[http://dx.doi.org/10.1016/S0022-5223(19)38162-0] [PMID: 376953]

[17]   Peña A, Pérez L, Nurko S, Dorenbaum D. Pectus carinatum and pectus excavatum: are they the same disease? Am Surg 1981; 47(5): 215-8.
[PMID: 7235385]

[18]   Hebra A, Thomas PB, Tagge EP, *et al.* Pectus carinatum as a sequela of minimally invasive pectus excavatum repair. PediatrEndosurgInnovatTechn 2002; 6: 41-4.
[http://dx.doi.org/10.1089/10926410252832456]

[19]   Fonkalsrud EW. Surgical correction of pectus carinatum: lessons learned from 260 patients. J Pediatr Surg 2008; 43(7): 1235-43.
[http://dx.doi.org/10.1016/j.jpedsurg.2008.02.007] [PMID: 18639675]

[20]   Currarino G, Silverman FN. Premature obliteration of the sternal sutures and pigeon-breast deformity. Radiology 1958; 70(4): 532-40.
[http://dx.doi.org/10.1148/70.4.532] [PMID: 13542801]

[21]   Chidambaram B, Mehta AV. Currarino-Silverman syndrome (pectus carinatum type 2 deformity) and mitral valve disease. Chest 1992; 102(3): 780-2.
[http://dx.doi.org/10.1378/chest.102.3.780] [PMID: 1516402]

[22]   Martinez-Ferro M, Fraire C, Bernard S. Dynamic compression system for the correction of pectus carinatum. Semin Pediatr Surg 2008; 17(3): 194-200.
[http://dx.doi.org/10.1053/j.sempedsurg.2008.03.008] [PMID: 18582825]

[23]   Cohee AS, Lin JR, Frantz FW, Kelly RE Jr. Staged management of pectus carinatum. J Pediatr Surg 2013; 48(2): 315-20.
[http://dx.doi.org/10.1016/j.jpedsurg.2012.11.008] [PMID: 23414858]

[24]   Abramson H, D'Agostino J, Wuscovi S. A 5-year experience with a minimally invasive technique for pectus carinatum repair. J Pediatr Surg 2009; 44(1): 118-23.
[http://dx.doi.org/10.1016/j.jpedsurg.2008.10.020] [PMID: 19159728]

[25]   Allwyn JS, Shetty L, Pare VS, *et al.* Chondro-manubrial deformity and bifid rib, rare variations seen in pectus carinatum: A radiological finding. Surg Radiol Anat 2012. Epub ahead of print
[PMID: 23196368]

[26]   Kelly RE Jr, Quinn A, Varela P, *et al.* Dysmorphology of chest wall deformities: Frequency distribution of subtypes of typical pectus excavatum and rare subtypes. Arch Bronconeumol 2012. Epub ahead of print
[PMID: 23218256]

[27]   Shamberger RC, Welch KJ. Surgical correction of chondromanubrial deformity (Currarino Silverman syndrome). J Pediatr Surg 1988; 23(4): 319-22.
[http://dx.doi.org/10.1016/S0022-3468(88)80197-0] [PMID: 3385582]

[28]   Freire-Maia N, Chautard EA, Opitz JM, Freire-Maia A, Quelce-Salgado A. The Poland syndrome-

clinical and genealogical data, dermatoglyphic analysis, and incidence. Hum Hered 1973; 23(2): 97-104.
[http://dx.doi.org/10.1159/000152560] [PMID: 4356989]

[29]   Poland A. Deficiency of the pectoralis muscles. Guys Hosp Rep 1841; 6: 191-3.

[30]   Froriep R. BeobachtungeinesFalles Von Mangel derBrustdrüse. NotizenausdemGebietederNaturund-Heilkinde 1839; 10: 9-14.

[31]   Lallemand LM. Ephermerides. MedicalesdeMontpellier 1826; 1: 144-7.

[32]   Seyfer AE, Icochea R, Graeber GM. Poland's anomaly. Natural history and long-term results of chest wall reconstruction in 33 patients. Ann Surg 1988; 208(6): 776-82.
[http://dx.doi.org/10.1097/00000658-198812000-00017] [PMID: 2848462]

[33]   Shamberger RC, Welch KJ, Upton J III. Surgical treatment of thoracic deformity in Poland's syndrome. J Pediatr Surg 1989; 24(8): 760-5.
[http://dx.doi.org/10.1016/S0022-3468(89)80532-9] [PMID: 2549232]

[34]   Welch KJ, Vos A. Surgical correction of pectus carinatum (pigeon breast). J Pediatr Surg 1973; 8(5): 659-67.
[http://dx.doi.org/10.1016/0022-3468(73)90404-1] [PMID: 4753002]

[35]   Samarrai AA, Charmockly HA, Attra AA. Complete cleft sternum: classification and surgical repair. Int Surg 1985; 70(1): 71-3.
[PMID: 4019089]

[36]   Shamberger RC, Welch KJ. Sternal defects. Pediatr Surg Int 1990; 5: 156-64.
[http://dx.doi.org/10.1007/BF00179653]

[37]   Knox L, Tuggle D, Knott-Craig CJ. Repair of congenital sternal clefts in adolescence and infancy. J Pediatr Surg 1994; 29(12): 1513-6.
[http://dx.doi.org/10.1016/0022-3468(94)90198-8] [PMID: 7877011]

[38]   Amato JJ, Douglas WI, Desai U, Burke S. Ectopia cordis. Chest Surg Clin N Am 2000; 10(2): 297-316, vii.
[PMID: 10803335]

[39]   Groner JI. Ectopia cordis and sternal defects. In: Zeigler MM, Azizkhan RG, Weber TR, Eds. Operative Pediatric Surgery. New York: McGraw-Hill 2003; pp. 279-93.

[40]   Amato JJ, Zelen J, Talwalkar NG. Single-stage repair of thoracic ectopia cordis. Ann Thorac Surg 1995; 59(2): 518-20.
[http://dx.doi.org/10.1016/0003-4975(94)00586-V] [PMID: 7847981]

[41]   Engum SA. Embryology, sternal clefts, ectopia cordis, and Cantrell's pentalogy. Semin Pediatr Surg 2008; 17(3): 154-60.
[http://dx.doi.org/10.1053/j.sempedsurg.2008.03.004] [PMID: 18582820]

[42]   Campbell RM Jr, Smith MD, Mayes TC, *et al.* The characteristics of thoracic insufficiency syndrome associated with fused ribs and congenital scoliosis. J Bone Joint Surg Am 2003; 85(3): 399-408.
[http://dx.doi.org/10.2106/00004623-200303000-00001] [PMID: 12637423]

[43]   Jeune M, Carron R, Beraud C, Loaec Y. Polychondrodystrophie avec blocage thoracique d'évolution fatale. Pediatrie 1954; 9(4): 390-2.
[PMID: 13185703]

[44]   Borland LM. Anesthesia for children with Jeune's syndrome (asphyxiating thoracic dystrophy). Anesthesiology 1987; 66(1): 86-8.
[http://dx.doi.org/10.1097/00000542-198701000-00020] [PMID: 3800042]

[45]   Tahernia AC, Stamps P. Jeune's syndrome (asphyxiating thoracic dystrophy). Chin Pediatr 1977; 16: 903-7.

[46] Williams AJ, Vawter G, Reid LM. Lung structure in asphyxiating thoracic dystrophy. Arch Pathol Lab Med 1984; 108(8): 658-61.
[PMID: 6547593]

[47] Finegold MJ, Katzew H, Genieser NB, Becker MH. Lung structure in thoracic dystrophy. Am J Dis Child 1971; 122(2): 153-9.
[PMID: 5564158]

[48] Langer LO. Thoracic pelvic phalangeal dystrophy: Asphyxiating thoracic dystrophy of the newborn, infantile thoracic dystrophy. Radiology 1968; 91: 447-56.
[http://dx.doi.org/10.1148/91.3.447]

[49] Oberklaid F, Danks DM, Mayne V, Campbell P. Asphyxiating thoracic dysplasia. Clinical, radiological, and pathological information on 10 patients. Arch Dis Child 1977; 52(10): 758-65.
[http://dx.doi.org/10.1136/adc.52.10.758] [PMID: 931421]

[50] Campbell RM. The incidence of proximal cervical spine stenosis in Jeune's asphyxiating dystrophy.

[51] Jarcho S, Levin PM. Hereditary malformations of the vertebral bodies. Bull Johns Hopkins Hosp 1938; 62: 216-26.

[52] Roberts AP, Conner AN, Tolmie JL, Connor JM. Spondylothoracic and spondylocostal dysostosis. Hereditary forms of spinal deformity. J Bone Joint Surg Br 1988; 70(1): 123-6.
[http://dx.doi.org/10.1302/0301-620X.70B1.3339042] [PMID: 3339042]

[53] Phillips JD, van Aalst JA. Jeune's syndrome (asphyxiating thoracic dystrophy): congenital and acquired. Semin Pediatr Surg 2008; 17(3): 167-72.
[http://dx.doi.org/10.1053/j.sempedsurg.2008.03.006] [PMID: 18582822]

[54] Ramirez N, Flynn JM, Emans JB, et al. Vertical expandable prosthetic titanium rib as treatment of thoracic insufficiency syndrome in spondylocostal dysplasia. J Pediatr Orthop 2010; 30(6): 521-6.
[http://dx.doi.org/10.1097/BPO.0b013e3181e78e6c] [PMID: 20733413]

[55] Gadepalli SK, Hirschl RB, Tsai WC, et al. Vertical expandable prosthetic titanium rib device insertion: does it improve pulmonary function? J Pediatr Surg 2011; 46(1): 77-80.
[http://dx.doi.org/10.1016/j.jpedsurg.2010.09.070] [PMID: 21238644]

[56] Mah VK, Zamakhshary M, Mah DY, et al. Absolute vs relative improvements in congenital diaphragmatic hernia survival: what happened to "hidden mortality". J Pediatr Surg 2009; 44(5): 877-82.
[http://dx.doi.org/10.1016/j.jpedsurg.2009.01.046] [PMID: 19433161]

[57] Colvin J, Bower C, Dickinson JE, Sokol J. Outcomes of congenital diaphragmatic hernia: a population-based study in Western Australia. Pediatrics 2005; 116(3): 356-63.

[58] Lally KP, Lasky RE, Lally PA, et al. Standardized reporting for congenital diaphragmatic hernia--an international consensus. J Pediatr Surg 2013; 48(12): 2408-15.
[http://dx.doi.org/10.1016/j.jpedsurg.2013.08.014] [PMID: 24314179]

[59] Dott MM, Wong LY, Rasmussen SA. Population-based study of congenital diaphragmatic hernia: risk factors and survival in Metropolitan Atlanta, 1968-1999. Birth Defects Res A Clin Mol Teratol 2003; 67(4): 261-7.
[http://dx.doi.org/10.1002/bdra.10039] [PMID: 12854661]

[60] Botden SM, Heiwegen K, van Rooij IA, et al. Bilateral congenital diaphragmatic hernia: prognostic evaluation of a large international cohort. J Pediatr Surg 2017; 52(9): 1475-9.
[http://dx.doi.org/10.1016/j.jpedsurg.2016.10.053] [PMID: 27894762]

[61] Stoll C, Alembik Y, Dott B, Roth MP. Associated malformations in cases with congenital diaphragmatic hernia. Genet Couns 2008; 19(3): 331-9.
[PMID: 18990989]

[62] Harting MT, Lally KP. The congenital diaphragmatic hernia study group registry update. Semin Fetal

Neonatal Med 2014; 19(6): 370-5.
[http://dx.doi.org/10.1016/j.siny.2014.09.004] [PMID: 25306471]

[63]   Akinkuotu AC, Cruz SM, Cass DL, *et al.* An evaluation of the role of concomitant anomalies on the outcomes of fetuses with congenital diaphragmatic hernia. J Pediatr Surg 2016; 51(5): 714-7.
[http://dx.doi.org/10.1016/j.jpedsurg.2016.02.008] [PMID: 26987711]

[64]   Kluth D, Keijzer R, Hertl M, Tibboel D. Embryology of congenital diaphragmatic hernia. Semin Pediatr Surg 1996; 5(4): 224-33.
[PMID: 8936651]

[65]   Iritani I. Experimental study on embryogenesis of congenital diaphragmatic hernia. Anat Embryol (Berl) 1984; 169(2): 133-9.
[http://dx.doi.org/10.1007/BF00303142] [PMID: 6742452]

[66]   Alamo L, Gudinchet F, Meuli R. Imaging findings in fetal diaphragmatic abnormalities. Pediatr Radiol 2015; 45(13): 1887-900.
[http://dx.doi.org/10.1007/s00247-015-3418-5] [PMID: 26255159]

[67]   Grivell RM, Andersen C, Dodd JM. Prenatal interventions for congenital diaphragmatic hernia for improving outcomes. Cochrane Database Syst Rev 2015; (11): CD008925.
[http://dx.doi.org/10.1002/14651858.CD008925.pub2] [PMID: 26611822]

[68]   Burgos CM, Frenckner B, Luco M, Harting MT, Lally PA, Lally KP. Prenatally diagnosed congenital diaphragmatic hernia: optimal mode of delivery? J Perinatol 2017; 37(2): 134-8.
[http://dx.doi.org/10.1038/jp.2016.221] [PMID: 28055024]

[69]   Morini F, Lally KP, Lally PA, Crisafulli RM, Capolupo I, Bagolan P. Treatment strategies for congenital diaphragmatic hernia: change sometimes comes bearing gifts. Front Pediatr 2017; 5: 195.
[http://dx.doi.org/10.3389/fped.2017.00195] [PMID: 28959686]

[70]   Burgos CM, Frenckner B, Luco M, Harting MT, Lally PA, Lally KP. Right *versus* left congenital diaphragmatic hernia - What's the difference? J Pediatr Surg 2017; S0022-3468(17)30649-8. Epub ahead of print
[PMID: 29122292]

[71]   Jani J, Keller RL, Benachi A, *et al.* Prenatal prediction of survival in isolated left-sided diaphragmatic hernia. Ultrasound Obstet Gynecol 2006; 27(1): 18-22.
[http://dx.doi.org/10.1002/uog.2688] [PMID: 16374756]

[72]   Jani J, Nicolaides KH, Keller RL, *et al.* Observed to expected lung area to head circumference ratio in the prediction of survival in fetuses with isolated diaphragmatic hernia. Ultrasound Obstet Gynecol 2007; 30(1): 67-71.
[http://dx.doi.org/10.1002/uog.4052] [PMID: 17587219]

[73]   Zamora IJ, Olutoye OO, Cass DL, *et al.* Prenatal MRI fetal lung volumes and percent liver herniation predict pulmonary morbidity in congenital diaphragmatic hernia (CDH). J Pediatr Surg 2014; 49(5): 688-93.
[http://dx.doi.org/10.1016/j.jpedsurg.2014.02.048] [PMID: 24851749]

[74]   Oluyomi-Obi T, Van Mieghem T, Ryan G. Fetal imaging and therapy for CDH-Current status. Semin Pediatr Surg 2017; 26(3): 140-6.
[http://dx.doi.org/10.1053/j.sempedsurg.2017.04.002] [PMID: 28641751]

[75]   Deprest J, Brady P, Nicolaides K, *et al.* Prenatal management of the fetus with isolated congenital diaphragmatic hernia in the era of the TOTAL trial. Semin Fetal Neonatal Med 2014; 19(6): 338-48.
[http://dx.doi.org/10.1016/j.siny.2014.09.006] [PMID: 25447987]

[76]   Chandrasekharan PK, Rawat M, Madappa R, Rothstein DH, Lakshminrusimha S. Congenital Diaphragmatic hernia - a review. Matern Health Neonatol Perinatol 2017; 3: 6.
[http://dx.doi.org/10.1186/s40748-017-0045-1] [PMID: 28331629]

[77]   Dassinger MS, Copeland DR, Gossett J, Little DC, Jackson RJ, Smith SD. Early repair of congenital

diaphragmatic hernia on extracorporeal membrane oxygenation. J Pediatr Surg 2010; 45(4): 693-7.
[http://dx.doi.org/10.1016/j.jpedsurg.2009.08.011] [PMID: 20385272]

[78]   Putnam LR, Tsao K, Lally KP, *et al.* Minimally invasive *vs* open congenital diaphragmatic hernia repair: is there a superior approach? J Am Coll Surg 2017; 224(4): 416-22.
[http://dx.doi.org/10.1016/j.jamcollsurg.2016.12.050] [PMID: 28147253]

[79]   Tsao K, Lally PA, Lally KP. Minimally invasive repair of congenital diaphragmatic hernia. J Pediatr Surg 2011; 46(6): 1158-64.
[http://dx.doi.org/10.1016/j.jpedsurg.2011.03.050] [PMID: 21683215]

[80]   Colvin J, Bower C, Dickinson JE, Sokol J. Outcomes of congenital diaphragmatic hernia: a population-based study in Western Australia. Pediatrics 116(3): 356-63.2005;

[81]   Morini F, Valfrè L, Capolupo I, Lally KP, Lally PA, Bagolan P. Congenital diaphragmatic hernia: defect size correlates with developmental defect. J Pediatr Surg 2013; 48(6): 1177-82.
[http://dx.doi.org/10.1016/j.jpedsurg.2013.03.011] [PMID: 23845604]

[82]   Putnam LR, Harting MT, Tsao K, *et al.* Congenital diaphragmatic hernia defect size and infant morbidity at discharge. Pediatrics 2016; 138(5): e20162043.
[http://dx.doi.org/10.1542/peds.2016-2043] [PMID: 27940787]

[83]   Menon SC, Tani LY, Weng HY, Lally PA, Lally KP, Yoder BA. Clinical characteristics and outcomes of patients with cardiac defects and congenital diaphragmatic hernia. J Pediatr 2013; 162(1): 114-119.e2.
[http://dx.doi.org/10.1016/j.jpeds.2012.06.048] [PMID: 22867985]

[84]   Tsao K, Allison ND, Harting MT, Lally PA, Lally KP. Congenital diaphragmatic hernia in the preterm infant. Surgery 2010; 148(2): 404-10.
[http://dx.doi.org/10.1016/j.surg.2010.03.018] [PMID: 20471048]

[85]   Brindle ME, Cook EF, Tibboel D, Lally PA, Lally KP. A clinical prediction rule for the severity of congenital diaphragmatic hernias in newborns. Pediatrics 2014; 134(2): e413-9.
[http://dx.doi.org/10.1542/peds.2013-3367] [PMID: 25022745]

[86]   Stocker JT. Sequestrations of the lung. Semin Diagn Pathol 1986; 3(2): 106-21.
[PMID: 3303232]

[87]   Yoon HM, Kim EA, Chung SH, *et al.* Extralobar pulmonary sequestration in neonates: The natural course and predictive factors associated with spontaneous regression. Eur Radiol 2017; 27(6): 2489-96.
[http://dx.doi.org/10.1007/s00330-016-4594-x] [PMID: 27659701]

[88]   Chien KJ, Huang TC, Lin CC, Lee CL, Hsieh KS, Weng KP. Early and late outcomes of coil embolization of pulmonary sequestration in children. Circ J 2009; 73(5): 938-42.
[http://dx.doi.org/10.1253/circj.CJ-08-0914] [PMID: 19276609]

[89]   Konan Blé R, Coste K, Blanc P, *et al.* [Congenital lobar emphysema: a rare etiology of hyperechoic lung]. Gynécol Obstét Fertil 2008; 36(5): 529-31.
[PMID: 18462976]

[90]   Perea L, Blinman T, Piccione J, Laje P. Bilateral congenital lobar emphysema: staged management. J Pediatr Surg 2017; 52(9): 1442-5.
[http://dx.doi.org/10.1016/j.jpedsurg.2017.01.056] [PMID: 28189445]

[91]   Depaepe A, Dolk H, Lechat MF. The epidemiology of tracheo-oesophageal fistula and oesophageal atresia in Europe. Arch Dis Child 1993; 68(6): 743-8.
[http://dx.doi.org/10.1136/adc.68.6.743] [PMID: 8333763]

[92]   Robert E, Mutchinick O, Mastroiacovo P, *et al.* An international collaborative study of the epidemiology of esophageal atresia or stenosis. Reprod Toxicol 1993; 7(5): 405-21.
[http://dx.doi.org/10.1016/0890-6238(93)90085-L] [PMID: 8274816]

[93]   Harris J, Källén B, Robert E. Descriptive epidemiology of alimentary tract atresia. Teratology 1995; 52(1): 15-29.
[http://dx.doi.org/10.1002/tera.1420520104] [PMID: 8533109]

[94]   Shaw-Smith C. Oesophageal atresia, tracheo-oesophageal fistula, and the VACTERL association: review of genetics and epidemiology. J Med Genet 2006; 43(7): 545-54.
[http://dx.doi.org/10.1136/jmg.2005.038158] [PMID: 16299066]

[95]   Clementi M, Di Gianantonio E, Pelo E, Mammi I, Basile RT, Tenconi R. Methimazole embryopathy: delineation of the phenotype. Am J Med Genet 1999; 83(1): 43-6.
[http://dx.doi.org/10.1002/(SICI)1096-8628(19990305)83:1<43::AID-AJMG8>3.0.CO;2-C] [PMID: 10076883]

[96]   Ramírez A, Espinosa de los Monteros A, Parra A, De León B. Esophageal atresia and tracheoesophageal fistula in two infants born to hyperthyroid women receiving methimazole (Tapazol) during pregnancy. Am J Med Genet 1992; 44(2): 200-2.
[http://dx.doi.org/10.1002/ajmg.1320440216] [PMID: 1456292]

[97]   Szendrey T, Danyi G, Czeizel A. Etiological study on isolated esophageal atresia. Hum Genet 1985; 70(1): 51-8.
[http://dx.doi.org/10.1007/BF00389459] [PMID: 3997151]

[98]   Nora AH, Nora JJ. A syndrome of multiple congenital anomalies associated with teratogenic exposure. Arch Environ Health 1975; 30(1): 17-21.
[http://dx.doi.org/10.1080/00039896.1975.10666626] [PMID: 1109267]

[99]   Chen H, Goei GS, Hertzler JH, *et al.* Family studies in congenital esophageal atresia with and without tracheoesophageal fistula. In: Epstein CJ, Curry CJR, Packman S, Eds. Risks, Communication, and Decision Making in Genetic Counseling. New York: Alan R. Liss for the National Foundation March-of-Dimes 1979.

[100]   Martínez-Frías ML, Rodríguez-Pinilla E. Tracheoesophageal and anal atresia in prenatal children exposed to a high dose of alcohol. Am J Med Genet 1991; 40(1): 128.
[http://dx.doi.org/10.1002/ajmg.1320400129] [PMID: 1887844]

[101]   Lipson A, Beuhler B, Bartley J, *et al.* Maternal hyperphenylalaninemia fetal effects. J Pediatr 1984; 104(2): 216-20.
[http://dx.doi.org/10.1016/S0022-3476(84)80995-6] [PMID: 6694013]

[102]   Geneviève D, de Pontual L, Amiel J, Sarnacki S, Lyonnet S. An overview of isolated and syndromic oesophageal atresia. Clin Genet 2007; 71(5): 392-9.
[http://dx.doi.org/10.1111/j.1399-0004.2007.00798.x] [PMID: 17489843]

[103]   Kluth D. Atlas of esophageal atresia. J Pediatr Surg 1976; 11(6): 901-19.
[http://dx.doi.org/10.1016/S0022-3468(76)80066-8] [PMID: 1003302]

[104]   Harmon C, Coran GC. Congenital anomalies of the esophagus.Pediatric Surgery. 6th ed. Philadelphia: Mosby 2006; pp. 1051-81.
[http://dx.doi.org/10.1016/B978-0-323-02842-4.50070-X]

[105]   Goh DW, Brereton RJ, Spitz L. Esophageal atresia with obstructed tracheoesophageal fistula and gasless abdomen. J Pediatr Surg 1991; 26(2): 160-2.
[http://dx.doi.org/10.1016/0022-3468(91)90898-4] [PMID: 2023073]

[106]   Kane TD, Atri P, Potoka DA. Triple fistula: management of a double tracheoesophageal fistula with a third H-type proximal fistula. J Pediatr Surg 2007; 42(6): E1-3.
[http://dx.doi.org/10.1016/j.jpedsurg.2006.11.009] [PMID: 17560187]

[107]   Touloukian RJ. Membranous esophageal obstruction simulating atresia with a double tracheoesophageal fistula in a neonate. J Thorac Cardiovasc Surg 1973; 65(2): 191-4.
[http://dx.doi.org/10.1016/S0022-5223(19)40790-3] [PMID: 4684997]

[108] Laffan EE, Daneman A, Ein SH, Kerrigan D, Manson DE. Tracheoesophageal fistula without esophageal atresia: are pull-back tube esophagograms needed for diagnosis? Pediatr Radiol 2006; 36(11): 1141-7.
[http://dx.doi.org/10.1007/s00247-006-0269-0] [PMID: 16967270]

[109] Centini G, Rosignoli L, Kenanidis A, Petraglia F. Prenatal diagnosis of esophageal atresia with the pouch sign. Ultrasound Obstet Gynecol 2003; 21(5): 494-7.
[http://dx.doi.org/10.1002/uog.58] [PMID: 12768564]

[110] Has R, Günay S. Upper neck pouch sign in prenatal diagnosis of esophageal atresia. Arch Gynecol Obstet 2004; 270(1): 56-8.
[http://dx.doi.org/10.1007/s00404-002-0463-8] [PMID: 12827385]

[111] Kalache KD, Chaoui R, Mau H, Bollmann R. The upper neck pouch sign: a prenatal sonographic marker for esophageal atresia. Ultrasound Obstet Gynecol 1998; 11(2): 138-40.
[http://dx.doi.org/10.1046/j.1469-0705.1998.11020138.x] [PMID: 9549842]

[112] Replogle RL. Esophageal atresia: plastic sump catheter for drainage of the proximal pouch. Surgery 1963; 54: 296-7.
[PMID: 14048024]

[113] Tönz M, Köhli S, Kaiser G. Oesophageal atresia: what has changed in the last 3 decades? Pediatr Surg Int 2004; 20(10): 768-72.
[http://dx.doi.org/10.1007/s00383-004-1139-1] [PMID: 15148614]

[114] Chittmittrapap S, Spitz L, Kiely EM, Brereton RJ. Anastomotic leakage following surgery for esophageal atresia. J Pediatr Surg 1992; 27(1): 29-32.
[http://dx.doi.org/10.1016/0022-3468(92)90098-R] [PMID: 1552439]

[115] Yanchar NL, Gordon R, Cooper M, Dunlap H, Soucy P. Significance of the clinical course and early upper gastrointestinal studies in predicting complications associated with repair of esophageal atresia. J Pediatr Surg 2001; 36(5): 815-22.
[http://dx.doi.org/10.1053/jpsu.2001.22969] [PMID: 11329597]

[116] Spitz L, *et al.* Oesophageal atresia and tracheoesophageal fistula. In: Freeman NV, Ed. Surgery of the Newborn. New York: Churchill Livingstone 1994; pp. 353-73.

[117] Millar AJ, Cox SG. Caustic injury of the oesophagus. Pediatr Surg Int 2015; 31(2): 111-21.
[http://dx.doi.org/10.1007/s00383-014-3642-3] [PMID: 25432099]

[118] Peters NJ, Mahajan JK, Bawa M, Chabbra A, Garg R, Rao KL. Esophageal perforations due to foreign body impaction in children. J Pediatr Surg 2015; 50(8): 1260-3.
[http://dx.doi.org/10.1016/j.jpedsurg.2015.01.015] [PMID: 25783392]

[119] Wei Y, Chen L, Wang Y, Yu D, Peng J, Xu J. Proposed management protocol for ingested esophageal foreign body and aortoesophageal fistula: a single-center experience. Int J Clin Exp Med 2015; 8(1): 607-15.
[PMID: 25785035]

[120] Rybojad B, Niedzielska G, Niedzielski A, Rudnicka-Drozak E, Rybojad P. Esophageal foreign bodies in pediatric patients: a thirteen-year retrospective study. ScientificWorldJournal 2012; 2012: 102642.
[http://dx.doi.org/10.1100/2012/102642] [PMID: 22593662]

[121] Hurtado CW, Furuta GT, Kramer RE. Etiology of esophageal food impactions in children. J Pediatr Gastroenterol Nutr 2011; 52(1): 43-6.
[http://dx.doi.org/10.1097/MPG.0b013e3181e67072] [PMID: 20975581]

[122] Sperry SL, Crockett SD, Miller CB, Shaheen NJ, Dellon ES. Esophageal foreign-body impactions: epidemiology, time trends, and the impact of the increasing prevalence of eosinophilic esophagitis. Gastrointest Endosc 2011; 74(5): 985-91.
[http://dx.doi.org/10.1016/j.gie.2011.06.029] [PMID: 21889135]

[123] Soprano JV, Mandl KD. Four strategies for the management of esophageal coins in children. Pediatrics 2000; 105(1): e5.
[http://dx.doi.org/10.1542/peds.105.1.e5] [PMID: 10617742]

[124] Muir AB, Merves J, Liacouras CA. Role of endoscopy in diagnosis and management of pediatric eosinophilic esophagitis. Gastrointest Endosc Clin N Am 2016; 26(1): 187-200.
[http://dx.doi.org/10.1016/j.giec.2015.08.006] [PMID: 26616904]

[125] El-Matary W, El-Hakim H, Popel J. Eosinophilic esophagitis in children needing emergency endoscopy for foreign body and food bolus impaction. Pediatr Emerg Care 2012; 28(7): 611-3.
[http://dx.doi.org/10.1097/PEC.0b013e31825cf7bb] [PMID: 22743755]

CHAPTER 4

Abdomen

Fatima H. Naeima[1], Zainab H. Ibrahim[1], Sarah N. Ahmed[1], Hayder D. Abbas[2], Karrar Z. Sadoun[2], Houreleen H. Salman[3] and Sultan M. Ghanim[4,*]

[1] *6ᵗʰ Grade Medical College, Faculty of Medicine, University of Kufa, Iraq*

[2] *5ᵗʰ Grade Jabir ibn Hayyan Medical University Najaf, Iraq*

[3] *6ᵗʰ Grade Medical College, Faculty of Medicine, University of Kufa, Iraq*

[4] *ME Unit, Medical College, Faculty of Medicine, University of Kufa, Iraq*

Abstract: In this chapter we discuss common and unusual conditions of the abdomen that are treated surgically, related to the stomach, small intestine and colon. Such as Hypertrophic pyloric stenosis, is one of the most common surgical conditions of the newborn. Congenital intestinal obstruction occurs in approximately 1 in 2000 live births and is a common cause of admission to a neonatal surgical unit. Normal rotation of the intestine requires transformation from a simple, straight alimentary tube into the mature fixed and folded configuration normally present at birth. Through precise embryologic events, the duodenojejunal junction become fixed in the left upper abdomen while the cecum is anchored in the right lower quadrant. The midgut, defined as the portion of the intestine supplied by the superior mesenteric artery (SMA), is thus suspended from a wide mesenteric base.

Keywords: Intestine, Stomach, Surgery.

HYPERTROPHIC PYLORIC STENOSIS

HPS is one of the most common surgical conditions of the newborn [1]. It occurs in approximately 1 in 300 live births and commonly in infants between 3 and 6 weeks of age. Male-to-female ratio is nearly 5:1, and there are several risk factors for HPS include family history, gender, younger maternal age, being a first-born infant, and maternal feeding patterns [2, 3].

Etiology

1. Genetic

* Corresponding author Sultan M. Ghanim: ME Unit, Medical College, Faculty of Medicine, University of Kufa, Iraq; Tel: +9647816669997; E-mail: sultanmalsaadi@uokufa.edu.iq

2. Environmental factors such as (method of feeding (breast *vs.* formula), seasonal variability, and exposure to erythromycin, environmental pesticides, and Trans pyloric feeding in premature infants).

Clinical Presentation

Infants with hypertrophic pyloric stenosis (HPS) typically present with non-bilious vomiting that becomes increasingly projectile, over the course of several days to weeks due to progressive thickening of the pylorus muscle.

Physical Examination

The neonate usually appears well if the diagnosis is made early depending on the duration of symptoms and degree of dehydration, the neonate may be gaunt and somnolent. Visible peristaltic waves may be present in the mid to left upper abdomen. So, the pylorus is palpable in 70–90% of patients [4, 5]. To palpate the pyloric mass (*i.e.* , "olive"), the neonate must be relaxed. Techniques for relaxing the patient include bending the newborn's knees and flexing the hips, using a pacifier with sugar water. These techniques should be attempted after the stomach has been decompressed with 10 French to 12 French oro-gastrictubes,after palpating the liver edge, the examiner's fingertips should slide underneath the liver in the midline. Slowly, the fingers are pulled backdown, trying to trap the "olive. " Palpating the pylorus requires patience and an optimal examination setting. If palpated, no further studies are needed.

Imaging

By ultrasound, the diagnostic criteria for pyloric stenosis are a muscle thickness of ≥4 mm and a pyloric length of ≥16 mm (Fig. **4.1**) [6]. A thickness of >3 mm is considered positive if the neonate is younger than 30 days of age.

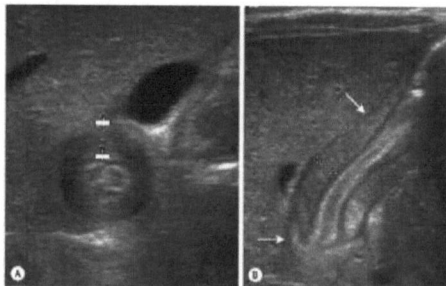

Fig. (4.1). Ultrasonography has become the standard imaging study for diagnosing pyloric stenosis and has supplanted physical examination at most institutions. The (A) transverse and (B) longitudinal views of hypertrophic pyloric stenosis are seen here. Muscle thickness ≥4 mm on the transverse view or a length ≥16 mm on the longitudinal view is diagnostic of pyloric stenosis. On this study, the pyloric wall thickness was 5 mm and the length (arrows) was 20 mm.

Treatment

The mainstay of therapy is typically resuscitation followed by pyloromyotomy (Fig. **4.2**). There are reports of medical treatment with atropine and pyloric dilation, but these treatments require long periods of time and are often not effective [7, 8].

Preparation for Surgery

Feedings should be withheld. Gastric decompression is usually not necessary but occasionally may be required in extreme cases. If a barium study was performed, it is important to remove all of the contrast material from the stomach to prevent aspiration. The hallmark metabolic derangement of hypochloremic, hypokalemic metabolic alkalosis is usually seen to some degree in most patients. Profound dehydration is rarely seen today, and correction is usually achieved in <24 hours after presentation. A basic metabolic panel should be ordered, and the resuscitation should be directed toward correcting the abnormalities. Most surgeons use the serum carbon dioxide (<30 mmol/L), chloride (>100 mmol/L), and potassium (4.5–6. 5 mmol/L) levels as markers of adequate resuscitation. Initially, a 10- to 20-mL/kg bolus of normal saline should be given if the electrolyte values are abnormal. Then D5/½NS with 20–30 mEq/L of potassium chloride is started at a rate of 1. 25–2 times the calculated maintenance rate. Electrolytes should be checked every 6 hours until they normalize and the alkalosis has resolved. Subsequent fluid boluses are given if the electrolytes remain abnormal. Then the patient can safely undergo anesthesia and operation. It is important to appreciate that HPS is not a surgical emergency and resuscitation is of the utmost priority. Inadequate resuscitation can lead to postoperative apnea due to decreased respiratory drive secondary to metabolic alkalosis [9].

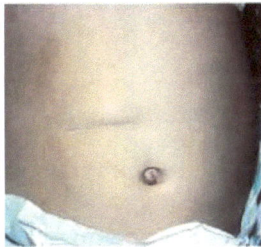

Fig. (4.2). This child underwent opens pyloromyotomy through a right upper quadrant transverse incision. Over time, the cosmetic appearance of his incision is not as attractive as that seen after the laparoscopic operation.

Types of Surgery

- **Open pyloromyotomy**
- **Laparoscopic pyloromyotomy**

Postoperative Care

IV fluids are continued for several hours. After which Pedialyte is offered, followed by formula or breast milk, which is gradually increased to 60 cc every 3 hours. Most infants can be discharged home within 24 to 48 hours following surgery. Recently, several authors have shown that ad lib feeds are safely tolerated by the neonate and result in a shorter hospital stay.

Complications

1. mucosal perforation
2. wound infection
3. incision hernia
4. prolonged postoperative emesis
5. incomplete myotomy
6. duodenal injury

Intestinal Obstruction

Duodenal and Intestinal Atresia and Stenosis

The duodenum is the most common site for intestinal obstruction in neonate, occurs in 1 per 500010,000 live births, affecting boys more commonly than girls [10]. Trisomy 21 is found in almost half the cases. About 20% of patients with duodenal atresia have cardiac anomalies. Esophageal atresia may accompany duodenal atresia. In congenital duodenal atresia, the obstruction is distal to the ampoule of Vater in 85% of patients. A complete obstruction may be a luminal web (most common), an atresia connected by a fibrous cord, or complete separation of proximal and distal segments. The ampoule is located close to the medial wall of the web, and care must be taken to avoid injuring it during repair. A fenestrated duodenal Fig. (**4.5**) web with incomplete obstruction may not be noted at birth but can be seen later with feeding intolerance or obstruction when solid foods are started.

Etiology

Congenital duodenal obstruction can occur due to an intrinsic or extrinsic lesion [11]. The most common cause of duodenal obstruction is atresia and other causes are duodenal web, duodenal stenosis, annular pancreas, duodenal duplication cyst, preduodenal portal vein may cause obstruction of the duodenum. A "windsock" deformity can suggest a more distal obstruction.

Classification System

Anatomically, duodenal obstructions are classified as either atresia or stenosis. An incomplete obstruction, due to a fenestrated web or diaphragm, is considered a stenosis. Most stenosis involves the third and/or fourth part of the duodenum. Atresia is a complete obstruction.

Atresia is classified into three morphologic types (Fig. **4.3**).

- Type I atresia account for >90% of the atresia that are represented by duodenal obstructions, containing a luminal diaphragm or distally ballooned diaphragm [12].
- Type II atresia are characterized by a dilated proximal and collapsed distal segment connected by a fibrous cord.
- Type III atresia have an obvious gap separating the proximal and distal duodenal segments [13].

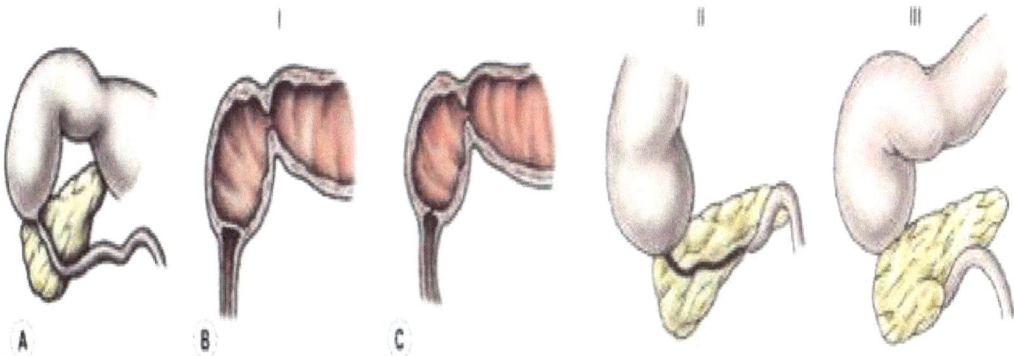

Fig. (4.3). Duodenal atresia (and stenosis) is depicted. In type I (A), either a membrane (B) or web (C) causes the intrinsic duodenal obstruction. There is no fibrous cord, and the duodenum remains in continuity. Type II is characterized by complete obliteration of a segment of the duodenum with the proximal and distal portions attached *via* a fibrous cord. Type III is associated with complete separation of the dilated proximal duodenum from the collapsed distal duodenum.

Clinical Presentation

The presentation of the neonate with duodenal obstruction varies depending on whether the obstruction is complete or incomplete and the location of the ampoule of Vater in relation to the obstruction. In pre-ampullary atresia and non bilious emesis, the cardinal symptom of intestinal obstruction in the newborn is bilious emesis. Abdominal distention is yet to be diagnosed. In neonates exhibiting duodenal atresia, the abdomen is scaphoid. Aspiration through a nasogastric (NG) tube of >20 mL of gastric contents in a newborn suggests intestinal obstruction as the normal aspirate is <5 mL [14]. In neonates with stenosis, the diagnosis is not made until the neonate starts taking food *via* mouth or GIT and feeding intolerance has been evaluated.

Diagnosis

The diagnosis can often be suggested by prenatal ultrasound (US). Sonographic evaluation in fetuses of mothers with a history of Polyhydraminous can detect two fluid-filled structures consistent with a double bubble in up to 44% of cases (Fig. **4.4**). The diagnostic radiographic presentation of duodenal atresia is that of a double bubble sign with no distal bowel gas. The proximal left-sided bubble represents the air- and fluid-filled stomach while the dilated proximal duodenum represents the second bubble to the baby's right of midline [15]. In almost all cases of duodenal atresia, the distal bowel is gasless; the presence of distal gas does not necessarily exclude the diagnosis of atresia as there is a report of a biffed common bile duct with insertion of one of the ducts proximal and the other distal to the atretic segment, which allowed the air to bypass the atresia. At our institution, neonates who present with bilious emesis and a decompressed stomach on plain abdominal films receive a limited upper GI contrast study to exclude malrotation and volvulus. With duodenal stenosis, a double bubble sign is often not present and the diagnosis is usually made with a contrast study. The more distal the obstruction, the more distended the abdomen becomes, and the greater the number of obstructed loops on upright abdominal films.

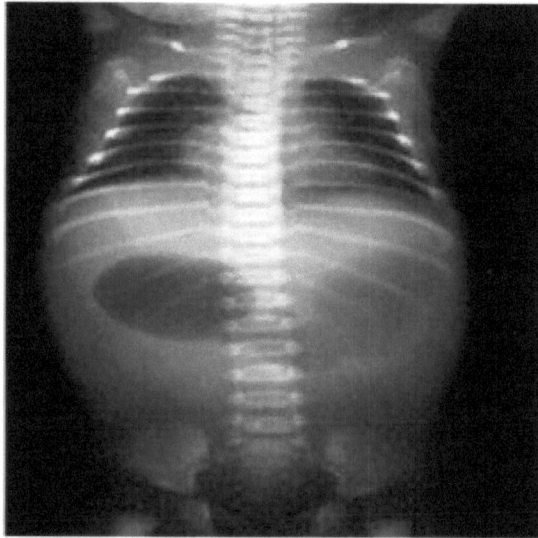

Fig. (4.4). Classic "double bubble" sign shown in abdominal radiograph of a neonate.

Treatment

An orgiastic tube is inserted to decompress the stomach and duodenum, the infant is given IV fluids to maintain adequate urine output. All neonates diagnosed with duodenal obstruction receive a complete metabolic profile, complete blood count, coagulation studies, an abdominal and spinal US, and two-dimensional echocardiography prior to any operation.

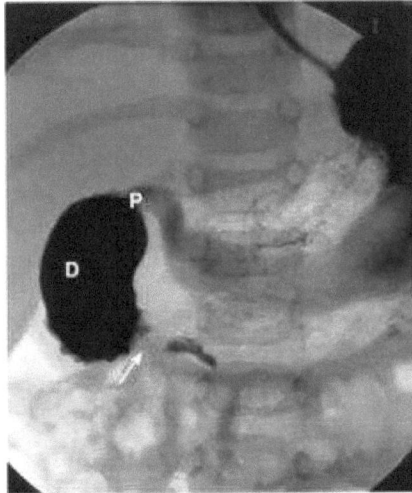

Fig. (4.5). An upper gastrointestinal contrast study is shown illustrating a duodenal web. Contrast medium outlines the markedly dilated proximal duodenum (D) with a collapsed distal segment. Note the absence of contrast agent at the location of the tiny web (arrow) P,pylorus.

If the infant appears ill, or if abdominal tenderness is present, a diagnosis of malrotation and midget volvulus should be considered, and surgery should not be delayed. A mutely one-third of newborns with duodenal atresia have associated Down syndrome (Trisomy 21).

These patients should be evaluated for associated cardiac anomalies. Once the workup is complete and the infant is stable, he or she is taken to the operating room, and repair is performed either *via* an open approach or laparoscopically [16].

Types of Surgery

- Duodenojejunostomy
- side-to-side duodenoduodenostomy
- diamond-shaped duodenoduodenostomy
- partial web resection with Heineke–Mikulicz-typeduodenoplasty

- Duodenoplasty
- Currently, the preferred technique is either laparoscopic or open duodenoduodenostomy.

Postoperative Care

Prophylactic antibiotics are discontinued within 24 hours. Patients are intubated in the operating room unless comorbdities such as cardiac anomalies require continued ventilator support. Nasogastric decompression is continued until output decreases and feedings can begin. Feedings may have to advance slowly because of poor emptying of the dilated stomach and proximal duodenum. Long-term outcome is good unless cardiac or chromosomal anomalies impact survival. Complications requiring reoperation are uncommon.

Intraoperative Complications

There are several intraoperative judgmental and technical pitfalls that will lead to postoperative difficulties. Incorrect identification of the site of obstruction most commonly when a long, floppy web (windsock deformity) is present, the proximally based web fills with gastrointestinal secretions and balloons out into the obstruction to appear much more distal than it actually is. The unwary surgeon, not recognizing the true attachment of the web, may then construct a bypass anastomosis entirely distal to it. Rarely, there will be more than one obstruction present. A distal web is easily missed because of the lack of any obvious adjacent proximal dilatation. The careful passage and withdrawal of balloon catheters both proximally into the stomach and distally into the jejunum before starting an anastomosis should prevent both of these situations.

Postoperative Complications

Prolonged feeding intolerance is the most common complication after surgery to relive duodenal obstruction. There is great deal variability in the time required for a bypass anastomosis or web excision to function adequately, persistent poor peristalsis leads to prolonged poor function. Late duodenal obstruction may occasionally be noted in older infants and children; this may occur after successful neonatal bypass procedure excision of web or de novo when a diagnosis of partial duodenal obstruction was initially missed. A piece of fibrous food or a foreign body may become impacted at the site of a partially resected web or relatively narrow anastomosis that was either constructed to an inadequate size, has become structured overtime or has failed to grow with the child.

Jejunoileal Atresia and Stenosis

Jejunoileal atresia and stenosis is a major cause of neonatal intestinal obstruction. Atresia refers to a congenital obstruction caused by a complete occlusion of the intestinal lumen and accounts for 95% of cases. Stenosis is defined as a partial intraluminal occlusion resulting in an incomplete intestinal obstruction, and accounts a 5% of Jejunoileal obstructions. The occurance of Jejunoileal atresia is reported in 1 out of 5000 live births with equal cases in both males and females, occurs as a result of an intrauterine ischemic insult to the midget, affecting single or multiple segments of the already developed intestine. Intrauterine vascular disruption can lead to ischemic necrosis of the bowel with subsequent resorption of the affected segment,additionally, atrasias seen in association with other intrauterine vascular insults such as intussusceptions, midget volvulus, thromboembolic occlusions, transmesenteric internal hernias, and incarceration or snaring of bowel in an omphalocele or gastroschisis. Since Jejunoileal atresia occurs in late stages of fetal life and has localized nature of vascular insult that is why usually low extra-abdominal organ complications are reported in it [17]. The development of Jejunoileal atresia is shown in Fig. (**4.6**)

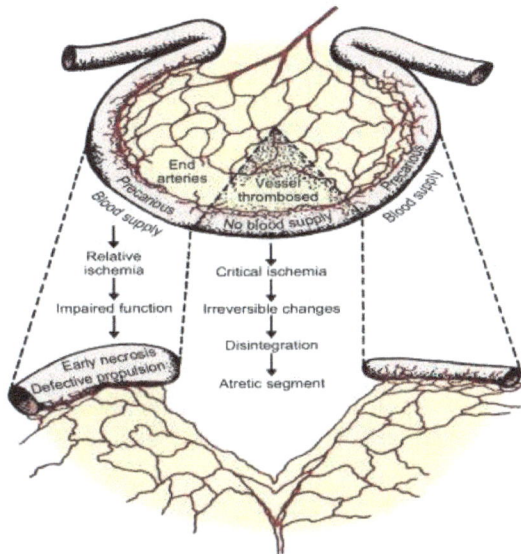

Fig. (4.6). The proposed mechanism of vascular compromise and subsequent development of Jejunoileal atresia is depicted.

Methylene blue, previously used for amniocentesis in twin pregnancies, has been implicated in causing small bowel atresia as well. The mothers on vasoconstrictive medications and with smoking habits in the first trimester of pregnancy increase the chances of risk of small bowel atresia [18]. The risk for development of small intestinal atresia is increased after maternal use of pseudoephedrine alone and in combination with acetaminophen and in mothers with migraine headaches receiving ergotamine tartarate and caffeine during pregnancies. Chromosomal abnormalities are seen in less than 1% of the babies born with Jejunoileal atresia. Most Jejunoileal atresia is separated by a cordlike segment or V-shaped mesenteric gap defect. Clinical observation like bile pigments, squames and lanugo hairs were often found distal to atretic segments strongly suggested that some factors other than epithelial plugging were involved. Fetal bile secretions and swallowing of amniotic fluid begin in the 11th and 12th weeks of intrauterine life may be a cause. Intrauterine intussusceptions are an infrequently reported cause of atresia, postnatal intussusceptions as a cause of jejunal atresia in a premature infant.

Clinical Presentation

The cases of midget volvulus or an internal hernia with subsequent ischemia may lead to Prompt finding of intestinal obstruction in the neonate and prenatal US is helpful in detecting duodenal atresia by showing dilated loops of bowel and Polyhydraminous. These symptoms may not be present in gestation. In neonates with atresia or stenosis, the presenting symptoms are bilious vomiting, abdominal distention, jaundice and failure to pass the meconium in the first day. Occasionally, meconium and necrotic tissue may be passed per rectum. Severe abdominal distention may be associated with respiratory distress due to elevation of diaphragm, easily visible veins and intestinal patterning characterized by visible loops of bowel, noted on abdominal wall by physical examination. Abdominal distention noted immediately at birth suggests the presence of giant cystic meconium peritonitis.

Prenatal US Findings

Prenatal US in mothers with Polyhydraminous have identified small bowel obstruction associated with atresia; volvulus and meconium peritonitis [19]. Prenatal US is more reliable in detection duodenal atresia than more distal lesions. Appearance of multiple distended loops of bowel with vigorous peristalsis Intestinal atresia is also suspected in fetuses with gastroschisis. The with intestinal dilatation.

Radiographic Findings

Erect and recumbent abdominal radiographs are obtained in each case. Thumb-sized intestinal loops (role of thumb) and fluid-air levels are highly suggestive of intestinal obstruction in the newborn. Peritoneal calcification is seen in 12% of cases and signifies presence of meconium peritonitis, a sign of intrauterine intestinal perforation. Intraluminal calcification indicates to antenatal volvulus. Large air-fluid levels seen in meconium pseudocyst. Colonic haustral markings rarely demonstrate on a plain abdominal radiograph (Fig. **4.7**). A barium enema should be performed in each instance of suspected neonatal intestinal obstruction. The contrast enema serves three purposes, to distinguish between small and large bowel distention, to determine if the colon used or not used, and locate the position of the cecum in regard to possible the presence of anomalies of intestinal rotation and fixation The great majority of infants with Jejunoileal atresia that demonstrate a micro-colon. A small bowel contrast entero lysis study has a higher diagnostic yield than a routine small bowel series. There is a need for exclusion of associated cystic fibrosis that can be done by Special investigations. This evaluation may include GI contrast study, contrast enema, rectal biopsy, and a $\Delta F508$ gene deletion assay or sweat test.

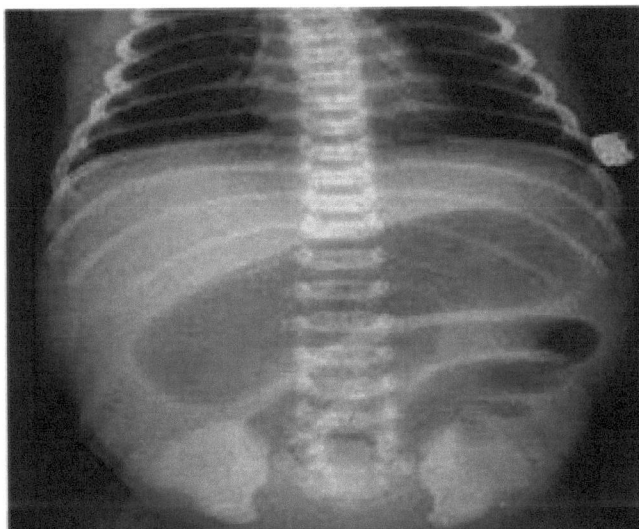

Fig. (4.7). Several proximally dilated intestinal loops consistent with jejunal atresia as shown in abdominal radiograph in this neonate.

Differential Diagnosis

- Colonic atresia.
- Midget volvulus.
- Meconium ileus.
- Duplication cysts.
- Internal hernias.
- Ileus due to sepsis.
- Birth trauma.
- Maternal medications.
- Prematurity.

• Hypothyroidism.

Management

The complications arising due to delay in diagnosis may include intestinal viability (50%), frank necrosis and perforation (10–20%), fluid and electrolyte abnormalities, and sepsis. Gastric decompression and fluid resuscitation is required as a preoperative measure. This ensures the correction of electrolyte abnormalities. In case of risk of perforation or infection, antibiotic is administered. During initial evaluation, the infant is maintained in warm humidified environment to avoid hypothermia (either isolate or overhead warmer). Orogastric tube is passed to avoid aspiration during transportation the infant weight determined, blood sample for baseline laboratory data (CBC, platelet count, blood urea, serum bilirubin, glucose, calcium, ph, blood gas tensions, serum electrolyte), and for type of blood and matching, urinary volume, specific gravity and osmolality. Percutaneous insertion IV lines of a short 22-24gauge silicone catheters. The infant's fluid deficits are evaluated and replacement therapy is initiated. In instances of peritonitis or severe distention, lactated ringer's solution is administrated at rate 20ml/kg over 30min. In instances of obstruction without perforation an empirical infusion of 10ml/kg to correct hypovolemic. Additional fluid in necessary to maintain the infant's blood pressure above 50mmHg and urine flow1-2ml/kg/hr Vitamin **k** oxide is routinely given.

Surgical Considerations

The location of the lesion, anatomic findings, and associated conditions marked at the time of operation, and the length of the remaining intestine are key factors required in operative management [20]. Resection of the dilated and hypertrophied proximal bowel, see (Fig. **4.8**), with primary end-to-end anastomosis with or without tapering of the proximal bowel, is the most common technique. Several approaches may be taken for the repair of small intestine, one such is laparoscopic approach. This approach may require subsequent resection and anastomosis performed in an extracorporeal fashion.

Postoperative Care

Parenteral nutrition can be useful in selecting patients. Parental nutrition should be initiated as soon as possible and continued, until the infant is tolerating full enteral feeds. Enteral feedings can be initiated when the gastric aspirate is clear, output is minimal, and the infant is stooling. Enteral feeding through a feeding tube is initiated at a rate of 20 mL/kg/day of breast milk or formula. The feed is gradually increased at a rate of 20–30 mL/kg/day. The feed is initiated orally if the baby has developed the sucking power and is able to tolerate at least 8 mL of tube feeds per hour. Infants with jejunal and ileal atresia may show the symptoms of Transient GI dysfunction. The etiology of this dysfunction is multifactorial. Infants with repair of type III (b) atresia, or having short bowel syndrome may develop some problems like Lactose intolerance, malabsorption and diarrhea, thus may require Regular monitoring for these clinical signs as well as some other that include Water-loss stools and its increasing frequency, hematochezia, fecal-reducing substances, or a decreased stool pH warrant or monosaccharide intolerance. Sugars, high-osmolality feeds, oral medications, and bacterial or viral infections may cause some injury to the mucosa. The decrease in the intestinal peristalsis activity can be noticed with the use of Lope amide hydrochloride. Cholestyramine is also beneficial as it binds to the bile salts but it should be avoided until the water-loss stools appear. The vitamin B12 is supposed to prevent megaloblastic anemia in the patient without a terminal ileum. The following factors are critical for the functional outcome: the location of the atresia, the maturity of the intestine and its length. If the residual small bowel length is shorter, ileocecal valve is responsible for more rapid intestinal adaptation, thus it is very important.

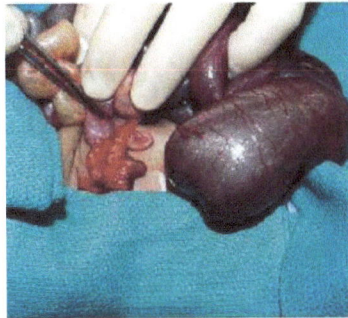

Fig. (4.8). A type III (a) distal atresia found at the time of surgery.

Colonic Atresia

Colonic atresia is a rare and may cause only 2–15% of intestinal obstruction among all GI atresia. Usually one case of colonial atresia is reported in 5000 to 1 in 60,000 live births, and may have various classification.

Type I this mucosal atresia may cause an intact bowel wall and mesentery.
Type II in this atresia the atretic ends are separated by a fibrous cord.
Type III the atretic ends are separated by a V-shaped mesenteric gap.

Type III lesions are the most common lesion while while types I and II are usually distal to the splenic flexure. Usually, a vascular insult is accepted as etiology for all types of colonic atresia like small bowl atresia. The abdominal distention, bilious emesis, and failure to pass meconium are the symptoms of colonic atresia. The "ground-glass" appearance of meconium may sometime be associated with the dilated intestinal loops of large bowel. Sometime the massive dilation may mimic the pneumoperitoneum as shown in Fig. (**4.9**). The abrupt halt at the level of the obstruction at distal colon as shown in Fig. (**4.10**) may lead to the diagnosis. Once the colonic atresia is diagnosed, it may require urgent surgical procedure. The operative preparation can be done by taking into account the level of the atresia and its associated small intestine atresia. The patency of the bowel distal to the atresia is also considered as an important factor. The solution lies in a staged approach consisting of colostomy with mucous fistula. If there is no delay in diagnosis, the mortality rate is below 10%, but a delay of more than 72 hours may increase the risk up to 60%. The reason for such a high mortality is a closed loop obstruction between an intact ileocecal valve and the atresia, this results in massive colonic distention and perforation.

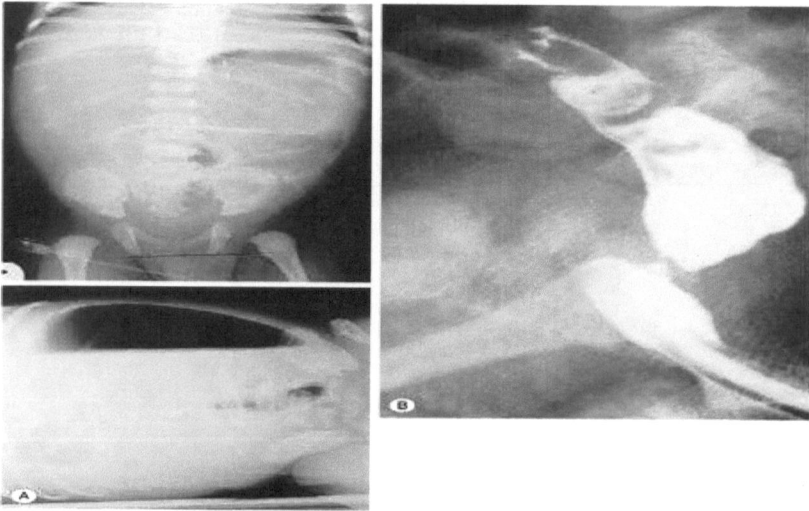

Fig. (4.9). (A) Abdominal flat (top) and cross-table lateral (bottom) radiograph of colonic atresia (B) Right colonic atresia with rectal stenosis as seen by this contrast enema.

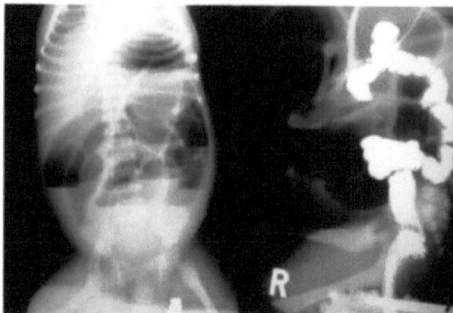

Fig. (4.10). In a patient with a distal intestinal obstruction (left), the contrast enema on the right.

Meconium Ileus

9–33% of neonatal intestinal obstructions is caused by MI which is characterized by extremely viscid, protein-rich, and inspissated meconium [21]. This may cause an intraluminal obstruction in the distal ileum at the ileocecal valve. The delayed treatment or diagnosis may lead to cystic fibrosis (CF) [22]. The pancreatic aplasia and total colonic aganglionosis may sometimes be associated with the CF. the meconium in CF is different to that of normal meconium with respect to abnormalities of exocrine mucous secretion and pancreatic enzyme deficiency. Less water content (65% *vs* 75%), lower sucrase and lactase level, increased albumin, and decreased pancreatic enzymes are other deviations than normal meconium. The associated abnormalities may include the reduction of concentrations of sodium, potassium, magnesium, heavy metals, and carbohydrates in CF. In contrast, there is rise in the concentration of protein nitrogen and abnormal mucoproteins. Thus, the absence of degrading enzymes may lead into meconium that is thick and dehydrated leading to the obstruction the intestine. A clinician treating and managing MI must be well-versed in understanding of CF. It is also known that CF locus is associated with human chromosome 7q31, and that mutations in the CF transmembrane (conductance) regulator (CFTR) gene result in CF. Infants with cystic fibrosis have characteristic pancreatic enzyme deficiencies and abnormal chloride secretion in the intestine that result in the production of viscous, water-poor meconium. Meconium ileus can be either uncomplicated, in which there is no intestinal perforation or complicated, in which prenatal perforation of the intestine has occurred or vascular compromise of the distended ileum develops. Antenatal US may reveal the presence of intra-abdominal or scrotal calcifications, or distended bowel loops. These infants present shortly after birth with progressive abdominal distention and failure to pass meconium with intermittent bilious emesis. Abdominal radiographs show dilated loops of intestine, because the enteric contents are so viscous air-fluid levels do not form, even when obstruction is complete. Small bubbles of gas become entrapped in the inspissated meconium in the distal ileum, where they produce a characteristic "ground glass" appearance. The abnormal transport of chloride ions across apical membranes of epithelial cells result in mucoviscidosis of exocrine secretions throughout the body, a characteristic of CF. This transport takes place *via* calcium-activated chloride channels. The role of intracellular Ca 2+ concentration on these channels may impact the pathophysiology of CF. There is also Abnormal bicarbonate transport in CF, which affects the mucin formation. There is chronic obstruction of the respiratory tract caused by the infection, insufficiency of the exocrine pancreas, and elevated sweat chloride levels. There may occur some variations in CF as well and these include patients with chronic sinusitis or adult males with congenital bilateral absence of the vas deferens (CBAVD) *etc.*

Clinical Presentation

The MI may be simple or complicated. The thickened meconium in utero obstructs the mid-ileum leading to proximal bowel dilatation and thickening accompanied with congestion. Almost 50% of the newborn may have this simple MI [23], The complicated MI may be caused by the complications of MI, including volvulus, gangrene, atresia, and/or perforation leading to meconium peritonitis and giant cystic meconium peritonitis. The symptoms of complicated MI appear within 24 hours of the birth in newborn. Some of these infants are symptomatic immediately after the birth showing signs of in utero perforation or bowel compromise. The initial examination of the newborn may reveal Signs of peritonitis, including distention, tenderness, abdominal wall edema and erythema, and clinical evidence of sepsis, there is a possibility of severe abdominal distention leading to the respiratory distress. So far there are four types of meconium peritonitis that include adhesive meconium peritonitis, giant cystic meconium peritonitis or pseudocyst, meconium ascites, and infected meconium peritonitis [24].

Diagnosis

The antenatal diagnosis of MI may be *via* high-risk group and a low-risk group. In low risk group, if a mother with a negative CF carrier is found on Sonographic appearances of MI and routine prenatal ultrasound (US) is conducted. If the parents are carriers of CF, give birth to a CF-affected child, it is included in high risk group. Research conducted with the passage of time has helped in the development of an algorithm Fig. (**4.10**) that is useful in managing the fetus suspected of having MI (Fig. **4.11**).

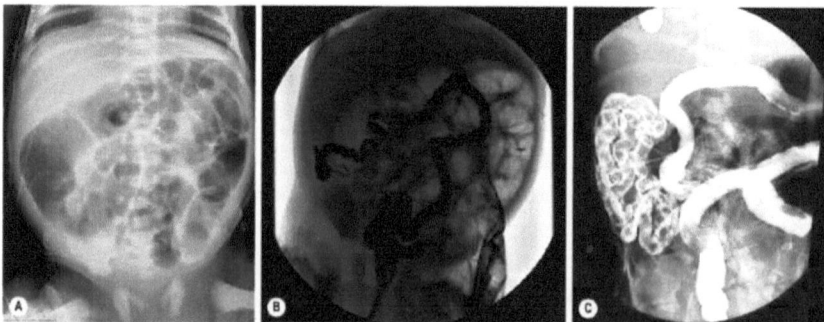

Fig. (4.11). (A) Classic radiographic findings of meconium ileus (B) A"microcolon of disuse" is seen with a small unused colon (C) Inspissated pellets (filling defects) of meconium found in the proximal small bowel.

The sonography of a patient with MI may reveal a hyperechoic, intra-abdominal mass (inspissated meconium), dilated bowel, and nonvisualization of the gallbladder. Usually the normal fetal meconium appears in second and third trimester that too is usually hypoechoic or isoechoic to adjacent abdominal structures.

A hyperechoic bowel has been reported with Down syndrome, intrauterine growth retardation, prematurity, in utero cytomegalovirus infection, intestinal atresia, abruptio placenta, and fetal demise. The finding of dilated bowel on prenatal US, in association with a family history of CF. The inability to visualize the gallbladder on fetal US has also been associated with CF. Caution should be exercised in the interpretation of an absent gallbladder as the differential diagnosis also includes biliary atresia, omphalocele, diaphragmatic hernia, chromosomal abnormalities, and a normal pregnancy. Fetal magnetic resonance imaging has been suggested as an additional tool for prenatal diagnosis of the underlying cause of echodense bowel because it can differentiate between meconium ileus, atresia, bowel duplication, and other pathologic conditions. Contrast enema that typically demonstrates a microcolon. Radiographic findings in complicated MI vary with the complication. Neonatal radiographs may show peritoneal calcifications, free air, and/or air–fluid levels (related to atresia). Speckled calcification on abdominal plain films is highly suggestive of intrauterine intestinal perforation and meconium peritonitis. The definitive study to confirm the diagnosis of CF is the sweat test. The test is typically performed at several weeks of life to obtain an adequate sample size. A sodium concentration of 60 mmol/L in 100 mg of sweat is diagnostic of CF, with 40–60 mmol/L being intermediate (but more likely to be diagnostic in infants) and <40 mmol/L being normal. Genetic testing for CFTR mutations is a able; however, commercial assays test for a limited number of mutations. Stool analyses for albumin, trypsin, and c trypsin are available, and abnormal values coupled with the operative findings suggest CF.

Treatment

Initially, the intestinal obstruction in neonates is achieved by volume resuscitation and ventilator support. Any coagulation disorders is treated by Gastric decompression and it prevents the progressive abdominal distension, aspiration, and pulmonary compromise. Initial management may also include an isotonic water-soluble contrast enema under fluoroscopic control and an antibiotic coverage. There could be some other causes of neonatal intestinal obstruction that should be excluded in water-soluble enema. An adequate supply of intravenous fluid is provided to the neonate before the water soluble enema is performed to avoid hypovolemia and receive appropriate electrolyte repletion. This is also necessary for being normothermic and getting fluoroscopic control [26]

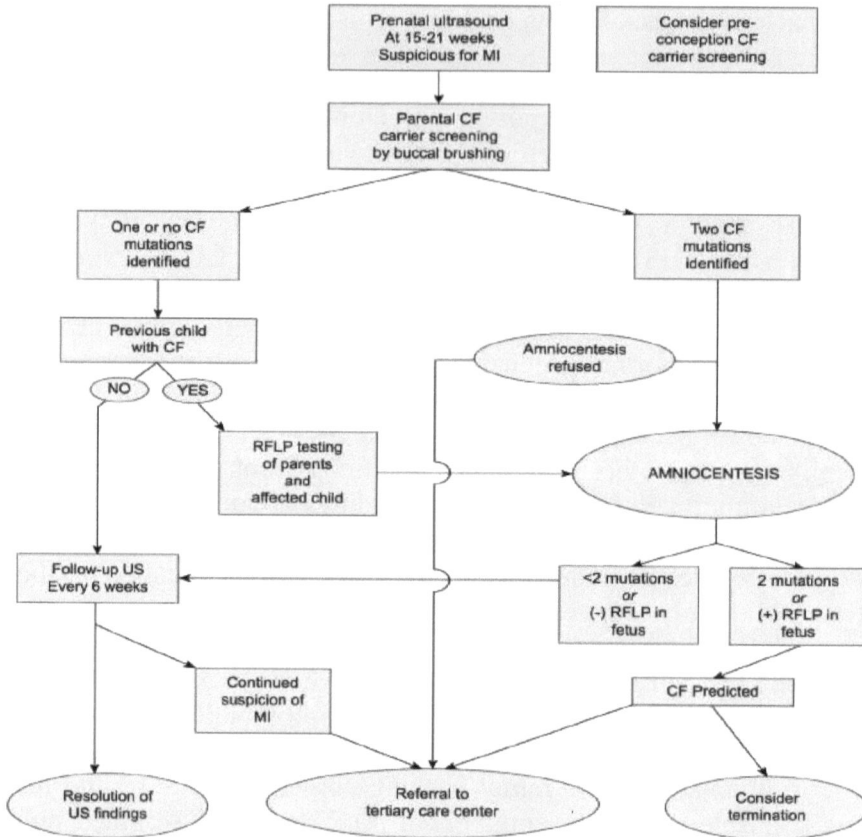

Fig. (4.12). Antenatal management of suspected meconium ileus (MI) and cystic fibrosis (CF) as shown by an algorithm as modified by the Joint Society of Obstetricians and Gynecologists of Canada (SOGC) – Canadian College of Medical Geneticists (CCMG) Opinion for Reproductive Genetic Carrier Screening. Wilson RD, De Bie I, Armour CM, et al. Joint SOGC-CCMG Opinion for Reproductive Genetic Carrier Screening: An update for all Canadian providers of maternity and reproductive healthcare in the era of direct-to-consumer testing. J ObstetGynacol Can 2016:38(8):742–762 e3.)

Operative Management

Inadequate meconium evacuation or any abnormality associated with contrast enema (*e. g.* , perforation, peritonitis, persistent intestinal obstruction, enlarging abdominal mass and ongoing sepsis) could be the possible indications for operative management in patients with simple MI. Failure in advancing the column of enema fluid into the ileum or an unsuspected associated intestinal atresia may result in the failure of non-operative treatment. Appendectomy and irrigation is conducted in neonates which don't show any signs of improvement through non-operative measures. Operative management is almost always required in patients with complicated MI. Indications of operation include:

peritonitis, persistant intestinal obstruction, enlarging abdominal mass and ongoing sepsis. The thick and tanacious meconium at the time of operation is shown in Fig. (**4.13**).

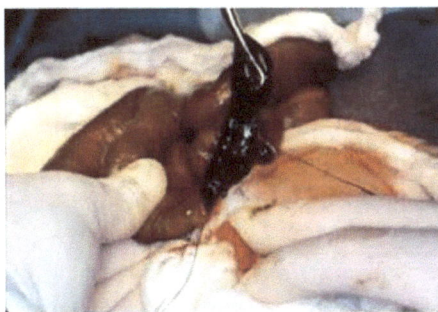

Fig. (4.13).   At operation, the meconium in a neonate with cystic fibrosis is very thick and tenacious.

Postoperative Care

Neonatology and pulmonary specialists are critical. If an enema was successful in evacuating the viscous meconium, N-acetylcysteine (Mucomyst) is started (5 mL per NG tube every 6 hours). Pancreatic enzymes are started when feeds are started beginning with a dose of 450 to 900 units of lipase per gram of fat. Breast milk or easily absorbed infant formulas such as Pregestimil are preferred. Residual meconium can be evacuated postoperatively by instilling N-acetylcysteine through the NG tube or, if a T-tube was placed, through the T-tube. As soon as spontaneous defecation is established, an elemental formula should be ordered and pancreatic enzymes started.

Necrotizing Enterocolitis

Necrotizing enterocolitis (NEC) is the most frequent and lethal gastrointestinal disorder affecting the intestine of the stressed, preterm neonate, it is primarily a disease of premature neonates. (VLBW, birth weight <1500 g) [27]. NEC is a significant risk factor for more severe respiratory distress in premature infants. Multiple risk factors have been associated with the development of NEC. These include prematurity, initiation of enteral feeding, bacterial infection, and intestinal ischemia resulting from birth asphyxia, umbilical artery cannulation, persistence of a patent ductus arteriosus, cyanotic heart disease, and maternal cocaine abuse. NEC may involve single or multiple segments of the intestine, most commonly the terminal ileum, followed by the colon. It is now is the most common newborn surgical emergency. Formulas with high osmolality have been shown increase the incidence of NEC. Compromise of intestinal epithelial mucosal barrier appears to be the first event leading to activation of the inflammatory cascade.

Clinical Diagnosis

NEC is typically diagnosed when characteristic radiologic findings are noted in the appropriate clinical setting (Fig. **4.14**). Clinically, NEC presents clinically with feeding intolerance manifested as vomiting or high gastric residuals and abdominal distention. Early signs may be even more nonspecific and include apnea, bradycardia, lethargy, and temperature instability. Hematochezia or occult fecal blood may also occur. Abdominal distention is the most common finding on exam. Visual inspection may reveal bowel loops projecting through the skin. Skin color changes should be noted. Duskiness of the abdominal wall may reflect underlying discoloration of bowel or stool through thin soft tissue. Erythema may suggest peritonitis with inflammation transmitted through the wall. Confirmation of the diagnosis of NEC combines signs and symptoms with radiologic findings. These findings have been combined into the clinical staging system proposed by Bell that aids in describing the severity of disease is seen in Table **4.1**.

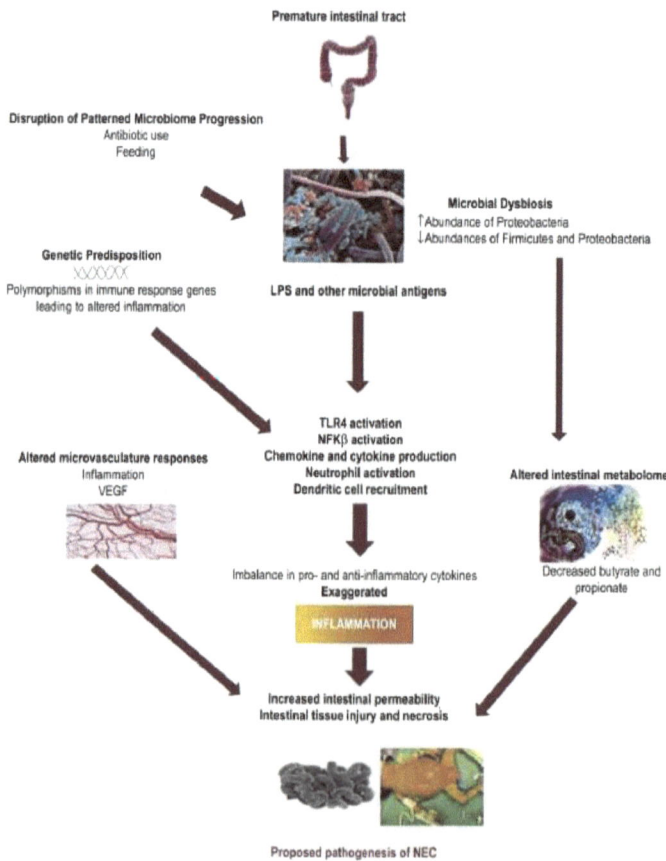

Premature intestinal tract

Disruption of Patterned Microbiome Progression
Antibiotic use
Feeding

Microbial Dysbiosis
↑Abundance of Proteobacteria
↓Abundances of Firmicutes and Proteobacteria

Genetic Predisposition
Polymorphisms in immune response genes leading to altered inflammation

LPS and other microbial antigens

TLR4 activation
NFKβ activation
Chemokine and cytokine production
Neutrophil activation
Dendritic cell recruitment

Altered microvasculature responses
Inflammation
VEGF

Altered intestinal metabolome

Imbalance in pro- and anti-inflammatory cytokines
Exaggerated

INFLAMMATION

Decreased butyrate and propionate

Increased intestinal permeability
Intestinal tissue injury and necrosis

Proposed pathogenesis of NEC

Fig. (4.14). This diagram summarizes the pathophysiology of NEC.

Table 4.1 Modified Bell Classification for NEC

Stage	Clinical findings	Radiological findings	Gastrointestinal finding
I	Apnea, bradycardia and Temperature instability	Normal gas pattern or mild ileus	Mild abdominal distension, Stool occult blood, gastric residuals
II A	Apnea, bradycardia and Temperature instability	Ileus with dilated loops and focal pneumatosis	Moderate abdominal distension, hematochezia, absent bowel sounds
II B	Metabolic acidosis and thrombocytopenia	Widespread pneumatosis, Portal venous gas, ascites	Abdominal tenderness and edema
IIIA	Mixed acidosis, coagulopathy, hypotension, oliguria	Moderate to severely dilated bowel loops, ascites, no free air	Abdominal wall edema, erythema, and induration
IIIB	Shock worsening vital signs	pneumoperitoneum	Bowel perforation

The diagnosis of NEC is not made with laboratory tests, but they may aid in establishing the degree of the infant's systemic illness. The degree of metabolic acidosis may reflect bowel and/or whole body perfusion. Leukocytosis with bandemia or leucopenia may be present. Worsening thrombocytopenia, especially a precipitous drop, may be an ominous sign [28]. Certain serum acute phase proteins and cytokines are elevated in NEC. Increased levels of IL-6, IL-10, and C-reactive protein (CRP) have been documented in premature infants with NEC. Fecal Calprotectin is a marker of intestinal inflammation that has been shown to differentiate limited NEC from NEC with system illness (Bell III) with 76% sensitivity and 92% specificity. Pneumatosis intestinal is seen on plain film is the hallmark radiologic finding in NEC. US is more sensitive than plain films for the diagnosis of NEC given its greater ability to identify smaller air or fluid collections, and to more completely characterize the bowel wall. Septic ileus may present with near-identical findings to early NEC and is the most clinically relevant diagnosis in the differential.

Medical Management

The primary management of medical NEC is supportive. The suspicion of NEC typically prompts treatment with bowel rest, gastric decompression, intravenous fluid, and parenteral nutrition [29]. Most clinician will add broad-spectrum antibiotics with anaerobic and Gram-negative coverage early in the process. Cardiopulmonary support focuses on delivering oxygen *via* appropriate resuscitation with fluids and blood products, adequate oxygenation and ventilation, and vasopressor support when necessary.

Surgical Management

Absolute indication for operative intervention is pneumoperitoneum on an abdominal radiograph (Fig. **4.15**). Paracentesis has been used in the diagnostic algorithm for NEC. A tap that is positive for enteric contents within the abdomen is also considered a clear reason for operation, neonates with severe NEC without obvious evidence of perforation should undergo an operation remains difficult. A prospective multicenter study found that clinical factors alone could not predict which infants will need surgical therapy [30]. Tepas and colleagues identified seven clinical and laboratory findings that were indicative of significant metabolic derangement in neonates with NEC. Positive blood culture, pH < 7. 25, bandemia with I/T >0. 2, sodium <130, platelets <50,000, mean arterial pressure less than gestational age or on vasopressors, absolute neutrophil count <2000/mm3). Presence of 3 of the 7 is a relative surgical indication.

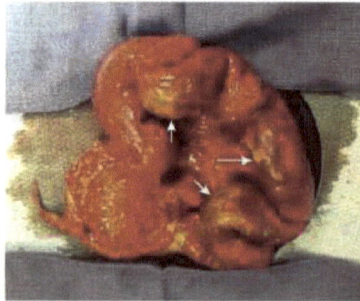

Fig. (4.15a). This infant was explored for pneumoperitoneum. As is evident, there is diffuse involvement of the bowel and pneumatics (arrows) is readily visualized. However, much of this bowel looks uninvolved, so the bowel was returned to the abdominal cavity and a second look operation performed 48 hours later, at which time segmental resections were performed.

Operative approach; Exploratory Laparotomy and Primary Peritoneal Drainage

Complications

• Intestinal stricture

• Intestinal malabsorption and short bowel syndrome

• Choleaststic liver disease

- Neurodevelopment complications

- Recurrent NEC

- Anastomotic ulceration

Appendicitis

Inflammation of appendix is most common surgical emergencies in children. It ranges from simple inflammation to gross perforation, obstruction of the lumen from many causes like fecal material (fecolith), lymphoid hyperplasia, foreign body, or parasites. You should distinguish neonatal appendicitis from necrotizing enterocolitis confined to the appendix [31]. Obstruction will lead to distention of appendix and then accumulation of mucus and bacterial proliferation then lymphatic and venous obstruction, lead to local edema and the result is necrosis and perforation. In children with cystic fibrosis, obstruction may be due to abnormal production of mucus leading to painful distention with or without inflammation [32].

Clinical Manifestation

Vague abdominal pain in periumbilical region (activation of visceral pain fibers) then radiate to right lower quadrant. Nausea, vomiting, diarrhea and anorexia may also present. Fever, tachycardia, and leukocytosis develop as a consequence of systemic inflammatory mediators released by ischemic tissues, white blood cells, and bacteria. The inflamed appendix then irritates the overlying peritoneum, typically by direct contact. This leads to focal peritonitis and localized right lower quadrant pain. This explains the migrating pain from umbilicus to right lower quadrant. Any movement of the peritoneum will lead to an exacerbation of the pain. Thus, children will often demonstrate voluntary guarding of the right lower quadrant during the exam. Furthermore, children will usually resist walking and jumping due to the increased pain associated with such movement. On examination, focal tenderness in the right lower quadrant. Palpating a mass is difficult and often impossible due to the level of discomfort and guarding. So it can be done after induction of anesthesia.

Laboratory Investigations

Mild leukocytosis (if it's very high so think about perforation) [33]. A left-shifted differential count may be a better diagnostic indicator. Inflammatory markers like C-reactive protein (greater than 3mg/dL) procalcitonin and d-lactate have also been investigated. Urine analysis (which is free of bacteria but red or white blood cell can be found because of inflammatory response of appendix can affect bladder or ureter).

Radiological Imaging

Plain radiography: On ultrasound, a fecolith may be visualized in the appendix.

Ultrasound: fluid-filled, no compressible appendix, a diameter greater than 6 mm, appendiceal wall thickening more than 1mm, appendicolith, periappendiceal or pericecal fluid, periappendiceal fat Fig. (**4.15**) stranding, and appendiceal wall enhancement. Ct scan can confirm the diagnosis in three different presentations as shown in Fig. (**4.16**) [34].

Differential Diagnosis

Causes of acute right lower quadrant pain that are often indistinguishable from appendicitis include tubo-ovarian pathologic processes, Crohn disease, mesenteric adenitis, cecal diverticulitis, Meckel diverticulitis, constipation, viral gastroenteritis, and regional bacterial enteritis (Yersinia and Campylobacter in particular). Lower abdominal pain or vague Non-focal pain can result from a urinary tract infection, kidney stone, ureteropelvic junction obstruction, uterine pathologic process, right lower lobe pneumonia, sigmoid diverticulitis, cholecystitis, pancreatitis, gastroenteritis, vasculitis, bowel obstruction, and malignancy (lymphoma). The most common diagnosis made in the presence of missed appendicitis is reported to be gastroenteritis [35]

Management

The definitive treatment for acute appendicitis is appendectomy.

Preoperative Preparation

NPO, intravenous fluids and broad-spectrum antibiotics. If it's uncomplicated (non-perforated) appendicitis, so perform appendectomy. Most surgeons will perform a laparoscopic appendectomy, which may have some advantage over removing the appendix through a single larger incision. During the laparoscopic appendectomy, a small incision is made at the umbilicus, and two additional incisions are made in the lower abdomen. The appendix is typically delivered through the umbilicus, and all incisions are then closed with dissolvable sutures then prophylactic antimicrobial agents should be given for 24 hours. Also some data shows administration of antibiotics without appendectomy may be sufficient to treat uncomplicated appendicitis (but recurrence rate is high). If it's complicated (perforated) appendicitis (can closely mimic those of gastroenteritis and include abdominal pain, vomiting, and diarrhea), an individualized approach is necessary. The choice of nonoperative *versus* operative treatment depends on the preoperative diagnosis of perforation. Fluid resuscitation and administration of broad-spectrum antibiotics before surgery should be given. Then do appendectomy after 6-10 weeks. If there is abscess formation so, manage as non operative way. Primary treatment of the abscess with antibiotics alone, or antibiotics and percutaneous drainage with or without drain placement for larger fluid collections, is a widely accepted treatment strategy. Interval appendectomy is then performed after the inflammation has subsided. The majority of patients with complicated appendicitis can be safely managed with appendectomy. Specifically, patients with a phlegmonous mass, appendicolith, or absence of a well-formed abscess on imaging have a higher risk of failure of nonoperative management.

Postoperative Care

If the appendix is not ruptured, the patient may start drinking liquids shortly after waking up from the operation and may be advanced to eat a solid diet the next day. Additional postoperative antibiotics for acute appendicitis are not necessary or recommended. However, it may be reasonable to administer additional antibiotics for patients with suppurative or gangrenous appendicitis during the first 24 hours after appendectomy or longer based on the patient's clinical status. The patient can return to school 1 week after surgery and usually is allowed to return to full physical activity after 2 to 3 weeks. During the recovery period, the patient can use painkiller. Patients with perforated appendicitis should receive postoperative antibiotics until clinical resolution has occurred. This includes normalization of leukocyte count and differential, full return of gastrointestinal function, resolution of fever, and normalization of physical exam. Antibiotic regimen employed for perforated appendicitis has traditionally been triple antibiotic therapy (ampicillin, gentamicin, and Clindamycin or metronidazole) [36]. However recently there has been a shift towards more simple antibiotic regimens. Single agent therapy with piperacillin/tazobactam or cefotaxime, or double agent therapy with ceftriaxone and metronidazole, has been shown to be efficacious and cost effective [37]. The most common complication after appendectomy is a surgical site infection. Others like bleeding or damage to other structures inside the abdomen are extremely rare.

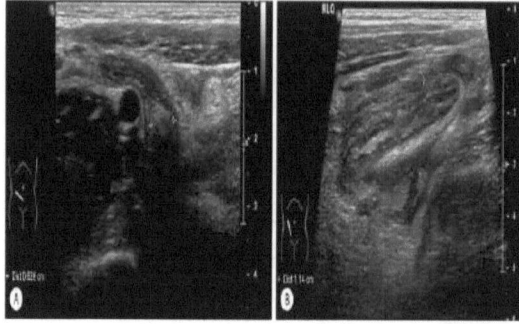

Fig. (4.15b). These ultrasound studies from two different patients depict evidence of appendicitis. On the axial view (A), an appendicolith measuring 6. 3 mm in diameter is depicted. The appendix is also larger than 6 mm in diameter, which meets criteria for appendicitis. On the right (B), in this longitudinal ultrasound view, the enlarged appendix measures 11 mm in diameter.

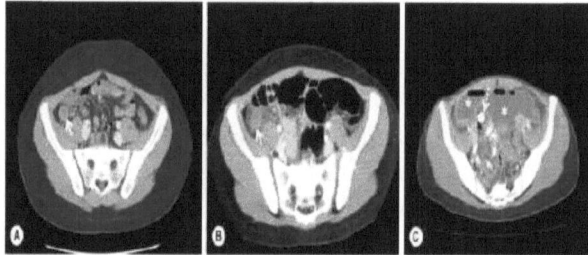

Fig. (4.16). These three CT scans show differing presentations for appendicitis. (A) The appendix (arrow) is enlarged and has a thickened wall. There are no inflammatory changes such as peri appendiceal fat stranding seen on this study. (B) The appendix (arrow) is enlarged, and there is free fluid and inflammatory changes medially indicating likely perforation. (C) The patient presented with a 1-week history of pain and the appendix has perforated with the development of two abscesses (asterisks). In addition, a fecalith is seen medially (dotted arrow). This patient was initially managed nonoperative with drainage of the abscesses and intravenous antibiotics. She underwent laparoscopic interval appendectomy 10 weeks following the initial admission.

Hirschsprung Disease

Congenital mega-colon is caused by a malformation in the pelvic parasympathetic system which results in the absence of ganglion cells in Auerbach's plexus of a segment of distal colon [38]. Approximately 1:5,000 live births. It happens more in 'transition zone' in the rectum or rectosigmoid colon then proximal colonic involvement then total colonic aganglionosis with variable involvement of the distal small intestine, and rarely near-total intestinal aganglionosis.

Box (4.1). Congenital anomalies and conditions commonly associated with Hirschprung disease.

Down syndrome (Trisomy 21) Neurocristopathy syndromes Waardenberg–Shah syndrome Yemenite deaf-blind-hypo pigmentation Piebaldism Other hypo pigmentation syndromes Goldberg–Shprintzen syndrome Smith–Lemli–Opitz syndrome Multiple endocrine neoplasia 2 Congenital central hypoventilation syndrome (Ondine's curse) Isolated congenital anomalies Congenital heart disease Malrotation Urinary tract anomalies Central nervous system anomalies Other

Etiology

Ganglion cells are derived from the neural crest. By 13 weeks' post-conception, the neural crest cells have migrated from proximal to distal through the gastrointestinal tract, after which they differentiate into mature ganglion cells. This is normal process. In this disease there are two theories: The first is failure of migration of ganglion cells, the second is the cell migrate but fail to differentiate neural crest into mature cells. Genetic basis plays role like Ret and GDNF.

Clinical Manifestation

Neonatal period, abdominal distention, bilious vomiting, feeding intolerance, delayed passage of meconium beyond the first 24 hours. If there is: fever, abdominal distention, dehydration, and diarrhea so this is Hirschsprung - associated enterocolitis (HAEC), which can be life-threatening. On rectal examination, forceful expulsion of foul-smelling liquid feces is typically observed and represents the accumulation of stool under pressure in an obstructed distal colon. Treat it by rehydration, systemic antibiotics, nasogastric decompression, and rectal irrigations while the diagnosis of Hirschsprung's disease is being confirmed . If no response so do a decompressive stoma (in ganglion containing bowel which is confirmed by frozen section at time of stoma creation).

Investigations

At plain radiographs, dilated bowel loops throughout the abdomen and in water-soluble contrast enema: Transition zone between the normal and aganglionic bowel can be shwon in Fig. (**4.17**) (which is pathognomonic finding of HD) [39]. Rectal biopsy which confirms the diagnosis, takes mucosa and submucosa at least 1. 0–1. 5 cm above dentate line shows absence of ganglion cells in the submucosal and myenteric plexuses and maybe hypertrophied nerve trunks on histological examination (gold standard) (Fig. **4.18**). Anorectal manometry is screening technique shows presence of a recto-anal inhibitory reflex (reflex relaxation of the internal anal sphincter in response to balloon distention of the rectum).

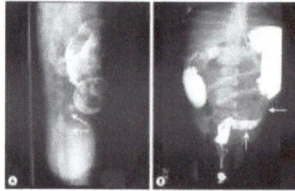

Fig. (4.17). (A) and (B) represent contrast enema examinations in different infants demonstrate Hirschsprung disease. The aganglionic rectum (arrows in both studies) is small and contracted. The proximal aganglionic colon is dilated. A transition zone between the aganglionic and aganglionic colon is nicely seen in both studies.

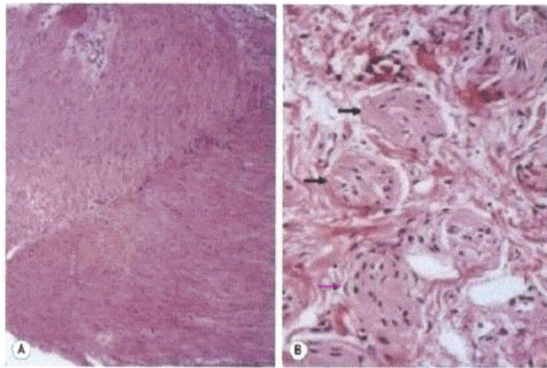

Fig. (4.18). Histological findings in children with Hirschsprung disease. (A) Absence of ganglion cells in the enteric plexus. (B) Hypertrophied nerve trunks are marked with arrows.

Management

Resuscitation with intravenous fluids and giving broad-spectrum antibiotics, nasogastric drainage, and rectal decompression using rectal stimulation and/or irrigation, then after stabilization of condition perform operation. The classic surgical approach consisted of a multiple-stage procedure. This included; A colostomy in the newborn period, followed by a definitive pull-through operation after the child was over 10 kg. We confirm the location in the bowel where the transition zone between ganglionic and aganglionic bowel exists, then resecting the aganglionic segment of bowel, and performing an anastomosis of ganglionated bowel to either the anus or a cuff of rectal mucosa, Swenson, Duhamel, Soave procedures or laparoscopic pull through (Fig. **4.19**) [40].

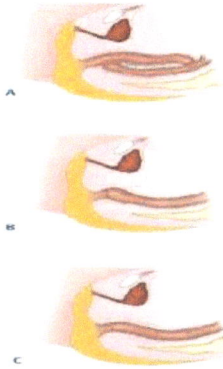

Fig. (4.19). The three operations for surgical correction of Hirschsprung's disease. A Duhamel procedure leaves the rectum in place and brings aganglionic bowel into the retro rectal space. B. the Swenson procedure is a resection with end-to-end anastomosis performed by exteriorizing bowel ends through the anus. C. the Soave operation is performed by end rectal dissection and removal of mucosa from the aganglionic distal segment and bringing the aganglionic bowel down to the anus within the neuromuscular tunnel.

Postoperative Care

They can be fed immediately and discharged within 24–48 hours. Parents should be instructed to protect the buttocks with barrier cream to prevent perineal skin breakdown, and parents should be educated about the signs and symptoms of postoperative enterocolitis. This can result in rapid severe illness and even death in a few patients [41].

Box 4. 2. Causes of obstructive symptoms following operation for Hirschsprung disease.

Mechanical obstruction
Recurrent or residual aganglionosis
Motility disorder involving the ganglionated bowel
Internal anal sphincter achalasia
Functional megacolon (stool-holding behaviour)

Intussusception

It is an acquired invagination of the proximal bowel (intussusceptum) into the distal bowel (intussuscipiens), it is the most frequent cause of bowel obstruction in infants and toddlers, its highest incidence between 4-9 month [42], and uncommon before 3 months and more than 3years. The abdominal radiograph in a patient with intussusception is shown in Fig. (**4.21**) while Fig. (**4.22**) shows the transverse Sonographic image.

Etiology

It is unclear but it can be classified into: Primary (idiopathic) when there is no lead point and it can be attributed to upper respiratory tract infection or gastroenteritis that leads to hypertrophy of peyer's patch [43] and secondary: there is lead point that drawing the proximal bowel into the distal bowel by peristaltic activity like Meckel diverticulum, polyps and duplications. Other benign lead points like appendix, hemangiomas, carcinoid tumors, foreign bodies, ectopic pancreas or gastric mucosa, lipomas, hamartoma from Peutz–Jeghers syndrome. Malignant lead point (rare) like lipomas and small bowl tumors, some diseases that can be found with intussusceptions like Henoch–Schönlein purpura, cystic fibrosis, celiac disease and Clostridium difficile colitis.

Pathophysiology

It begins in the terminal ileum and extends distally into the ascending, transverse, or descending colon and rarely may prolapse through the rectum. Due to peristaltic action of the intestine that causes the bowel distal to the lead point to invaginate into itself. So it will be compressed, resulting in venous obstruction and bowel wall edema; then arterial insufficiency will ultimately lead to ischemia and bowel wall necrosis.

Clinical Manifestation

Intermittent, crampy abdominal pain. Between attacks the baby looks comfortable then eventually lethargic, bilious vomiting and "currant jelly' stools (bloody mucus) due to ischemia that compress on mucus gland and cause mucosal sloughing (late sign). The vital signs are usually normal. Examination between the attacks reveals no finding; the attack repeats every 15 to 30 minutes and re examination is difficult. Sausage-shaped mass Fig. (**4.20**) anywhere in abdomen maybe felt, and dance sign (right lower quadrant emptiness)maybe noticed. Regarding ractal examination, blood stained mucus that is late sign and prolapse of intussusception through anus which can misdiagnose with anal prolapse maybe shown. To distinguish it use a lubricated tongue blade alongside the protruding mass if it's inserted so this is intussusception, if not so this is the tissue of anus and so this is anal prolapse.

Diagnosis

Plain flat and upright abdominal X-ray (abdominal mass, abnormal distribution of gas and fecal contents, air fluid level) [44] also it can be demonstrated by air enema. Ultrasound can show target sign or doughnut lesion in cross-section or pseudo-kidney in longitudinal section (Fig. **4.23**). CT scan and MRI are not routinely done but can confirm the diagnosis and see the malignant causes. Laparoscopy can help in diagnosis.

Management

Nasogastric tube to decompress the stomach, and the patient should be assessed for peritonitis. Bowel rest and IV fluid resuscitation. CBC and electrolyte should be checked. There are two approach of treatment, non operative and surgical approach.

Non Operative Approach

The first line treatment is non operative approach by air enema [unless there are contraindications like intestinal perforation (free intra-abdominal air), peritonitis, or persistent hypotension]. Air is insufflated into the rectum through specific pressure. The successful trail is known if there is free reflux of air into multiple loops of small bowel and symptomatic improvement as the infant suddenly becomes pain free. If it fails a second trail should be attempted [45]. If it's succeeded so observe the baby for abdominal pain (bowl ischemia or recurrent), bowel rest and give IV fluid.

Drawback of Air Enema

Tension pneumoperitoneum (treated by immediate cessation of enema and release of pneumoperitoneum), and poor visualization of lead points.

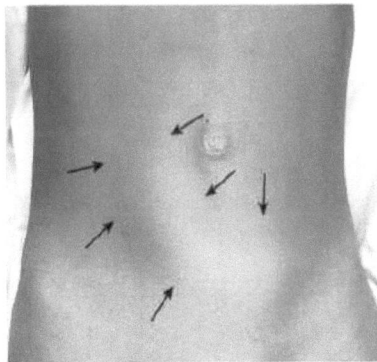

Fig. (4.20). This 10-year-old boy has a palpable sausage-shaped mass (arrows) due to an intussusception.

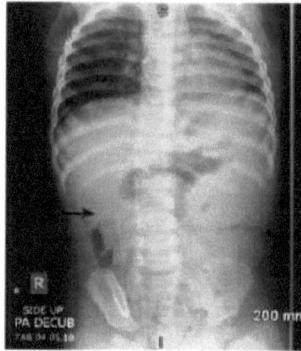

Fig. (4.21). This abdominal radiograph in a patient with intussusception shows dilated loops of small bowel in the right lower quadrant and a right upper quadrant soft tissue mass density in the vicinity of the transverse colon near the hepatic flexure (arrow).

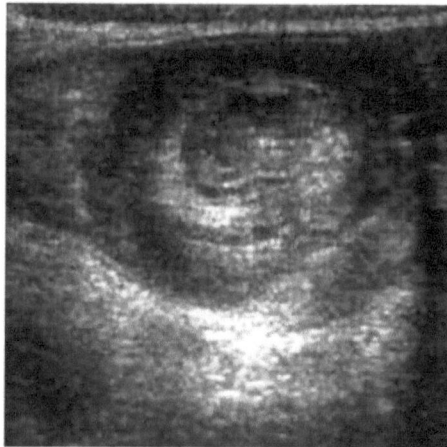

Fig. (4.22). This transverse Sonographic image shows the alternating rings of low and high echogenicity due to intussusception. This finding has been called a "target" sign.

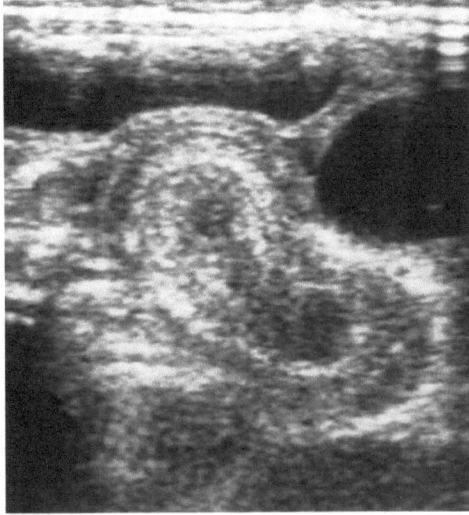

Fig. (4.23). Sonogram showing the "pseudo kidney" sign seen with intussusception on longitudinal section.

The surgical approach (open *vs* laparoscopic);

Open surgery is indicated if non operative approach is failed, or there is peritonitis, the presence of a lead point, and radiographic evidence of pneumoperitoneum. Preoperative preparation includes: Administration of broad-spectrum antibiotics, intravenous fluid resuscitation, insertion of a urinary catheter, and placement of a nasogastric tube for gastric decompression. Then when we open the abdomen and once the intussusceptions is identified, gently manipulate it back toward its normal position in the terminal ileum. Inspect the bowel for viability, lead point, and perforation. Then do appendectomy (location of scar is similar to open appendectomy). Remember, if manually reduction is failed, ischemic bowel or identification of a lead point, so resection then do bowel anastomosis.

Laparoscopy: bowel is inspected, and if it appears to be viable, reduction is performed by milking the bowel or using gentle traction. Contraindications of laparoscopic approach; peritonitis, hemodynamic instability and severe bowel distention that precludes adequate visualization.

Recurrent Intussusception

It is less common after operative approach [46], and treated by air enema which is successful in most cases. If it recurs more than 3times; so lead point should be taken in mind.

Postoperative Intussusception

It occurs 10 days after procedures like: ileocolic intussusception reduction and resection, retroperitoneal dissections, long intra abdominal procedures, a Ladd procedure, extra abdominal operations [47].

Malrotation

The congenital malrotation of the bowel may occur where the caecum remains high and the midgut mesentery is narrow, and drags across the duodenum. This may also lead to obstruction. Incidence is 1 in 6000 live births. Associated with other anomalies.

Normal development of midgut involves four distinct stages: herniation; rotation; retraction; fixation [48]. At 4th week of gestation the intestinal loop herniated into extraembryonic coelom. Then bowel rotates 270 counterclockwise allowing the cephalic limb to be positioned to the left of the SMA while the caudal limb is on the right, failure of this process allowing a range of rotational disorder like non rotation, incomplete rotation and reversed rotation.

Pathophysiology

The most common forms of rotational disorders include non rotation, incomplete rotation and reversed rotation, right and left mesocolic hernias can also occur. In non rotation, there is failure of the normal intestinal 270° counter clockwise rotations around the SMA. Thus, the duodenojejunal limb lies in the right hemi-abdomen with the cecocolic limb in the left hemi-abdomen. Midgut volvulus due to a narrow mesenteric pedicle and extrinsic duodenal obstruction secondary to abnormally positioned cecal attachments are the most common symptomatic consequences. In cases of incomplete rotation, normal rotation has been arrested at or near 180°. The cecum will usually reside in the right upper abdomen. Obstructing peritoneal bands over the duodenum are present. With reversed rotation, an errant 90° clockwise rotation occurs, which leaves a tortuous transverse colon to the right of the SMA, passing through a retroduodenal tunnel dorsal to the artery and in the small bowel mesentery. The duodenum will assume an anterior position. Reverse rotation with volvulus may occur with obstruction of the transverse colon. Paraduodenal hernias are rare and result from failure of the right or left mesocolon to fuse to the posterior body wall. A potential space is created. Subsequently, the small intestine may become sequestered and potentially obstructed.

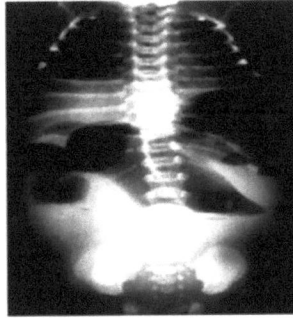

Fig. (4.24). Upright abdominal film in an infant demonstrating proximal small bowel dilatation. This infant had a midgut volvulus.

Clinical Manifestation

It needs high index of suspicion (previously healthy baby who presents with bilious vomiting). Occur at any age, but common in first few weeks of life. Up to 75% of patients present during the first month of life, while another 15% will present within the first year [49]. Bilious vomiting (all infant with this symptom must be evaluated for malrotation with volvulus, irritability, bloody stool (from vascular compromise) eventually, circulatory collapse, erythema then edema of abdominal wall as a result of advanced ischemia of the intestine), scaphoid abdomen or only mild upper abdominal wall distention. Abdominal distention (obstructed bowel develops), abdominal wall erythema and shock (vascular compromise) can be seen. Patients with chronic obstruction will present with nonspecific presenting problems such as failure to thrive, gastroesophageal reflux, early satiety, and mild abdominal discomfort.

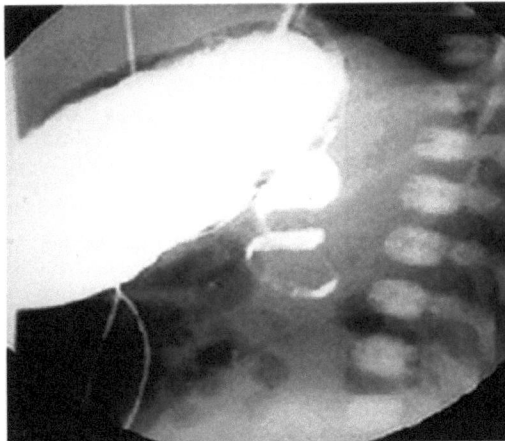

Fig. (4.25). Lateral image on upper gastrointestinal series in an infant with malrotation and midgut volvulus showing the "corkscrew" appearance of the obstructed duodenum.

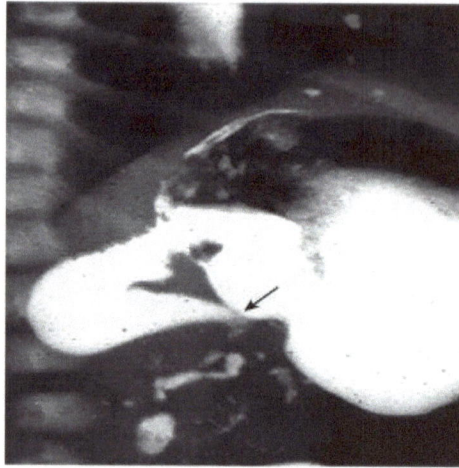

Fig. (4.26). Lateral image on upper gastrointestinal series in infant with malrotation and midget volvulus showing the "beak" (arrow) appear-ance of the obstructed duodenum. Note that a small amount of contrast agent has progressed through the volvulus.

Diagnosis

Fetal ultrasonography (US) may show the sequelae of prenatal midgut volvulus, such as bowel dilatation, meconium peritonitis, and/or fetal ascites.

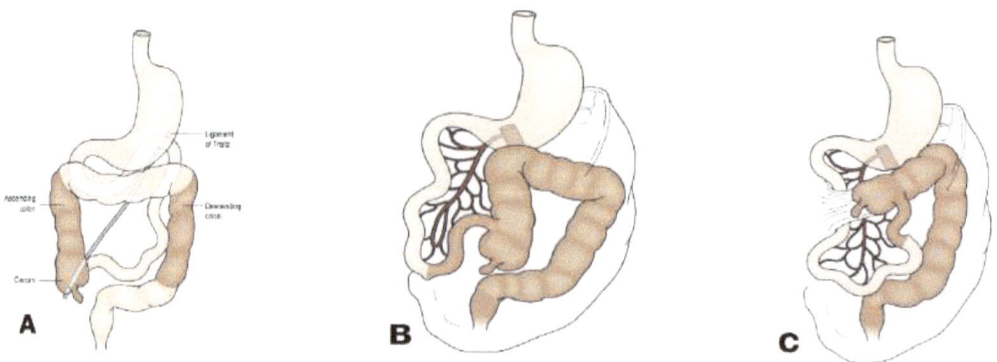

Fig. (4.27). A- Normal intestinal anatomy results in fixation of the duodenoje-junal junction in the left upper quadrant and the cecum in the right lower quadrant. This allows a wide breadth to the mesentery of the small bowel. B- Nonrotation. The prearterial midgut (lightly shaded) is found on the right side of the abdomen, while the postarterial midgut (darkly shaded) remains on the patient's left. Neither segment has undergone appropriate rotation. Volvulus is a risk. C- Incomplete rotation. Both the prearterial (lightly shaded) and postarterial (darkly shaded) segments have undergone partial, yet not complete, rotation. Ladd bands are seen attaching the cecum to the right posterior abdominal wall. The duodenum becomes compressed and possibly obstructed. Volvulus is a risk.

Initial evaluation will usually begin with a plain anteroposterior abdominal film combined with a lateral decubitus or upright view (Fig. **4.24**). Nonspecific findings ranging from gastric distention to a gasless abdomen are common. The upper gastrointestinal (UGI) contrast study remains the gold standard and is needed to document the position of the ligament of Treitz to the left of the spinal pedicles, and rising to the level of the gastric outlet. If volvulus has d oped, the contrast study may show the "coilspring" or "corkscrew" configuration with incomplete obstruction and the "beak" appearance in the duodenum with complete obstruction (Figs. **4.25**, **4.26**). Color Doppler US imaging may reveal a dilated duodenum with inversion of the SMA and vein (the whirlpool sign) in cases of acute volvulus.

Management

Patients with suspected or confirmed midgut volvulus may be dehydrated and demonstrate electrolyte imbalances. They should be aggressively resuscitated. Given intravenous broad-spectrum antibiotics, decompressed with an oro- or nasogastric tube, and taken to the operating room for immediate exploration,If there are no signs of volvulus or obstruction, there is no need of a nasogastric tube postoperatively. After the laparoscopic approach, it may take 1-2 days in the resumption of normal bowel function. Since old patients may have prolonged ileus, there is a need for nasogastric drainage and parenteral support in such cases. There is no need for Postoperative antibiotics and the surgeon decides about the feeding also. The extended or subtotal small bowel resection is the major problem and such patients make a lot of complains. The parenteral nutrition must not be discontinued.

Box 4. 3. Operative correction of malrotation.

1. Entry into abdominal cavity and evisceration (open) 2. Counterclockwise detorsion of the bowel (acute cases) 3. Division of Ladd cecal bands 4. Broadening of the small intestine mesentery 5. Incidental appendectomy 6. Placement of small bowel along the right lateral gutter and colon along the left lateral gutter

Imperforate Anus

It means rectum fails to descend through the external sphincter complex. One out of every 4000 to 5000 newborns and is slightly more common in males [50]. Imperforate anus without fistula is found in both sex and often associated with Down syndrome. Well-developed sacrum and good muscles help in making a good prognosis in terms of bowel function.

Classification

It can be classified according to anatomical location of rectum to levator ani: If rectum ends above it so this is high type, if anus descends through it this is low type and according to fistoulus opening. Associated anomalies with imperforate anus are VACTREL (**V**-vertebral, **A**-anal, **C** -cardiac, **T** -tracheoesophagal, **R** -renal, **E**-ear and **L**-limb)

Box 4. 4. Classifications of infants with anorectal malformations.

Males
Rectoperineal fistula
Rectourethral bulbar fistula
Rectourethral prostatic fistula
Rectobladderneck fistula
Imperforate anus without fistula
Rectal atresia/rectal stenosis
Females
Rectoperineal fistula
Rectovestibular fistula
Cloaca
Complex malformations
Imperforate anus without fistula
Rectal atresia/rectal stenosis

Male

1-Rectourethral Fistulas

Most common type in male [51], Fistula may be located at the lower (bulbar) or the higher (prostatic) part of the urethra. Above the fistula, the rectum and urethra share a common wall. Lower urethral fistulas are usually associated with good-quality muscles, a well-developed sacrum, a prominent midline groove, and a prominent anal dimple, whereas higher urethral fistulas are more frequently associated with poor-quality muscles, an abnormally developed sacrum, a flat perineum, a poor midline groove, and a barely visible anal dimple.

2-Rectoperineal Fistulas

Other names (covered anus, anal membrane, anteriorly mislocated anus, and bucket-handle malformations),is the lowest defect. The rectum is located within most of the sphincter mechanism. The fistula follows a sub epithelial midline tract, opening somewhere along the midline perineal raphe, scrotum, or even at the base of the penis. The diagnosis is clinical.

3-Rectobladderneck Fistulas

Rectum opens into the bladder neck. It has poor prognosis for bowel control because the levator muscles, the striated muscle complex, and the external sphincter frequently are poorly developed. Sacrum is often deformed and short. In fact, the entire pelvis seems to be underdeveloped. The perineum is often flat, which is evidence of poor muscle development.

4-Rectal Atresia/Rectal Stenosis

Lumen of the rectum is totally (atresia) or partially (stenosis) interrupted. Upper pouch is represented by a dilated rectum, whereas the lower portion empties into a small anal canal that is in the normal location and is 1–2 cm long. Excellent functional prognosis because they have a well-developed anal canal, normal sensation in the anorectum, and normal voluntary sphincters. Must be screened for a presacral mass.

Female

1-Rectovestibular Fistulas

Most common defect in females with excellent functional prognosis, diagnosis is based on clinical examination. A meticulous inspection of the newborn's genitalia allows the clinician to observe a normal urethral meatus and a normal vagina, with a third whole in the vestibule. It can be repaired without a protective colostomy, however the complications of surgery (perineal infection followed by dehiscence of the anal anastomosis or perineal body, or recurrence of the fistula) provokes severe fibrosis that may interfere with the sphincter function. So the patient may lose the function of sphincter. Thus, a protective colostomy is still the best way to avoid these complications.

2-Rectoperineal Fistulas

Equivalent to the perineal fistula in male, rectum and vagina are well separated.

3-Persistent Cloaca

Rectum, vagina, and urinary tract meet and fuse into a single common channel. Diagnosis of a cloaca is a clinical one (single perineal orifice that opens in urethra, external genitalia are hypoplastic). Length of the common channel varies from 1–7cm, if it's less than 3cm defect can be repaired with a posterior saggital operation without opening the abdomen(good functional prognosis). If it's longer than 3 cm are more complex, abdominal approach must be utilized. Evaluation of the patient's Müllerian anatomy at time of repair or colostomy is important, and

Us for hydrocolpos . Sacral deformities can happen with anorectal malformation and the poor functional prognostic signs are: more than 2 absent sacral vertebrae and tethered cord.

Diagnosis

Patient is stable and abdomen is not distended. Perineal inspection must be performed, If meconium is seen on the perineum, a rectoperineal fistula is present. If there is meconium in the urine, a rectourinary fistula exists. The radiological imaging is not helpful (collapsed rectum). They can be used for evaluation of associated conditions, and after 24 hr do cross table lateral radiograph.

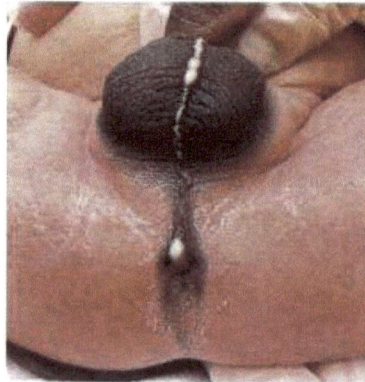

Fig. (4.28). This male infant has a rectoperineal fistula with a subepithelial tract filled with either mucus or meconium that extends into the scrotal raphe.

Management

In first 24 hours, the neonate should receive intravenous fluids, antibiotics, and nasogastric decompression, and be evaluated for associated defects. These include cardiac malformations, esophageal atresia, and urinary defects [52]. If persistent cloaca is present; the urinary tract needs to be evaluated at the time of colostomy formation, if low lesion is present, only a perineal operation without a colostomy, if high lesion requires a colostomy (descending or upper sigmoid) in the newborn period, followed by a pull-through procedure at approximately 2 months of age. If there is any doubt about the type of lesion, it is safer to perform a colostomy. After doing colostomy, the patient will undergo pull through procedure (posterior sagittal anorectoplasty (PSARP) procedure, this involves placing the patient in the prone jackknife position, dividing the levator ani and external sphincter complex in the midline posteriorly, dividing the communication between the gastrointestinal tract and the urinary tract, and bringing down the rectum after sufficient length is achieved. The muscles are then reconstructed and sutured to the rectum.

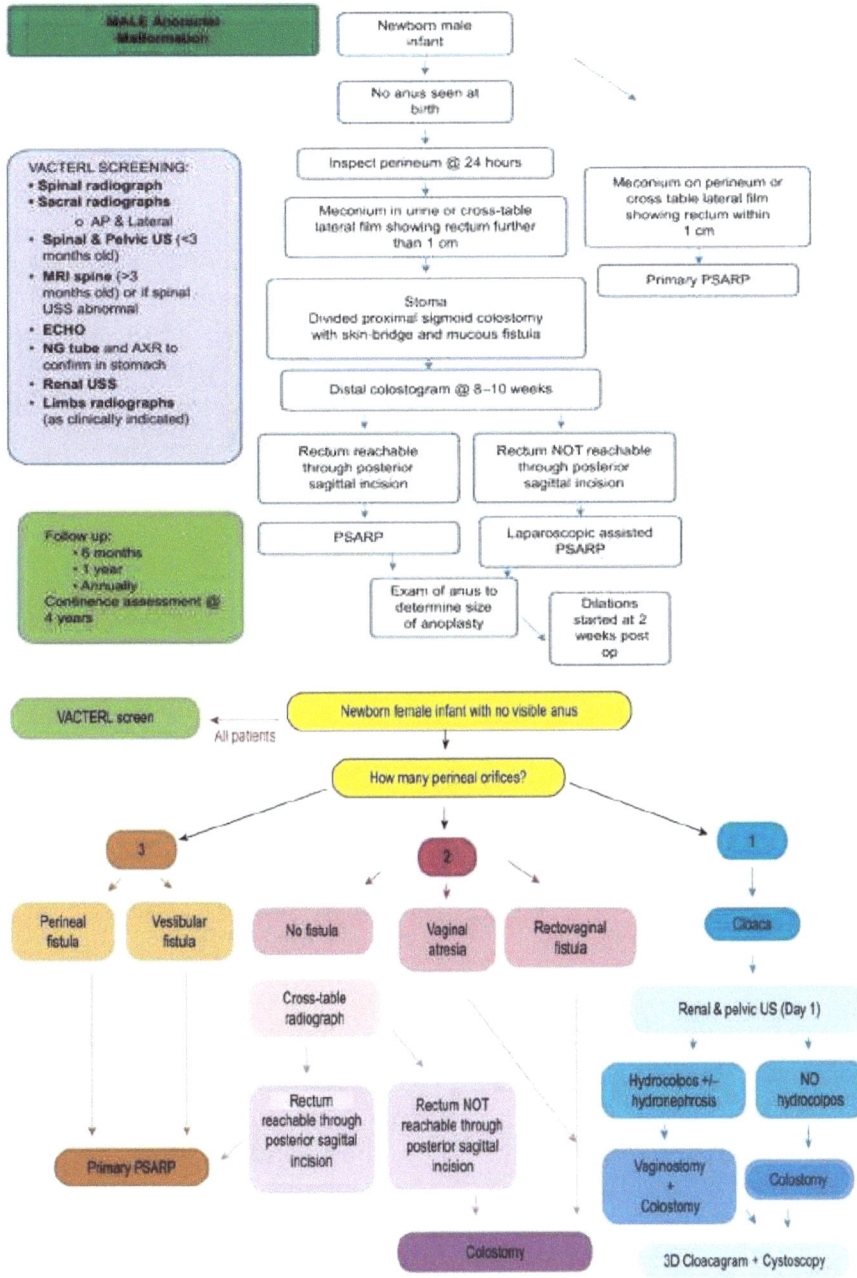

Fig. (4.29). Algorithm for the management of newborns with anorectal malformations based on the physical examination and radiographs.

Advantages of Early Operation

Less time with an abdominal stoma, less size discrepancy between the proximal and distal bowel at the time of colostomy closure, and easier anal dilation (because the infant is smaller).

Postoperative Care

IV antibiotics are administered for 24 hours and antibiotic ointment is applied to the perineal sutures for 7 days. Urinary catheterization and discharge 2-4 days after operation and anal dilatation until reach desire goal. Then do colostomy closure. Then perform endoscopy to evaluate the repair. After the colostomy is closed, the patient may have multiple bowel movements and may develop perineal excoriation. A constipating diet may be helpful in treating this problem. After several weeks, the number of bowel movements decreases and most patients will develop constipation and need laxatives [53]. After one to three months, the patient develops a more regular bowel movement pattern.

A good prognosis is: One to three bowel movements per day, remains clean between bowel movements, and shows evidence of feeling or pushing during bowel movements.

Biliary Atresia

Is a relatively rare obstructive condition of the bile ducts causing neonatal jaundice? The incidence: approximately 1 in 8000 to 1 in 18,000. Female > male (the ratio is 1. 4-1. 7: 1). Biliary atresia is associated with Congenital malformations occur in 11-20% [54]. Generally, biliary atresia (BA) is not considered an inherited disorder. However, genetic mutations that result in defective morphogenesis may be important in syndromic BA that is associated with other congenital anomalies, including interrupted inferior vena cava, preduodenal portal vein, intestinal malrotation, situs inversus, cardiac defects, annular pancreas and polysplenia [55]. Polysplenia is the most common associated anomaly and occurs in 7. 5% overall. Polysplenia syndrome is defined as: polysplenia, pre-duodenal portal vein, malrotation and abdominal situs inversus. It occurs in conjunction with maternal diabetes and may be associated with poorer outcomes [56].

Etiology

The biliary system originates from the hepatic diverticulum of the foregut at 4 weeks of embryonic life and differentiates into cranial and caudal components. The cranial component gives rise to the proximal extra-hepatic ducts and the majority of the intrahepatic biliary system, whereas the caudal component gives rise to the gallbladder, cystic duct and common bile duct. Genetic, immune-mediated and infectious causes have all been implicated in the pathogenesis of biliary atresia, but remain unproven, so the cause of biliary atresia remains unknown. A congenital origin of biliary atresia is theorized to result from failure of recanalization of extra-hepatic biliary system during embryo. Embryonic duct occlusion and subsequent vacuolization have not yet been confirmed [57]. It has also been suggested that failure of extra-hepatic biliary and intrahepatic biliary ducts to meet during the development may underlie certain types of biliary atresia with partial patency of ductal system. The ductal plate malformation theory: is suggested a failure of bile duct remodeling at hepatic hilum → these abnormal fetal bile ducts are poorly supported by mesenchyme and subsequent leak as perinatal bile flow increases→ this leakage of bile triggers intense local inflammatory reaction → obliteration of biliary tree. Additional speculative factors underlying biliary atresia include intrauterine or perinatal viral infection (including both rotavirus and reovirus type 3) [58], immunologically Mediated, exposure to toxins, a loss of blood supply, abnormal bile acid metabolism and pancreatic obiliary malunion. Biliary atresia is considered to be an acquired rather than congenital, this premise is supported by clinical observation that approximately 40% of patients pass normal meconium at birth and up 60% pass cholic stool initially and for a short period after birth [59].

Classification

Type I: atresia at common bile duct.

Type IIA: atresia at common hepatic duct.

Type IIB: atresia at common hepatic duct + cystic duct + common bile duct.

Type III: atresia of the common bile duct, cystic duct, and hepatic ducts up to the portahepatis. (Present in over 90% of patients with biliary atresia).

Clinical Features

Infants are initially active and their growth appears normal during the first few weeks to months after birth. Full term baby,the first meconium is usually normal. The pathologic jaundice typically appears within weeks after birth, Pale (acholic) stools and dark urine [60]. As biliary obstruction persists, the liver gradually increases in size and develops a firm consistency.

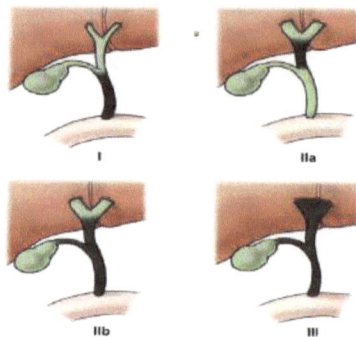

Fig. (4.30). Morphologic classification of biliary atresia based on macroscopic and cholangiographic findings. Type I, occlusion of common bile duct; Type IIa, obliteration of common hepatic duct; Type IIb, obliteration of common bile duct, hepatic and cystic ducts, with cystic dilatation of ducts at the portahepatis, and no gallbladder involvement; Type III, obliteration of common, hepatic, and cystic ducts without anastomosable ducts at the portahepatis (From Lefkowitch JH. Biliary atresia, Mayo Clin Proc 1998; 73:90–95).

Signs and symptoms of Malabsorption of fat soluble vitamins lead to anemia, malnutrition and growth failure. Cirrhosis will ultimately develop and mild splenomegaly may follow. If untreated, most children will die of hepatic decompensation, esophageal variceal bleeding or infection within 19 months. **Note**: jaundiced infants with pale stool, dark urine and hepatomegaly,biliary atresia should be strongly suspected.

Differential Diagnosis

Neonatal hepatitis, interlobular biliary hypoplasia, choledochal cyst and Inspissated bile syndrome.

Laboratory Studies

Pathological jaundice is suspected when the conjugated bilirubin >20% of total serum bilirubin [61]. Serologic evaluation can help distinguish between infection, hematologic problems, metabolic diseases and genetic disorders (*e. g.* α1-Antitrypsin deficiency).

Liver function tests alone cannot be used to diagnose BA.

γ-glutamyltranspeptidase (γ-GTP) are elevated. Coagulation profile, Hepatitis (A, B, C) serology, TORCH titers,α1-Antitrypsin level, Serum Lipoprotein-X, sweat chloride test or direct genetic analysis to rule out cystic fibrosis.

Hyaluronic Acid: Which has been considered a serum marker for liver function and biochemical marker for evaluating infants with BA [62].

Serum Bile Acids: Serum bile acid levels increase in infants with cholestatic disease, but both the total bile acid level and the ratio of chenodeoxycholic acid to cholic acid have no value for differentiating BA from other cholestatic diseases [63].

NOTE: Serum Lipoprotein-X is positive in all patients with BA, although it also may be positive in 20–40% of patients with neonatal hepatitis.

Imaging

Abdominal Ultrasound should be performed on all jaundiced infants. US will exclude other surgical causes of jaundice such as choledochal cyst and inspissated bile syndrome. In BA, the gallbladder is small, shrunken, and noncontractile, and there is increased echogenicity of the liver (Fig. **4.30**). The presence of other associated anomalies of the polysplenia syndrome is pathognomonic of BA [64], the "triangular cord" sign: well-defined triangular area of high-reflectivity echogenicity is seen at the portahepatisand corresponding to fibrotic ductal remnants. A recent meta-analysis found that the triangular cord signs and gallbladder abnormalities are the two most accurate and widely accepted US findings [65], whereas the absence of a common bile duct, enlargement of the hepatic artery and the presence of hepatic subcapsular blood flow are less valuable findings for diagnosis. Amniotic fluid digestive enzymes, which are synthesized by the biliary epithelium, gradually decrease until 24 weeks of gestation. As it is no longer possible to differentiate between abnormally low and physiologically low levels of the enzymes after 24 weeks of gestation, the prenatal diagnosis of BA is difficult [66].

Duodenal Aspiration

Aspiration of duodenal fluid by nasoduodenal intubation has been recommended as an inexpensive, noninvasive and rapid test. The diagnosis of biliary atresia is excluded if typical yellow bilirubin pigment is detected by either 24-hour collection or in serial duodenal intubations.

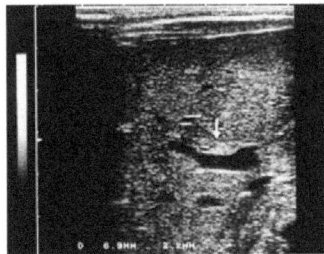

Fig. (4.30). Ultrasonography shows a well-defined triangular area of high echogenicity (arrow) at the portahepatis, corresponding to fibrotic ductal remnants (the "triangular cord" sign).

Hepatobiliary Scintigraphy

It uses Technetium labeled compound diisopropyliminodiacetic acid (DISDIA), is widely used to confirm ductal patency and help differentiate BA from other causes of infantile cholestasis. Pretreatment with phenobarbital (5 mg/kg/day) for 3-5 days before imaging will enhance excretion and thus increase discrimination between biliary atresia and nonobstructive causes of intrahepaticcholestasis. Visualization of the radionuclide in the intestine confirms ductal patency and excludes biliary atresia. Failure of the isotope to appear in the intestine after 24 hours, particularly after pretreatment with phenobarbital is highly suggestive of ductal obstruction as a result of biliary atresia. Isotope excretion maybe delayed because of hepatic dysfunction, so it is essential to obtain images 24 hours after injection if earlier images fail to confirm radionuclide in the intestine.

ERCP has a limited role in the evaluation of infantile jaundice and is not routinely performed. **Liver biopsy** is considered the most reliable preoperative test in the diagnosis of biliary atresia. Histologic findings consistent with biliary atresia include: preservation of basic hepatic architecture, bile ductular proliferation, bile duct plugsandinflammatory cell infiltrate, hepatocyte giant cell transformation, and edema and fibrosis of the portal tract. Uncorrected biliary atresia results in histologic evidence of cirrhosis as early as 3 to 4 months of age.

Laparoscopy-assisted Cholangiography
Intraoperative Cholangiogram
Complications

1. Malabsorption and growth retardation.
2. Cholestasis.
3. Secondary cirrhosis.
4. Liver failure.

Pre-operative Management

Preoperative blood test: should include complete blood count, coagulation profile and LFT. Patients should be nil by mouth for 24 hours prior to surgery. Bowel preparation should commence with oral kanamycin and glycerin enemas to decrease abundant colon microbiota to minimize intestinal gas. All infants should have parenteral vitamin K2 (1-2 mg/kg I. M) supplementation for several days before exploration. Parenteral broad-spectrum antibiotics should administered preoperatively just before the skin incision.

Kasai Procedure (Hepatic Portoenterostomy): is the standard operation for the treatment of biliary atresia. The infant is positioned supine for standard laparotomy. Surgical exploration commences through an upper abdominal transverse incision centered to the right, the incision can be extended across the midline if the biliary reconstruction is required. The extra-hepatic biliary structures are totally excised en bloc (as a whole), and the fibrous cone transected at the liver hilus is anastomosed to a Roux-en-Y jejunal limb [67].

Postoperative Manegement

Nasogastric drainage is continued until intestinal function returns normal, usually within 48 hours, the typically removed before discharge. Intravenous antibiotics are continued until a diet commences, at which time long term oral antibiotics are initiated. Length of stay averages 5 days. The use of steroid has been controversial. Steroids have been postulated to have a choleretic effect by stimulation of the bile flow through the bile salt-independent fraction induced by Na+/K+ ATPase activity. However, the salutary effect of steroid use in the management of biliary atresia has been difficult to prove.

Postoperative Complications

Nutritional complications: weight gain after surgery maybe retarded if hepatic dysfunction persists. Because the enterohepatic circulation has been impaired for several months, metabolic perturbations (disorders) involving fat, protein metabolism and vitamin and trace mineral absorption may occur [68]. Essential fatty acid deficiency and rickets may develop in up to 32%. The use of medium-chain triglyceride containing formulas is recommended when bile flow is absent or scanty.

Cholangitis: is the most common complication after hepatic portoenterostomy with incidence ranging from 33%-60%, occurs during the first 2 years in approximately 40% of infants can occur in the early postoperative period, especially before bilioenteric fistulae have developed. The cause and pathogenesis of cholangitis remain incompletely understood. Theories include direct contamination *via* reflux of intestinal contents through the Roux-limb, portal venous infection, impaired lymphatic drainage at portahepatis and systemic bacteria translocation. Predisposing factors may include biliary stasis caused by partial obstruction of the intrahepatic bile ducts and bacteria overgrowth of the intestinal conduit. It is defined as an elevated serum bilirubin (>2. 5 mg/ dL), leukocytosis, and a change from normal to acholic stools in a febrile patient (>38. 5°C). It must be treated by **intra-venous antibiotics immediately.** If stools remain acholic or revert to acholic, a pulse of corticosteroids should be trialed. It is important to note that cholangitis also may be **late-onset** and **precipitate liver failure**→necessitating emergency liver transplantation.

Portal hypertension is common after portoenterostomy, even in infants with good bile flow (Fig. **4.31**). The basic inflammatory process affecting the extra-hepatic ducts in BA also damages the intrahepatic branches, and evidence of persistent hepatic fibrosis has been found in some children despite successful portoenterostomy. Clinical manifestations of portal hypertension include **esophageal varices, hypersplenism** and **ascites.** The development of portal hypertension justifies a nonsurgical approach as long as hepatic function is preserved. However, in the presence of poor hepatic function, complications from portal hypertension are an indication for liver transplantation.

Intrahepatic bile lake cysts: biliary cysts or "lakes" can develop within the livers of short to long-term survivors at any time after portoenterostomy and cause recurring attacks of cholangitis (Fig. **4.32**). After percutaneous drainage of a bile lake, patients are usually anicteric and the lake cyst may disappear. Prolonged antibiotics and ursodeoxycholic acid may be helpful in preventing cholangitis. Persistent refractory infection is an indication for liver transplantation.

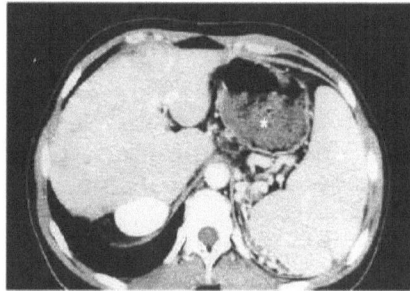

Fig. (4.31). CT scan of a 20-year-old woman in whom severe portal hypertension developed. Note marked atrophy of the left lobe of the liver, severe splenomegaly, and varices (asterisk) around the stomach.

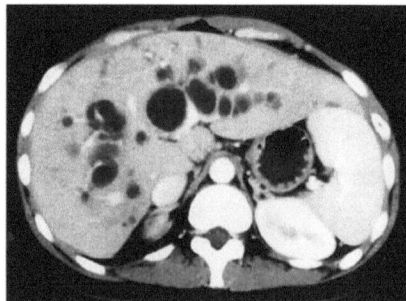

Fig. (4.32). CT scan of a 17-year-old patient with biliary atresia. Multiple biliary cysts or "lakes" have developed within the liver of this long-term survivor and caused recurrent attacks of cholangitis.

Hepato-pulmonary syndrome: is characterized by cyanosis, dyspnea on exertion, hypoxia, and finger clubbing. It appears to be more prevalent in children with syndromic BA. Diffuse intrapulmonary shunting can occur as a complication of chronic liver disease in children with BA as a result of vasoactive compounds from the mesenteric circulation not being able to be deactivated by the liver. Other complications are Porto pulmonary hypertension and Hepatic malignancy.

Prognosis

the Kasai hepatic portoenterostomy has greatly improved outcomes of infants with BA, and the results of surgical treatment have improved steadily over the past 30 years. The major determinants of satisfactory outcome after portoenterostomy are: age at initial operation; A favorable outcome is expected if hepatic portoenterostomy is performed before 60 days of age because cirrhosis will usually develop by 3–4 months of age. Outcomes are considerably worse if patients are older than 100 days at the time of portoenterostomy because obliterative cholangiopathy and hepatic fibrosis have likely already developed. successful achievement of postoperative bile flow presence of microscopic ductal structures at the portahepatis. the extent of liver parenchymal disease at the time of diagnosis, technical factors involving the portoenterostomy anastomosis.

Choledocal Cyst

Is congenital dilatation of the biliary tract, the dilatation can be found in any portion of biliary tract? The diameter of the bile duct varies according to the child's age (69), any diameter of the bile duct greater than the upper limit for age should be considered abnormal. The most common site is the choledochus. Incidence is Female > male (the ratio is 3. 2-1), it is minimal in infants and gradually becomes more significant as the patient gets older.

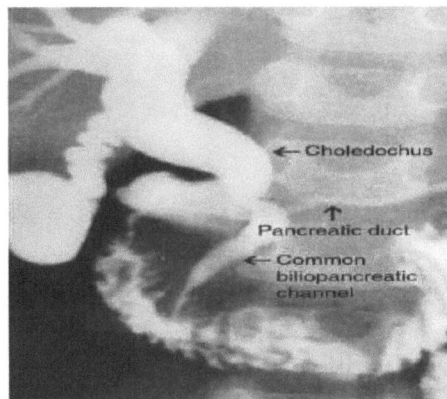

Fig. (4.33). This contrast study depicts a long common biliopancreatic channel that allows reflux of pancreatic secretions into the biliary tree. A long common biliopancreatic channel is thought to be the etiology of an acquired choledochal cyst.

Etiology

There are many theories to explain the development of a choledochal cyst (CC), but none of these can explain the formation of the five different types of CC. Choledochal cyst seem to be is either congenital or acquired. Congenital cysts develop during fetal life [70] as a result of a prenatal structural defect in the bile duct. Acquired choledochal cysts develop later in life. Normally, the terminal CBD and pancreatic duct unite to form a short common channel, which is well surrounded by the Oddi sphincter. This normal anatomic arrangement prevents the reflux of pancreatic fluid into the bile duct, If this common channel is long and part of it is not surrounded by the normal sphincter, pancreatic secretions can reflux into the biliary tree (Fig. **4.33**), Proteolytic enzymes from the pancreatic fluid are activated and can cause epithelial and mural damage that leads to mural weakness and dilatation of the choledochus.

Note: This theory is supported by the fact that high concentrations of activated pancreatic amylase and/or lipase have been found in patients with CC and long pancreaticobiliary channels [71].

Classification

Different classifications have been proposed for choledochal cyst (CC), the Todani classification has been the most widely accepted (Fig. **4.34**) [72].

Todani's classification

Type I:Ia: cystic dilatation of the CBD.

Ib: fusiform dilatation of the CBD.

Type II: diverticulum of the CBD.

Type III: choledochocele (dilatation of the terminal CBD within the duodenal wall).

Type IV: IVa: multiple cysts of the extra-hepatic and intrahepatic ducts.

IVb: multiple extra-hepatic duct cysts.

Type V: intrahepatic duct cyst (single or multiple, as in Caroli disease).

Type I CCs predominate. Together with type IVa cysts, they account for more than 90% of cases. **Forme fruste** is a special variant of CC characterized by pancreaticobiliary malunion, but little or no dilatation of the extra-hepatic bile duct [73]. Children present with symptoms similar to those in patients with a CC.

Excision of the extra-hepatic bile duct is recommended in these children because of the likely eventual development of cancer due to chronic pancreaticobiliary reflux.

Clinical Features

Patients with choledochal cyst usually are classified as **infantile** or adult in nature. In the infantile form patients ranging from 1-3 months of age present with: Obstructive jaundice, Pale (acholic) stools, Dark urine and Hepatomegaly. Patients with infantile form do not tend to have abdominal pain or palpable mass. Infants who have been diagnosed to have a choledochal cyst **prenatally** do not ordinarily become jaundiced until 1-3 weeks after birth. Low grade fever may be present as in patients with **biliary atresia**, but not with a pattern that suggests **cholangitis**. In the adult form of choledochal cyst, clinical manifestations do not generally become evident until after 2 years of age. Patients with adult form, mostly have fusiform deformity of common duct without high grade or complete obstruction (tend to have partial obstruction). Because only partial obstruction in adult form, symptoms are intermittent. So, they have **classic triad**: Abdominal pain (in the right upper quadrant and occasionally the back), Palpable mass and intermittent jaundice [74]. **Hepatomegaly** in adult form, it is less prominent than in infantile form in which biliary obstruction is not complete in adult form. Abdominal pain is similar to recurrent pancreatitis and is evidenced by elevation of serum amylase level but serum amylase is elevated because of abnormal amylase clearance.

Differential Diagnosis

In infantile form: Biliary atresia.

In adult form: Primary sclerosing cholangitis, congenital cirrhosis, congenital stricture of the common hepatic duct or common bile duct, congenital hepatic fibrosis and Caroli's disease with hepatic fibrosis.

Laboratory Tests

Laboratory studies performed in patients with choledochal cysts are often normal. Serum conjugated and unconjugated bilirubin and hepatocellular transaminase levels are within normal limits unless the patient has cholangitis or has developed cirrhosis. Serum amylase level: is elevated (if the patient is presented with pancreatitis). Coagulation profile: is abnormal if biliary is obstructed.

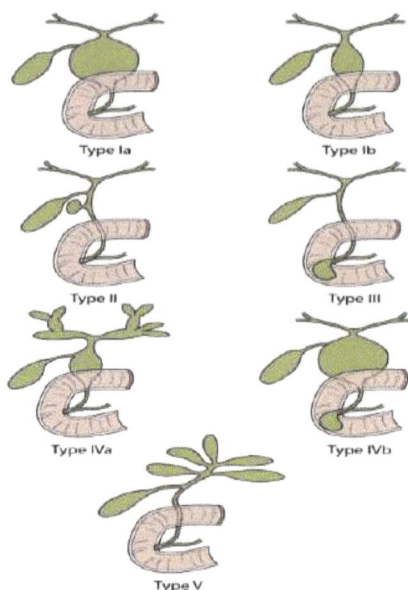

Fig. (4.34). These diagrams depict the five classifications for choledochal cyst according to Todani. (From Todani T, Watanabe Y, Narusue M, *et al*. Congenital bile duct cysts: classification, operative procedures, and review of thirty-seven cases including cancer arising from choledochal cyst. Am J Surg 1977; 134:263–269).

Imaging

Abdominal Ultrasonography: is the initial imaging method of choice. Contour and position of the CC, the status of the proximal ducts, vascular anatomy, and hepatic echo texture can be evaluated on US. Ultrasonography (US) is the best screening study. If a choledochal cyst is suspected on US screening, technetium-99m DISIDA Scintigraphy can confirm the diagnosis and provide information about drainage, obstruction and hepatic function. Other advantage of US as a screening study are that it is capable of demonstrating changes in caliber of the bile and pancreatic ducts and it can also provide information about the status of liver in terms of density and possible fibrosis. **ERCP** allows excellent definition of the cyst as well as the entire anatomy including the pancreatobiliary junction. ERCP is invasive and has complication such as pancreatitis, perforation of the duodenal or biliary tracts, hemorrhage and sepsis [75]. **MRCP** is highly accurate in the detection and classification of the cyst (Fig. **4.35**). The overall detection rate of MRCP for a CC is very high (96–100%) and should be considered a first-choice imaging technique for evaluation [76] and its replacement ERCP because it is noninvasive. **Intraoperative cholangiography** is indicated when the anatomic detail of the biliary tract cannot be demonstrated by MRCP or ERCP. Operative cholangiography may be performed either through the gallbladder or directly into dilated bile duct itself. **Contrast-enhanced CT** may be indicated in some patients with pancreatitis or if an associated tumor is suspected. **Operative liver biopsy** is useful to determine whether the cirrhosis is present or not.

Treatment of Choledochal Cyst

Treatment of a choledochal cyst is essential because it will cause recurrent episodes of cholangitis and may cause the development of biliary cirrhosis or evolve into a cholangiocarcinoma. All of these patients will require surgical intervention; but the type of procedure is performed according to the subtype of choledochal cysts. For a patient who presents with cholangitis or acute pancreatitis, surgical intervention is delayed until the inflammatory process has resolved.

Types I and IV Choledochal Cyst

the treatment of choledochal cyst is surgical excision followed by biliary-enteric reconstruction. The posterior plane between the cyst and portal vein must be carefully dissected to removal. Resection of the cyst requires circumferential dissection. Cyst excision is accomplished, and the proximal bile duct is anastomosed to the intestinal tract. Biliary drainage is achieved by an end-to-side hepaticojejunostomy *via* a **Roux-en Y** jejunal limb. Complete resection of the cyst is important because its division at the superior edge of the duodenum may leave residual cyst wall in the head of the pancreas, which could lead to a recurrence or a future malignancy. The pancreatic duct is vulnerable to injury during distal cyst excision but can be avoided by avoiding entry into the pancreatic parenchyma.

Type II Choledochal Cyst

excision of the diverticulum and the extra-hepatic biliary tract with a Roux-en-Y hepaticojejunostomy to re-establish drainage of the proximal bile ducts is the procedure of choice. Although simple excision of the diverticulum with ligation at its base can be performed. excision of the extra-hepatic biliary tract is generally recommended because of the risk of the development of a cholangiocarcinoma in the remaining extra-hepatic biliary tract.

Type III Choledochal Cyst

the recommendations for treatment vary according to the type of epithelium found within the choledochal cyst. An ERCP should be performed before surgical intervention. At the time of ERCP, biopsy of the mucosa lining the cyst should be performed. If the biopsy reveals mucosa of duodenal origin, the lesion can be treated by a sphincterotomy or meatotomy to enlarge the opening and to relieve the obstruction, This can be done endoscopically or with open surgery. In cases where the epithelium lining the lesion appears to be of biliary tract origin, excision of the cyst with reimplantation of both the bile duct and the pancreatic duct has been recommended. it is essential to excise all of the biliary epithelium so as to minimize the likelihood of the development of a cholangiocarcinoma.

Type V Choledochal Cyst (Caroli Disease)

The extent of disease dictates the type of surgical procedure performed. In patients with disease confined to one lobe of the liver, formal hepatic lobectomy is recommended. If a patient has bilobar disease, liver transplantation will be necessary.

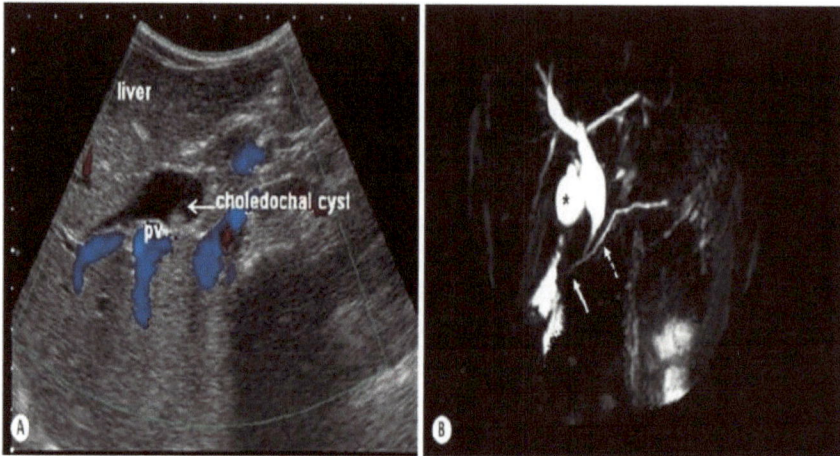

Fig. (4.35). (A) Ultrasound is the initial imaging method of choice for identifying a choledochal cyst. The cyst is identified as well as the portal vein (pv) lying posterior to it. (B) MRCP is highly accurate in the detection and classification of the cyst. On this MRCP image, note the fusiform choledochal cyst as well as the pancreatic duct (dotted arrow) and long common channel (solid arrow). The gallbladder is marked with an asterisk.

Postoperative Care

Oral feeding is initiated after the fluid from the gastric tube becomes clear, usually by postoperative day 2 or 3. The abdominal drain is removed on day 5 if there is no evidence of leak from the bilio-enteric anastomosis. Antibiotics are started and maintained for at least **6 months**. If no episodes of cholangitis occur during the 6-month period, antibiotics are discontinued.

Postoperative Complications

Early Complication: Bleeding, Anastomotic leak, pancreatic fistula and Intestinal obstruction.

Late complication: cholangitis, anastomotic stricture, intrahepatic calculi and bowel obstruction [77].

Inspissated Bile Syndrome

It is defined as partial or complete obstruction of the extra-hepatic system by impaction of thick bile or sludge in the distal common bile duct during the neonatal period. Inspissated bile syndrome can occur in infants with dehydration, hemolysis, impaired hepatic bile secretion, cystic fibrosis, receiving diuretic therapy [78] or total parenteral nutrition [79]. **A predisposition** in disorder that either increases the viscosity or decreases the solubility of bileinitially difficult to differentiate inspissated bile syndrome from **biliary atresia** because both are characterized by jaundice and pale (acholic) stools. Inspissated bile syndrome may precede **cholelithiasis.**

Investigation

Abdominal ultrasound demonstrates Mild to moderate proximal biliary dilatation, Sludge or stones in the distal common bile duct. Radionuclide scan shows hepatic concentration of isotope without excretion into the intestine.

Treatment

Inspissated bile syndrome usually resolves spontaneously [80] as the underlying disease or predisposing factors are treated. Persistent jaundice is evaluated and treated at surgical exploration by intraoperative cholangiography performed through the gallbladder fundus, which will confirm the diagnosis and exclude biliary atresia. Cholangiography is often curative and may be augmented by intraoperative saline irrigation. SSDuodenotomy or choledochotomy is rarely acquired.

Pancreas Conditions

EMBREOLOGY

Pancreas originate from two bud during 4th week of gestation, dorsal bud which give rise to body and tail of the pancreas, its minor duct (Santorini) and papilla, and the continuation of the major duct (Wirsung) into the body and tail. The ventral bud which give rise to the head of the pancreas as well as the proximal portion of the Wirsung duct (Fig. **4.36**), the two pancreatic buds fuse to form one pancreas at approximately 7 weeks' gestation, although it appears that complete fusion of the two ducts to form the main pancreatic duct is delayed until the perinatal period [81].

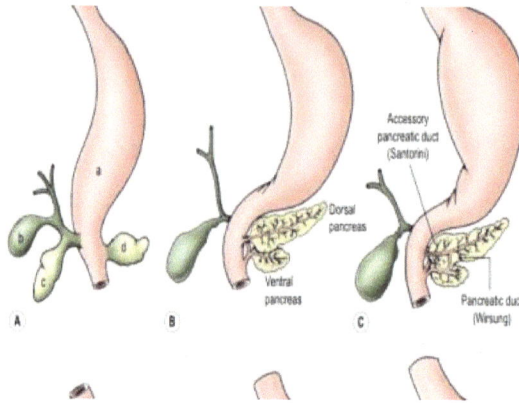

Fig. (4.36).   Pancreatic embryology. (A) Stomach (a), gallbladder (b), and ventral (c) and dorsal (d) pancreatic buds develop separately at embryologic week 4. The pancreas develops as an evagination of the developing foregut. The dorsal bud evaginates directly off of the duodenal anlage. (B) The ventral bud evaginates from the biliary bud and then swings around to the left, with gut rotation occurring simultaneously. (C) The main pancreatic duct of Wirsung and the minor accessory duct of Santorini are shown.

ANATOMY

Pancreas is retroperitoneal and is light pink in children. Pancreas is composed from head body and tail although these area have no distinct anatomic border, the head site to the right on L2, the body covers L1 and the tails rises to T12 on the Left. The main pancreatic duct together with common bile duct enter the duodenum at the site of the major papilla, the accessory pancreatic duct open into the minor papilla. The arterial supply of the pancreas is from the celiac and SMA arteries [90], which form the pancreaticoduodenal arcade. The pancreas also has anastomoses from the splenic artery [82].

ACUTE PANCREATITIS

Acute pancreatitis is an acute inflammation of the pancreas, varying in severity from mild abdominal pain to fulminant necrotizing pancreatitis and death, incidence between 3. 6 and 13. 2 cases per 100,000 children.

Etiology

The causes of acute pancreatitis include trauma, biliary tract stone disease, choledochal cyst, ductal developmental anomalies, drugs, metabolic derangements, and infections. Most commonly, the cause is not apparent and is termed idiopathic. As the pancreas is fixed against the lumbar spine, trauma to the upper abdomen can fracture the pancreas or injure the major duct at that point (Fig. **4.37**). Bilary stone disease, increasing in frequency in children, may lead to pancreatitis from transient pancreatic duct obstruction ductal developmental anomalies, drugs such as asparaginase and valproic acid [83]. Systemic illnesses and metabolic conditions, such as CF, Reye syndrome, Kawasaki disease, hyperlipidemias, and hypercalcemia, as well as viral infections (*e. g.*, coxsackie virus and rotavirus) and generalized bacterial sepsis, also can cause pancreatitis [84]. Choledochal cysts produce pancreatitis by pancreatic duct compression or bile reflux resulting from a long common biliary–pancreatic duct within the head of the pancreas.

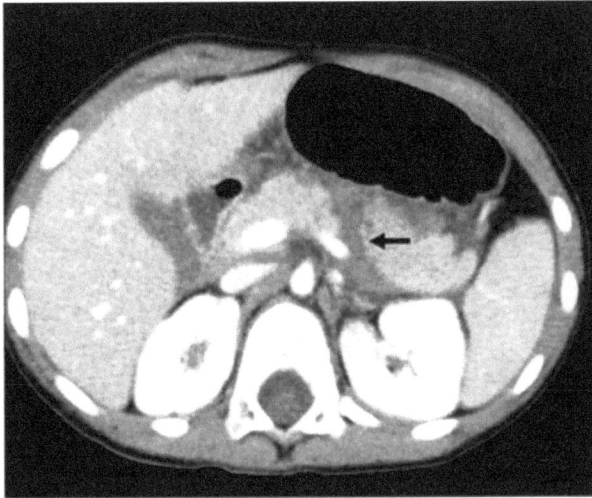

Fig. (4.37). This abdominal contrast-enhanced CT shows a complete transection (arrow) of the body of the pancreas following a bicycle handlebar injury tothe epigastrium. The patient underwent laparoscopic distal pancreatectomy and recovered uneventfully.

Diagnosis

Diagnostic criteria for acute pancreatitis include at least two of the following:

1. Acute abdominal pain (especially in the epigastria region).

2. Serum amylase or lipase more than three times the upper limit of normal, and imaging findings characteristic or compatible with acute pancreatitis [85]. The abdomen is diffusely tender with signs of peritonitis, and distention occurs with a paucity of bowel sounds. In severe cases of necrotizing or hemorrhagic pancreatitis, hemorrhage may spread away from the pancreas along tissue planes, appearing as ecchymosis either in the flanks (Grey Turner sign) or at the umbilicus (Cullen sign) (Fig. **38**). These ecchymoses generally take 1–2 days to develop.

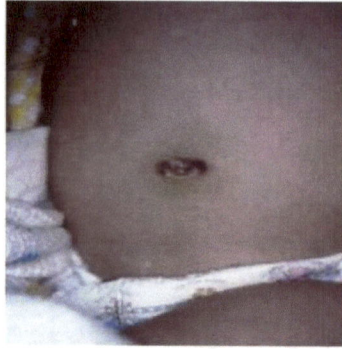

Fig. (4.38). Positive Cullen sign, with periumbilical ecchymosis, in a patient with hemorrhagic pancreatitis.

3. Elevated amylase levels are helpful in the diagnosis, although a normal serum amylase level does not exclude pancreatitis. Hyperamylasemia also may be caused by salivary inflammation/trauma, intestinal disease (such as perforation, ischemia, necrosis, or inflammation), and macroamylasemia. Lipase has been suggested as an alternative marker, but can be falsely elevated in pancreatic cancer, macrolipasemia, renal insufficiency, cholecystitis, esophagitis, intestinal perforation, and hypertriglyceridemia. Elevated lipase tends to be more sensitive in infants and toddlers and may also help differentiate pancreatitis from salivary trauma. The degree of enzyme elevation does not correlate with disease severity [86, 87]. Imaging the abdomen is important as part of the evaluation of the patient with abdominal pain. In the patient with pancreatitis, plain abdominal radiographs may reveal an isolated loop of intestine in the vicinity of the inflamed pancreas, termed the sentinel loop. Pancreatic calcifications suggest chronic pancreatitis. Plain chest radiographs should be performed in all patients with acute pancreatitis to look for evidence of pleural effusion and pulmonary edema. Abdominal ultrasound (US) is useful in the evaluation of the patient with pancreatitis, but has limited applications [88]. It is well established in the evaluation of biliary stone disease as the etiology for pancreatitis and can detect choledochal cysts and pancreatic pseudocysts as well. Abdominal computed tomography (CT) provides much better resolution of the pancreas than US. Its primary role is in the detection of early and late complications, such as pancreatic necrosis, pseudocysts, and fluid collections [89]. MRCP is a newer, noninvasive technique for evaluating the biliary tree and pancreatic duct by using resonance imaging (MRI). It is the initial imaging study of choice for the evaluation of pancreatic ductal anatomy in children with recurrent or unexplained pancreatitis. Studies comparing MRCP and ERCP show high concordance in diagnoses. Its disadvantages are that it does not allow for therapeutic intervention (though it may direct the type of intervention necessary). The most frequent indication for ERCP in children is in the diagnosis or treatment of acute, recurrent, or chronic pancreatitis [90, 91].

Management

Pain control, IV fluid resuscitation, pancreatic rest, and monitoring for complications, fluid resuscitation and maintenance should be guided toward a goal urine output of 2 mL/kg/h measured by an indwelling urinary catheter. Patients with severe acute pancreatitis may require nasogastric decompression. Most patients receive histamine-2 (H2) receptor antagonists to reduce exposure of the duodenal secretin-producing cells to gastric acid somatostatin in the treatment of pancreatitis is equivocal and probably serves more to mitigate complications of pancreatitis rather than to treat the disease itself. This therapeutic regimen is logical but empiric, because no studies have shown improvement in outcomes with these interventions. Enteral nutrition (EN) has become the preferred method over total parenteral nutrition (TPN). Mild to moderate cases of acute pancreatitis often resolve prior to requiring EN or TPN. More severe cases should be treated with EN *via* a nasojejunal tube, When EN is contraindicated, some advocate waiting as long as 5 days prior to starting TPN. Compared with TPN, EN has been shown to decrease length of stay, reduce the need for surgery, and reduce the risk of infectionAdequate analgesia is critical to minimizing the physiologic stress that develops from pain. Although meperidine (Demerol) was once advocated because morphine was thought to cause spasm of the Sphincter of Oddi, no clinical trials have shown superiority of meperidine over other narcotic analgesics. Large doses of meperidine, however, are associated with the risk of seizure, euphoria, and drug interactions, suggesting other narcotics such as morphine and fentanyl may be safer alternatives. The diagnosis of pancreatitis must be certain prior to initiating treatment with high doses of narcotics as these may mask signs of serious nonpancreatic pathology, such as intestinal or gastric perforations. In the management of severe acute pancreatitis, a major decision is whether and when surgery for pancreatic infection and necrosis is necessary [92].

CHRONIC PANCREATITIS

Chronic pancreatitis is distinguished from acute pancreatitis by the irreversibility of the changes associated with the inflammation. Chronic pancreatitis remains a substantial clinical problem, afflicting roughly 140,000 individuals in the United States alone. The disease entails several clinical problems: severe and intractable pain typically requiring narcotics, malabsorption due to loss of pancreatic digestive enzymes from the exocrine pancreas requiring chronic enzyme replacement for life. Life-threatening complications such as pancreatic pseudocyst, pancreatic ascites, biliary obstruction, *etc.* a 13-fold increased risk of pancreatic cancer and the development of insulinopenia and overt diabetes mellitus in over half of patients [93].

Causes

Obstructive pancreatitis is most often due to an anatomic or functional obstruction of the pancreatic duct. The most common anatomic causes are pancreas divisum followed by choledochal cysts, potential causes are the anatomic variant, structural narrowing of the minor papilla, sphincter of Oddi dysfunction, or the relatively high association with CFTR mutations (Table **4.2**) [94].

Clinical Picture

Chronic pancreatitis can manifest with a characteristic pain, diminished pancreatic function, and radiographic abnormalities. Increased stool fat, diabetes, and steatorrhea are signs of pancreatic insufficiency.

Blood Biochemistry The degree of permanent damage to the pancreas may be assessed by blood test (pancreatic enzyme), stool tests (pancreatic enzymes, Fecal fat), and noninvasive test of pancreatic function, such as the pancreatic stimulation (secretin) [95].

Diagnostic Imaging Frequently on a CT scan, the pancreas has microcalcifications throughout the parenchyma and calcified stones in the duct Fig. (4.39). Additionally, pancreatic pseudocysts or inflammation may be seen on the CT scan. ERCP and MRCP can evaluate the ductal anatomy and identify anatomic causes of chronic pancreatitis. Only ERCP provides a means for evaluating sphincter pressure measurements for functional obstruction [96].

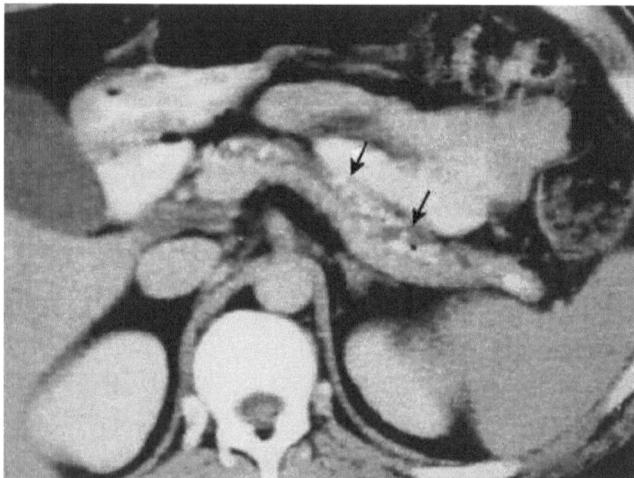

Fig. (4.39). CT scan of a pancreas with chronic calcifying pancreatitis. A dilated duct can be seen within the pancreas, further supporting the diagnosis of chronic pancreatitis. Calcified stones (arrows) can be seen in the dilated duct.

Surgical Treatment

Surgery of the pancreas is generally of three types:

1-Sphincteroplasty

2-Pancreatic drainage *via* longitudinal pancreaticijejunostomy (Puestow) or end to end pancreaticijejunostomy (Duval)

3-Pancreaticogastrostomy (smith) and pancreatectomy

Longitudinal Pancreaticojejunostomy (Puestow technique) in adult has been successful in eliminating or ameliorating pain from chronic pancreatitis in 70% to 97%of patients. In children some authors maintain that the Puestowprocedure improves pancreatic function, decrease hospitalization and increase body weight toward ideal. Others have reported that distal pancreatectomy and pancreaticojejunostomy is ineffective. Subtotal or total pancreatectomy is associated with considerable morbidity and mortality and is reserved for patients with intractable pain who have diffuse parenchymal damage without duct dilatation [97], the procedure is not generally indicated in children.

PANCREATIC PSEUDOCYST

Pancreatic pseudocyst is a complication of trauma or pancreatitis that forms after injury to the pancreatic ductal system. The acute pseudocyst has an irregular wall on CT scan, is tender, and usually develops shortly after an episode of acute pancreatitis or trauma (Fig. **4.40**). Chronic pseudocysts are usually spherical with a thick wall and are commonly seen in patients with chronic pancreatitis. The distinction is important because half of acute pseudocysts resolve without treatment, while chronic pseudocysts rarely spontaneously resolve.

Pseudocysts in children tend to resolve more frequently with medical therapy alone [98]. Pancreatic pseudocysts that persist or are symptomatic require either a drainage procedure or excision. Endoscopic treatment, well established in adults, has been reported to be safe and efficacious in children as well, other options include laparoscopic transgastric and intragastric drainage into the stomach or jejunum. Percutaneous drainage is the preferred approach for an infected pseudocyst because these cysts typically have thin, weak walls that are not amenable to internal drainage.

Table 4. 2. Causes of chronic relapsing pancreatitis in children.

Congenital anomalies of the pancreatic duct
Pancreaticobiliarymalunion
Pancreas divisum
Annular pancreas
Biliary tract disorder
Choledocholithiasis
Cholelithiasis
Trauma
Systemic infection
Hereditary pancreatitis
Hyperlipoproteinemia
Hyperparathyroidism and hypercalcemia
Cystic fibrosis
Inborn error of metabolism
Chronic inflammatory conditions
Crohn's disease
Ulcerative colitis
Systemic lupus erythematous
Chronic fibrosing pancreatitis
Juvenile tropical pancreatitis
Idiopathic chronic pancreatitis

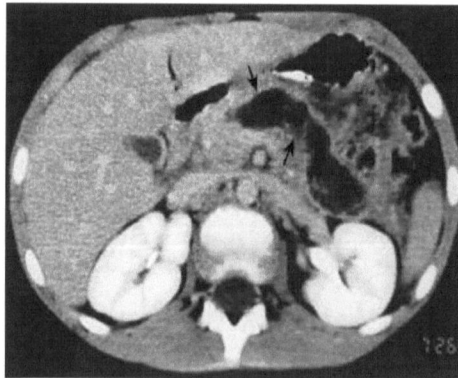

Fig. (4.40). CT scan of an acute pseudocyst in a patient after a severe motor vehicle accident. The wall (arrows) is irregular with nonloculated fluid inside.

The three major complications of pancreatic pseudocysts are hemorrhage, rupture, and infection. Patients with hemorrhage require emergency angiography with embolization, rupture or infection of a pseudocyst is uncommon. In both cases, external drainage is indicated.

CONGENITAL HYPERINSULINISM

CHI patients typically develop hypoglycemia shortly after birth, though it may manifest at a later age. Infants with CHI are often macrosomic. Symptoms may be subtle, such as lethargy and irritability, or severe with apnea, seizures, and coma. Simultaneous insulin and glucose measurements show a high ratio of insulin to glucose, keeping in mind that insulin levels may be normal but inappropriate in the presence of hypoglycemia. These patients differ from insulinoma patients, who usually have high absolute insulin levels. Another powerful indicator of CHI is a glucose requirement greater than 8 mg/kg/min. Owing to the much higher incidence of insulinoma, patients older than 1 year at the onset of hypoglycemia should be evaluated for both conditions. Mutations in seven genes are currently known to cause CHI, though roughly half of cases are caused by genetic malformations not yet understood. Initially discovered was the loss-of-function mutations in the SUR1 and Kir6. 2 components of the ATP-sensitive potassium channel (KATP) found in the cell membrane of the pancreatic β-cell. These mutations either impair the ability of Mgadenosine diphosphate (ADP) to stimulate channel activity or affect the expression of the KATP channels at the surface membrane, resulting in continuous depolarization of the β-cell membrane and dysregulated insulin secretion [99], Table **4.3**.

Medical Management

Stabilization of the CHI patient includes frequent intermittent or continuous feeding, with the addition of intravenous glucose as needed. Central venous access is advised because adequate venous access is lifesaving and high concentrations of intravenous glucose may be necessary. Maintaining normoglycemia is key to preventing potentially disabling hypoglycemic brain injury. Intramuscular glucagon can be used as a temporizing measure until definitive venous access is obtained. Treatment of CHI begins with medical management. Diazoxide remains a mainstay of therapy. Diazoxide binds the SUR1 component of the KATP channel and maintains it in a persistently open state, preventing insulin secretion. Patients with diazoxide-sensitive CHI who can tolerate fasting can be managed medically until they outgrow their condition. Those unresponsive to diazoxide should be managed with frequent feedings, glucose infusions, and somatostatin analogs. Somatostatin analogs inhibit pancreatic insulin secretion and can be administered subcutaneously either intermittently or continuously by a pump. Somatostatin analogs are associated with gallstones and biliary sludge, and have been implicated in cases of necrotizing enterocolitis. Medical failure to control hypoglycemia necessitates surgical intervention [100].

Table 4. 3. Classification of genetic forms of hyperinsulinemiahypoglycemia of infancy.

K $_{ATP}$ channel defect
SUR1 mutations
Kir6. 2 mutations
Loss of heterozygosity
Glucokinase-activating mutation
Glutamate dehydrogenase-activating mutation
Undefined
Autosomal dominant
Autosomal recessive
Sporadic
Beckwith-Wiedemann syndrome
Beta-cell adenoma-MEN1

Surgical Management

The goal of the surgery is to reduce excessive insulin production, but the procedure is unphysiologic and inexact. The current recommendation is a 95% resection with only a rim of tissue left on the duodenum and bile duct rather than the traditional 75% resection Fig. (**4.41**) serum glucose levels are monitored closely throughout the operation. The procedure is performed through an upper abdominal transverse incision the lesser sac is entered to expose and mobilize the entire pancreas, and a kocher maneuver is performed on the duodenum.

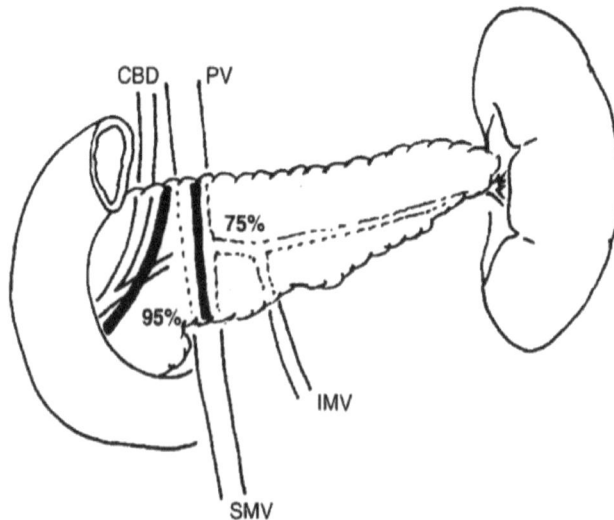

Fig. (4.41). Extent dissection of pancreas.

PANCREATIC TUMOR

The only pancreatic endocrine tumors seen in infants and children are insulinomas, gastrinomas, and VIPomas. VIPoma is a tumor of vasoactive intestinal peptide (VIP) producing cells and only case reports exist in children. **Insulinoma** is the most common of the three, though still quite rare among pediatric tumors in general. Only 10% of insulinomas are malignant, and these tend to spread to the liver and peripancreatic lymph nodes. Insulinomas cause symptoms of hypoglycemia, including dizziness, headaches, confusion, sweating, and seizures. The classic Whipple triad was described in patients with insulinoma and consists of symptoms of hypoglycemia with fasting, glucose levels less than half of normal when fasting, and relief of symptoms with glucose administration. Patients are typically in their adolescence; though younger children have been described with insulinoma. The lesions are usually solitary, except in multiple endocrine neoplasia type I (MEN I), in which multiple insulinomas may be found [101]. The gold standard test for insulinoma is the 72-hour fast, though studies have shown that a positive result is achieved in 80–90% of patients with insulinoma after a shorter 24 or 48-hour fast, respectively. While fasting, periodic blood glucose levels are obtained. When the patient's blood glucose falls below 50 mg/dL and symptoms are present, blood is drawn for plasma glucose, C-peptide, proinsulin, insulin, β-hydroxybutyrate, and sulfonylureas. Administration of exogenous insulin, followed by measurement of the Cpeptide level, can be suggestive of an insulinoma, but is not completely reliable. Measuring the insulin-to-glucose ratio is no longer needed. Most experts advocate for both transabdominal US and CT Magnetic resonance (MRI) is most useful for detecting liver metastases. If noninvasive studies fail to identify the tumor, intra-arterial calcium stimulation *via* a catheter in several visceral arteries with parallel venous sampling from the right hepatic vein has been reported to regionally localize insulinomas in 80–94% of cases. Intraoperative US is strongly advocated for identification of adjacent biliary and vascular structures. All patients with insulinoma should undergo resection. Insulinomas are pink, firm, encapsulated, and usually amenable to enucleation. In most cases, through preoperative and intraoperative analysis, the tumors can be localized, but in patients in whom they cannot be localized, blind distal pancreatic resection is no longer advised. The distinction between benign and malignant lesions is difficult and is based on tumor size (<2 cm tend to be benign) and the presence of metastases. Insulinomas that are hard, cause puckering of surrounding tissues, appear infiltrating, or cause distal pancreatic duct dilation should be assumed malignant and resected with a margin instead of enucleated. Malignant tumors can be treated with chemotherapy, biotherapy (such as octreotide), hepatic artery embolization/chemoembolization, radiation therapy, or radiofrequency ablation [102].

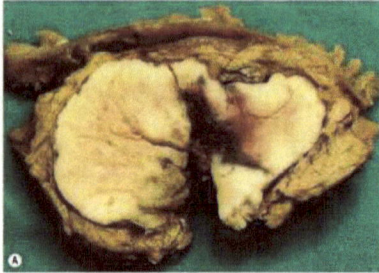

ADENOCARCINOMA AND PANCREATOBLASTOMA

Exocrine pancreatic cancers account for roughly half of pancreatic neoplasms in children. Whereas ductal adenocarcinoma is most common in adults, its embryonic counterpart pancreatoblastoma is more common in children. Pancreatoblastoma (Fig. **4.42**) is believed to result from the persistence of embryonic pancreatic progenitor cells beyond the eighth week of gestation. It tends to be diagnosed in early childhood and is more common in boys and those of Asian descent. An allelic loss on 11p is often associated and suggests a similar pathogenesis with Beckwith–Wiedemann syndrome and other embryonic tumors. A large multicenter review demonstrated that the tumor distribution was homogenous throughout the pancreas, most were larger than 5 cm at presentation, and over half had distant metastases [103].

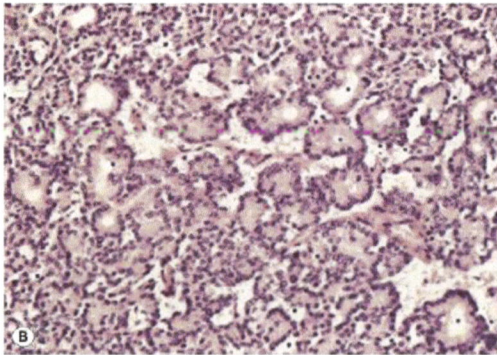

Elevation of serum α-fetoprotein was an inconsistent feature. The prognosis is relatively good with complete resection and with appropriate neoadjuvant and/or adjuvant chemotherapy and radiation therapy. Relapse is common, so continued monitoring is essential. Acinar cell carcinoma and ductal adenocarcinoma are less common pancreatic exocrine tumors. Ductal adenocarcinoma is infrequently reported in the pediatric literature, and no definitive recommendations are possible, acinar cell carcinoma is comparatively more common, Complete resection for both tumor types appears necessary with appropriate provision of neoadjuvant or adjuvant chemotherapy based on also known as a papillary-cystic tumor or Frantz tumor. It has a female preponderance and is derived from exocrine cells but without acinar or ductal structures. Presenting symptoms often include a palpable abdominal mass and abdominal pain. These tumors can be very large at the time of diagnosis (Fig. **4.43**). Pretreatment staging, Long-term survival improves with an earlier stage at presentation.

Occurring slightly less frequently than pancreatoblastoma is the solid pseudopapillary tumor, they are very slow growing, and there are reports of patients surviving 20 years after diagnosis without treatment [103]. Although these tumors are rarely metastatic, excision of regional and distal metastases greatly improves survival. Even with its indolent nature, an aggressive approach with complete resection is recommended as one retrospective study of patients with incomplete resections showed poor long-term survival [104].

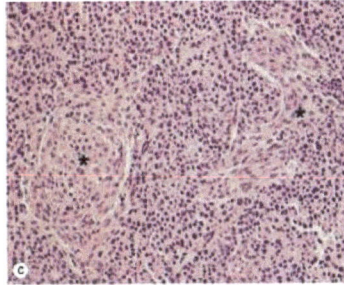

Fig. (4.42). Pancreatoblastoma surgical specimen (pancreaticoduodenectomy). Large solid mass (A) with clear margins with extensive involvement of the head of the pancreas and a central hemorrhagic area, at histopathology (B), prominent acinar differentiation is seen. Characteristic squamoid corpuscles (asterisks) are shown in (C) (From Malagò R, Capelli P, De Robertis R, *et al.* Rare neoplasms. In: D'Onofrio M, Capelli P, Pederzoli P, editors, imaging and Pathology of Pancreatic Neoplasms. New York: Springer; 2015; p. 397.

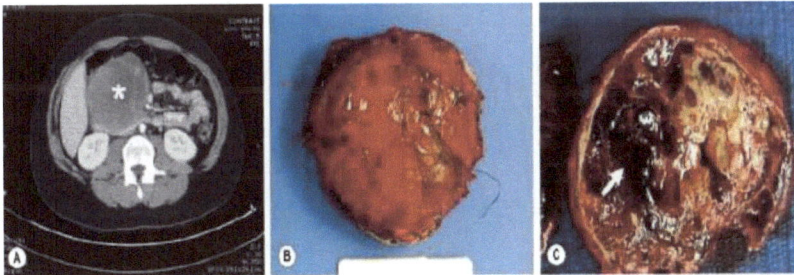

Fig. (4.43). this solid pseudopapillary tumor was found in a 14-year-old boy. **(A)** CT scan of the abdomen demonstrates a large, heterogeneous mass (asterisk) in the head of the pancreas. **(B)** The tumor is seen at excision. Note that the tumor appears encapsulated and well circumscribed. **(C)** Cut sec-tion of the mass demonstrates solid and cystic regions as well as an area of hemorrhagic necrosis (arrow). (From Speer AL, Barthel ER, Patel MM, *et al.* Solid pseudopapillary tumor of the pancreas: a single-institution 20-year series of pediatric patients. J Pediatr Surg 2012; 47:1217–122.

SPLENIC CONDITION

Embryology

A mesenchymal bulge in the dorsal mesogastrium between the stomach and the pancreas give rise to the splenic primordium. The spleen is associated with the production of WBCs and RBCs during fetal life although this production of WBCs and RBCs stops during later stages of gestation [105, 106].

Anatomy

The abdominal surface of the diaphragm separates the spleen from the lower left lung and pleura and the ninth to eleventh ribs. The visceral surface faces the abdominal cavity and contains gastric, colic, renal, and pancreatic impressions. Spleen size and weight vary with age. The average adult spleen is 7 to 11 cm in length and weighs 150 g (range, 70–250 g). The splenic artery give rise to segmental vessels, which divides into trabecular arteries. Their bifurcation give rise to small arteries enter the white pulp composed of lymphocytes and macrophages,, the red pulp destroys old and defective cells and it is consists of the endothelial cords of Billroth [106].

Physiology

The essential role of the spleen in the defense against bacterial organisms, is the immune response. As soon as antigen have contact with macrophages and helper T-cells, cytokine synthesis is initiated that activated T-cells and a humoral response is generated. The destruction of old and defective cells by the red pulp, Heinz bodies (denatured hemoglobin), and Pappenheimer bodies (iron granules) takes place in spleen which is a biological filter and a reservoir for platelets and factor VIII [106, 107].

ANATOMIC ABNORMALITIES

Asplenia and Polysplenia

Wandering spleen, it is mobile spleen.

Due to lack of ligamentous attachments to the diaphragm, colon, and retroperitoneum, splenic ligaments from the dorsal mesentery fails to develop. Children with an abdominal mass, episodic pain, torsion and infarction may be presented, requiring splenectomy [108, 109]. This condition can be treated by Splenopexy [110]. The use of an absorbable or nonabsorbable mesh with fixation in the left upper quadrant and placement of spleen in an extraperitoneal pocket is seen in Fig. (**4.44** and **4.45**) respectively [111].

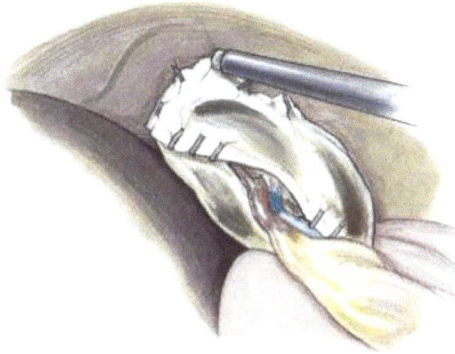

Fig. (4.44). Laparoscopic splenopexy.

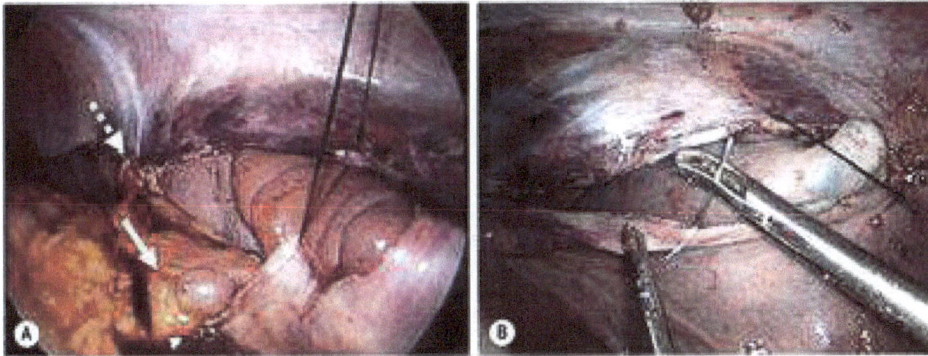

Fig. (4.45). (A) Spleen placement in the retroperitoneal pouch closed with interrupted sutures. Opening left in the pouch prevents the vessels from compressing on the closure of the pouch. (B) Interrupted silk sutures placement to approximate the peritoneal flaps over the spleen.

Accessory Spleens

These originate from mesenchymal remnants on its failure to fuse with the main splenic mass in 15–30% of children. Splenic hilum is the place where most of these are located as shown in Fig. (4.46). In almost 86% of the cases, these occur singly, 10% have two and 2-3% have three or more (112). An un-attended spleen at the time of total splenectomy may give rise to the recurrence of the primary disease process [113].

Splenic Gonadal Fusion

An early fusion between the left gonad and the spleen, prior to descent of the testis lead to their attachment [114].

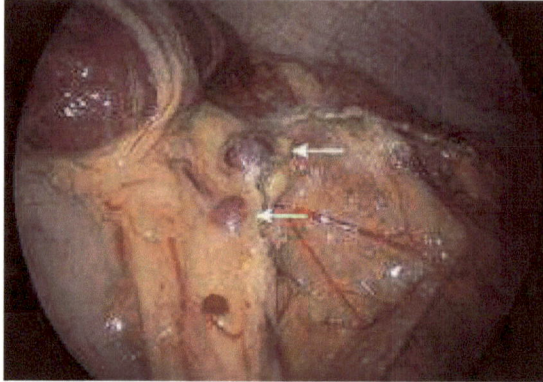

Fig. (4.46). In this child undergoing a laparoscopic splenectomy, two accessory spleens (arrows) are seen near the inferior edge of the spleen.

Splenic Cysts

Are divided into true cysts lined by epithelium and pseudocysts, (Fig. **4.47**). Are most frequently primary, true nonparasitic cysts, thought to be congenital and benignmosttrue parasitic cysts are due to Echinococcus. Pseudocysts are Post-traumatic occasionally seen [115]. Inclusion of surface mesothelium into the splenic parenchym could be the possible cause of origin of epithelial cysts. Patients may present with symptoms related to their size with gastric compression or pain, an abdominal mass, rupture, or infection with an abscess, early satiety, and back and shoulder pain. The diagnosis is best made with CT scan. Usually these cysts are larger than 8 cm and require treatment. A recent study showed percutaneous aspiration and sclerosis with alcohol caused disappearance in 20% of patients and 67% had symptom resolution with cysts larger than 5 cm [116]. Marsupialization and laparoscopic partial excision is the remedy but both of these may give rise to the recurrence if not removed properly [117]

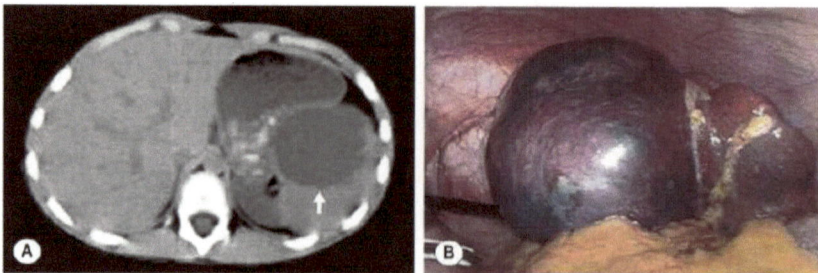

Fig. (4.47). (A) A large epithelial splenic cyst (arrow) is seen on the CT scan. (B) At laparoscopy, the large cyst (seen in [A]) is seen to occupy most of the spleen.

INDICATIONS FOR SPLENECTOMY

Hereditary Spherocytosis

This autosomal dominant condition is the inherited red cell disorder Northern European descendants. 25% of the affected children may represent new mutations, defects in red cell proteins ankyrin or spectrin that may lead to poorly deformable spherocytes. The children undergoing this disease may show symptoms like anemia, high reticulocyte count, and a mild elevation in bilirubin. The diagnosis is confirmed by the positive osmotic fragility test. The children undergoing this disease may show an aplastic crisis with parvovirus B19 infection giving rise to diminished production of the bone marrow red cell [118].

Moderate-to-severe anemia may give rise to the need of Splenectomy, but it can be delayed until the age of 5-6 years to prevent the risks of overwhelming postsplenectomy infection (OPSI). Splenomegaly is common in these patients. Gallstones are often found. Before the splenectomy is conducted, an ultrasound (US) of the gallbladder is critically evaluated. Instead of total splenectomy, Partial splenectomy should be performed to remove enough spleen to treat the anemia. This also preserves spleen and prevent OPSI [119].

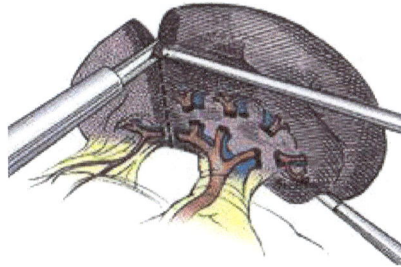

Fig. (4.48). Laparoscopic partial splenectomy

Immune Thrombocytopenic Purpura

ITP occurs when antiplatelet autoantibodies, usually IgG, bind with platelets, leading to destruction in the reticuloendothelial system. Treatment options include corticosteroids, which may function by inhibiting the reticuloendothelial binding of platelet-antibody complexes; intravenous immunoglobulin (IVIG), which competitively inhibits the Fc receptor binding of platelets by macrophages; use of Rho (D) immunoglobulin in Rh-positive children, which binds to red cells that then saturate the splenic capacity and spares the antibody-coated platelets; and splenectomy. Response to corticosteroids, IVIG, or both predicts response (97%) to splenectomy, whereas failure to respond to either predicts a 70% failure rate to splenectomy. Others have noted the response to IVIG to be a better predictor of response to splenectomy than corticosteroids. Childhood ITP is usually a self-limited, acute disorder, and splenectomy is only required in chronic cases [120].

Sickle Cell Disease

Elongated crescent-shaped erythrocytes are unable to deform within the microvasculature, resulting in thromboses and microinfarctions. Although most patients with sickle cell disease are autosplenectomized, some require splenectomy for acute sequestration crisis and hypersplenism.

Thalassemia

Are autosomal dominant defects in hemoglobin synthesis that result in hemolytic anemia, major (β-thalassemia) may cause anemia. Splenomegaly may lead to decrease in the RBC sequestration, such cases may require the need for transfusion. The possible solution is Total or partial splenectomy.

Gaucher Disease

This is associated with the excessive glucocerebroside in the macrophages of the spleen, liver, bone marrow, and lungs. This may give rise to severe splenomegaly and possibly both partial and total splenectomy may be required to solve the defect. This may avoid the destruction of red blood cells, leukocytes, and platelets [121].

SPLENECTOMY

Open Splenectomy

The massive splenomegaly when conducted in case of emergency may require left upper quadrant incision. This intial division of the splenorenal, splenocolic, and splenophrenic ligaments may lead the spleen to mobilise out of the abdominal cavity, through the left upper quadrant. Firstly, short gastric vessels and then the hilar vessels are divided. The accessory spleens is searched very carefully. A lateral muscle-splitting approach is very helpful in this regard [119 - 122].

Laparoscopic Splenectomy

The preferred approach for elective splenectomy due to less pain, shorter hospitalization, faster return to regular activities, and smaller incisions are better than open splenectomy. Splenectomy may require a long time in applying and its performing may not be easy in patients with splenomegaly, is usually not a cable for traumatic splenic injuries because children who require operation are usually unstable and hence require rapid control of bleeding . The basic concern is that the laparoscopic approach is correlated with the accessory spleen detection [122, 123].

Operation

A lateral approach is adopted by the surgeons across the globe for laparoscopy. This may require slight elevation of the left flank. The procedure may require an initial elevation of the left side and then is tilted to the patient's right side as shown in Fig. (**4.49**). While standing on the patient's right side, the surgeon with the help of assistant place incisions with several configuration. The upper midline instruments (3 mm) can be inserted without cannulas if the patient has small spleen or it is young child. The surgeon need to have the camera (5 mm, 30–45° telescope) in the left hand and the energy source in the right hand while doing this procedure. Initially, there is a division of splenocolic ligament, thus the splenic flexure falls away from the spleen. The inferior portion of the gastrosplenic ligament, and then short gastric vessels are divided while opening the lesser sac. An utmost care is required regarding the superior short gastric vessels as any injury to this may harm the stomach or diaphragm. The presence of accessory spleen is the next step for which the lesser sac is investigated. The splenophrenic ligament is divided to fully mobilize the upper pole, at this point, the hilum can be approached and a decision must be made to either staple across all the vessels or divide each individually with an energy device, if a stapler is utilized, it is often easiest to divide the splenorenal ligament to allow easy access to the entire hilum. Proximity of the hilum and pancreas is the main issue in terms of positioning the stapler, so may be occur Pancreatitis and pancreatic fistula, our current practice is to individually ligate secondary vessels distal to the pancreas (*i. e.* , secondary dissection) in adults to decrease splenic fever and pancreatic leakage, this technique has been advocated in adults to decrease splenic fever and pancreatic leakage.

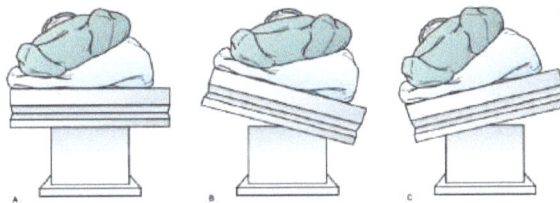

Fig. (4.49). *(A) initial positioning of the patient (B) The table has been tilted to the patient's left to achive the supine position of the patient. (C) The table is then rotated back to the patient's right to achieve a right lateral decubitus position* (Reprinted with permission.) The EnSeal and LigaSure have limited lateral thermal spread (<2 mm) and are relatively easy to use for dissection and ligation of the hilar vessels, The Endo Catch II (Covidien, Norwalk, CT) can be inserted through a 15-mm umbilical port with the telescope moved to one of the smaller ports. If a 12-mm port has been placed in the umbilicus, it can be removed and the bag can be introduced directly into the abdominal cavity.

Single-incision Laparoscopic Surgery and Single-incision Laparoendoscopic Surgery Splenectomy

In adults, preoperatively, patients appear to be primarily concerned with the safety of the surgery [127]. SILS/SIPES techniques may improve cosmesis by utilizing the umbilicus as a single-access site for surgery. Single-port access splenectomy has been reported utilizing either a multi-instrument port or separate umbilical fascial incisions after raising skin flaps [128].

Partial Splenectomy

Postsplenectomy infection has lead us to the concept of partial splenectomy that may result in the removal of 85–95% of the enlarged spleen and preserving almost 25% of the splenic size that is quite normal. The supply of the one or two short gastric vessels is also ensured to the remnant spleen in such cases. We prefer this technique for laparoscopic partial splenectomy. The spleen divided 1 cm onto the ischemic side to ensure lesser bleeding. We currently use cautery to divide the splenic parenchyma and then apply a topical hemostatic agent and omentum to the exposed parenchyma, the upper splenorenal and splenophrenic ligaments are left intact to avoid torsion. If there is no evidence of Howell–Jolly bodies on peripheral smear, and the numer of pitted red cells are also decreasing, it means splenic phagocytic function is preserved. Splenic regeneration happens in patient of all ages with any correlation with the hemolysis. Cholelithiasis may develop after partial splenectomy giving rise to the need of subsequent total splenectomy. A recent comparative study found that laparoscopic partial splenectomy patients had more pain and a longer hospitalization than those undergoing open partial splenectomy, we have also noted an increased hospitalization with laparoscopic partial splenectomy (2. 3 days) compared with an open operation (1. 2 days) [129].

COMPLICATIONS AND CONTROVERSIES ASSOCIATED WITH LAPAROSCOPIC SPLENECTOMY

Accessory Spleen Detection

Recently, laparoscopy has been shown to be better than preoperative CT for identification of accessory spleens. In reviewing several comparative pediatric series, accessory spleens were found in 20. 3% of patients undergoing an open splenectomy and 20. 2% at laparoscopy. Over 200 laparoscopic splenectomies indicated to a 19% accessory spleens. Laparoscopic removal of missed accessory spleens has shown a great success. Almost 26–75% cases reported that accessory splenectomy has improved the ITP ranges [123 - 130].

Conversion to Open Splenectomy

Bleeding and Splenomegaly may give rise to the need of conversion and have been reported in 1. 3–2. 8% of children. The obvious cause for this conversion is larger spleens, less surgeon experience, and obese patients [131].

OPERATIVE TIME

The laparoscopic approach may require more time in surgical procedure than open splenectomy [122].

COMPLICATIONS

An analysis of pediatric studies revealed that complication rate is 15. 5% and 26. 6% for laparoscopic and open splenectomy respectively, based on the data of surgeries conducted between 1991 and 2002. A few pulmonary, wound, and infectious complications were reported in cases of laparoscopy while more bleeding resulted due to this. . Symptomatic splenosis has been reported in ITP due to rupture of the endoscopic bag, with thrombocytopenia occurring 13 months after the initial laparoscopic splenectomy. Splenic vein or portal vein thrombosis though a rare complication may be common in patients of splenomegaly [132].

POSTSPLENECTOMY SEPSIS

May be fetal, the causative organism is likely Streptococcus pneumonia, Pneumococcus, Haemophilus influenza, meningococcus, and group A streptococcus. The latest researches has recommended a Routine immunization against *S. pneumoniae, H. influenzae*, and meningococcus, as well as postoperative antibiotic prophylaxis. There is no clear suggestions regarding the length of the antibiotic prophylaxis, but initial 2 years are very important with regard to the highest rate of OPSI. An adult study of sepsis in patients splenectomized as children noted an estimated frequency of late postsplenectomy infections of 0. 69 and deaths at 0. 46 per 1000 patient-years 134 of interest, one of the surviving patients had low antibody levels against pneumococcal serotypes despite pneumococcal meningitis and subsequent vaccinations, suggesting that non responders may be at increased risk for OPSI [133].

ABDOMINAL WALL DEFECTS

Gastroschisis

Gastroschisis occurs in 1 of 4000 live births [134]. An increased incidence in mothers younger than 21 years of age has been widely documented, although the reasons leading to the rising numbers are unclear [135]. The occurrence of gastroschisis in all maternal age groups has been increased in the past 10 to 20 years [136], giving rise to preterm delivery in such infants. It is also more prevalent 28% as compared to only 6% without abdominal wall defect [137]. The fourth week of gestation is the time when this wall is formed as a result of differential growth of the embryo leading to infolding in the craniocaudal and mediolateral directions. The 6th gestation week is the time when the rapid intestinal and liver growth leads to herniation of the midgut into the umbilical cord. The ensuing 4 weeks results in the elongation and rotation of the midgut. By the 10th gestation week, it returns to the abdominal cavity, where the first, second, and third portions of the duodenum and the ascending and descending colon assume their fixed, retroperitoneal positions. At the most basic level, an abdominal wall defect involves an interruption of these embryologic processes and results in abnormal development. Another theory advocates that possible failure of the mesoderm to form in the anterior abdominal wall may cause gastroschisis. Fig. (**4.50**) shows the difference between an omphalocele and gastroschisis.

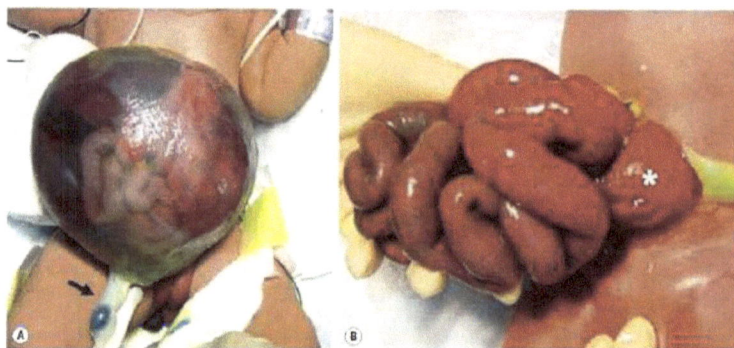

Fig. (4.50). The difference between an omphalocele and gastroschisis. (A) In an omphalocele both the liver and bowel may be herniated, a sac is present with an umbilical cord (arrow) inserts onto the sac. (B) With a gastroschisis, noherniation of the liver is present and a sac is absent.

Currently, The ventral body folds' theory that advocates the development of gastroschisis early in the gestation is the most accepted theory and before an omphalocele might develop. the size of the defect is usually<4 cm and it is located at the junction of the umbilicus and normal skin, and is almost always to the right of the umbilicus. A number of possible causative factors, including tobacco, certain environmental exposures (nitrosamines), cyclooxygenase inhibitor use (aspirin and ibuprofen), and decongestants (pseudoephedrine and phenylpropanolamine), have been suggested as etiologic agents [138 - 141]. The well-known association of lower maternal age and low socioeconomic status with a higher incidence of gastroschisis has been linked with violence against women during gestation as a potential factor.

PRESENTATION AND DIAGNOSIS

Sonography especially during the 20 weeks' of gestation may indicate the complications in pregnancy caused by gastroschisis [142-144]. Routine ultrasonography (US) often suggests the abnormality that is confirmed on a higher level US [143], Fig. (**4.51**). An abnormal maternal serum α-fetoprotein (AFP) level may give rise to the need of US. The elevated AFP level is accepted to be the cause of gastroschisis [142 - 144]. If bowel loops freely floating in the amniotic fluid are detected or there is a possible defect in the abdominal wall to the right of a normal umbilical cord, these are diagnostic for gastroschisis. Intrauterine growth restriction (IUGR) has been noted in a large number of these fetuses. Some fetuses with gastroschisis are not diagnosed prenatally and are discovered at the time of delivery, which can result in challenges with neonatal management. These neonates must be transferred to a center with the ability to care for gastroschisis.

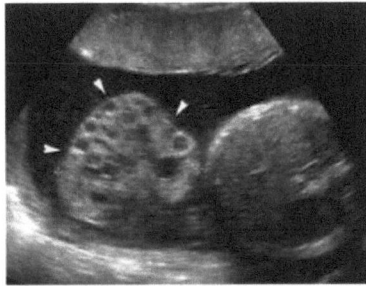

Fig. (4.51). Prenatal ultrasound of a 30-week gestation age fetus with a gastroschisis. Arrows point to the bowel outside within the amniotic fluid.

PRENATAL MANAGEMENT AND DELIVERY

The ideal prenatal test would be able to accurately differentiate gastroschisis fetuses at risk for complications such as intestinal loss or closing defects. Despite extensive use of US in fetal gastroschisis and the identification of multiple potential predictors of an adverse outcome (such as complex gastroschisis), there is no consensus on their use in selecting fetuses for early delivery [142 - 146]. Gastroschisis is associated with a variable degree of inflammatory thickening of the visceral bowel walls, which results in the characteristic appearance of "matted" intestinal loops. The reason for this inflammatory "peel" is unclear, but the presence of elevated levels of cytokines (interleukin-6 [IL-6], IL-8, tumor necrosis factor [TNF]-α) in the amniotic fluid, in addition to the effects of fetal urine, is thought to cause the abnormal collagen deposition [147 - 150]. One report noted a significant decrease in interstitial cells of Cajal (ICCs) in gastroschisis bowel in neonates compared with controls, further implicating the role of the proinflammatory state in utero [151, 152]. The possible mode and timing of delivery for a fetus with gastroschisis has been a matter of debate for many decades. The vaginal birth may lead to infection and sepsis, thus cesarean delivery (C-section) is recommended by its proponents [153].

POSTNATAL MANAGEMENT

Neonatal Resuscitation

Open abdominal cavity and exposed bowel lead to significant evaporative water loss in neonates with gastroschisis. Intravenous access is thus required for fluid resuscitation in the range of 160 to 190 cc/kg per day. Nasogastric (NG) decompression is important to prevent further gastric and intestinal distention. Routine endotracheal intubation is not necessary. Warm saline-soaked gauze wrapping may be required and placed in a central position on the abdominal wall. Kinking of the mesentery may result into bowel ischemia, and this should be prevented by positioning the neonate on the right side. The infant may also be wrapped into a plastic bag to prevent the evaporative loss and maintain the homeostasis as shown in Fig. (**4.52**). An excess fluid resuscitation may sometimes be harmful causing edema and abdominal compartment syndrome [136, 154]. Most of the time, infants with gastroschisis may have Concomitant bowel atresia.

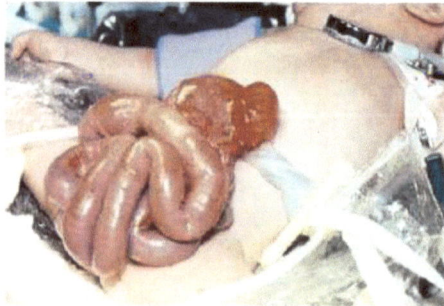

Fig. (4.52). Image showing an infant with gastroschisis wrapped and transported with a bowel bag. The untied bag allows inspection of the herniated bowel [156 - 162].

RISK STRATIFICATION

The literature revealed that infants born with gastroschisis rarely exhibited cardiac, pulmonary, nervous, musculoskeletal, genitourinary or chromosomal anomalies [140, 155]. Over the course of the last two decades, realization that there was a subset of gastroschisis neonates that were at higher risk for morbidity and mortality has led to the development of risk stratification [156 - 158]. This risk was based on the presence or absence of any intestinal complication (atresia, ischemia, perforation, or development of necrotizing enterocolitis [NEC]) and could be classified as complex or simple gastroschisis. Patients with complex defects have a higher mortality rate, require multiple operative interventions, and have a prolonged hospitalization, increased rates of sepsis, and higher rates of prolonged cholestasis and need for intestinal transplantation due to intestinal failure.

SURGICAL MANAGEMENT

The major goal is to return the viscera to the abdominal cavity expeditiously while minimizing the risk of damage due to intestinal injury or increased intra-abdominal pressure. The two main treatment options are primary repair and delayed closure with use of a temporary silo and serial reduction [135]. Obstructing bands, perforation, or atresia should require the inspection of the bowl in all cases. The subsequent intestinal obstruction can be avoided by lysing the bands crossing the bowl loops before silo placement or primary closure. The choice of which course to undertake is dependent on the presentation of the bowel, as well as surgeon and institution preferences, and is both variable and controversial [163, 164]. During reduction, the bladder or stomach pressure is the key in measuring the Intra-abdominal pressure and guiding the surgeon. A pressure higher than 10–15 mmHg may lead to decreased renal and intestinal perfusion, thus arising a need for a silo or patch, whereas above 20 mmHg they correlate with organ dysfunction and complications. There may need for silo placement or patch closure if the central venous pressure is greater than 4 mmHg. Reduction is also correlated with splanchnic perfusion pressure, the difference between mean arterial pressure and intra-abdominal pressure. If the splanchnic perfusion is below 44 mmHg implies a decrease in the blood flow. Urgent primary closure of gastroschisis was advocated in all cases, and in the situation in which this was not possible, the neonate would not survive. Definitive closure in the operating room is similar to that for primary closure with the choices for sutureless *versus* skin *versus* fascial closure; again, prospective trials and systematic reviews would suggest that sutureless repair is associated with a longer hospital stay. There has been recent success with the utilization of nonsurgical closure of gastroschisis. In this technique, the umbilical cord is placed over the defect, which is then covered with a transparent occlusive dressing. Over the ensuing days, the cord provides a tissue barrier, and the defect spontaneously closes. This approach allows for nonsurgical coverage in a majority of cases of gastroschisis, even in the setting of very large openings. Questions remain regarding the long-term presence of umbilical hernias in these children and the total hospitalization.

CLOSING GASTROSCHISIS

An intestinal atresia should be differentiated from "vanishing bowel" in infants with gastroschisis. A "closing gastroschisis" is when the defect size decreases prior to delivery (Fig. **4-53**) [165]. As the hole gets smaller, the blood supply to the viscera progressively diminishes and can result in an atresia. In extreme cases, the intestine outside the abdominal cavity completely disappears and results in congenital short bowel syndrome. There is no prenatal US finding that can reliably distinguish this condition. However, intra-abdominal bowel distention or dilation can occur, which can help in deciding to deliver early in some patients [146].

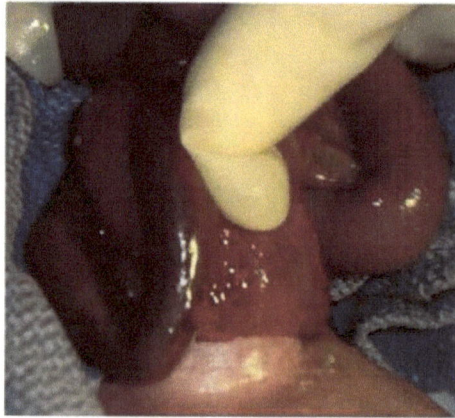

Fig. (4.53). Closing gastroschisis. In this infant, the defect is "closing" around the root of the small bowel mesentery and a finger cannot be introduced into the defect. This could potentially lead to vascular compromise of a significant length of bowel with necrosis and perforation. Note the edematous mesentery (Image courtesy Drs. PramodPuligandla and Jean-Martin Laberge).

POSTOPERATIVE COURSE

In cases in which primary closure has been performed, care must be directed to ensure there are no effects from increased abdominal pressure. These effects may range from perturbations in ventilation, renal function, and gastrointestinal ischemia. If an abdominal compartment syndrome is suspected, prompt laparotomy and silo placement should be performed. Gastroschisis" is when the defect size decreases prior to delivery. As the hole gets smaller, the blood supply to the viscera progressively diminishes and can result in an atresia. In extreme cases, the intestine outside the abdominal cavity completely disappears and results in congenital short bowel syndrome. There is no prenatal US finding that can reliably distinguish this condition. Gastroschisis is associated with abnormal intestinal motility and nutrient absorption, both of which gradually improve in most patients. Introduction of enteral feeding is often delayed for weeks while awaiting return of bowel function. The exact cause of the prolonged dysmotility is poorly understood but may be linked to the diminished number of ICCs in the intestine and the degree of peel. This waiting period may require nasogastric decompression and parenteral nutrition and after the beginning of the bowel activity, enteral feeds is suggested. Because progression to full enteral feeding can take weeks, central venous access is important. Due to risk of losing sucking reflex, Early oral stimulation is advised. A systematic review attempted to address the issue of early enteral feeding on outcomes and found that when feeds were initiated within 7 days of life or closure, there was an earlier attainment of full feeds, and each day delay in starting the feedings was associated with a 1. 4-day delay in attainment of full feeds. This study was unable to fully ascertain the effect of early feeding as the data were all retrospective and had confounding variables. Prokinetic medication may be helpful in the postoperative period. In a rabbit model of gastroschisis, the intestine contractility was enhanced with the help of cisapride, while erythromycin was helpful in improving motility in adult tissue only. However, a randomized controlled trial of erythromycin *versus* placebo found that enterally administered erythromycin did not improve time to full enteral feedings. Postoperative NEC has been found in full-term infants with gastroschisis in higher than expected frequencies (up to 18. 5%). Significant bowel loss from NEC can predispose to short bowel syndrome and its associated hepatic and infectious complications. On the other hand, another group found that the clinical course of babies with gastroschisis who developed NEC often followed an uncomplicated course. There are reports suggesting that infants with gastroschisis who were fed breast milk had a lower incidence of NEC than those who were fed formula.

LONG-TERM OUTCOMES

The infants born with with gastroschisis are generally have excellent long term outcomes. However, the presence of complex disease is the most important prognostic determinant for a poor outcome [160, 167].

Table 4. 4. Differentiating Characteristics Between Gastroschisis and Omphalocele.

Characteristic	Omphalocele	Gastroschisis
Herniated viscera	Bowel ± liver	Bowel only
Sac	Present	Absent
Associated anomalies Location of defect	Common (50%)	Uncommon (<10%)
Mode of delivery	Umbilicus	Right of umbilicus
Surgical management	Vaginal/caesarean	Vaginal
Prognostic factors	Nonurgent	Urgent
	Associated anomalies	Condition of bowel

OMPHALOCELE

Incidence, Embryology and Etiology

The incidence of omphalocele seen at 14–18 weeks is as high as 1 in 1100, but the incidence at birth drops to 1 in 4000–6000 [168]. Omphalocele can vary from a small defect with intestinal contents to giant omphalocele in which the abdominal wall defect measures 4 cm or more in diameter and contains liver. Omphalocele occurs in association with special syndromes such as exstrophy of the cloaca (vesicointestinal fissure), the Beckwith-Wiedemann constellation of anomalies (macroglossia, macrosomia, hypoglycemia, and visceromegaly and omphalocele) and Cantrell's Pentalogy (lower thoracic wall malformations [cleft sternum], ectopiacordis, epigastric omphalocele, anterior midline diaphragmatic hernia and cardiac anomalies). There is a 60% to 70% incidence of associated anomalies, especially cardiac (20–40% of cases) and chromosomal abnormalities. The current understanding of the etiology for an omphalocele has revealed that this defect is not caused by the failure in body wall closure or migration, but due to the failure of the viscera to return to the abdominal cavity [169]. The sac consists of the covering layers of the umbilical cord and includes amnion, Wharton jelly, and peritoneum. This defect may possibly be located in the mid-abdominal or central region or sometime in the the epigastric or hypogastric regions as well.

Prenatal Diagnosis and Management

Elevation of maternal serum AFP is also present in many pregnancies complicated by omphalocele, although not as common as in gastroschisis. The diagnosis of omphalocele can be made by two-dimensional US at the time of the normal 18-week US evaluation for dates. Early first-trimester detection is possible if three-dimensional US is utilized [170]. US evaluation is very useful for the detection of associated anomalies in these infants. This is important as an isolated omphalocele has a survival rate of over 90%, but those with other defects (such as cardiac) are much less likely to survive [168, 171]. Prenatal US and karyotyping are able to identify only 60–70% of the associated defects that are found postnatally [172]. The route of delivery of infants with an omphalocele should be dictated by obstetric considerations as C-section has not been shown to be advantageous.

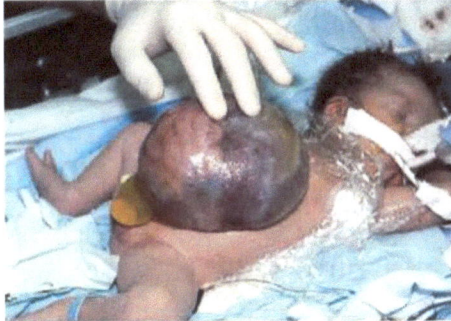

Fig. (4.54). This neonate was born with a large omphalocele. As is evident, the abdominal cavity is quite small. Primary closure is not possible in such a patient.

Neonatal Resuscitation and Management

After delivery, a thorough search for associated anomalies is important. All neonates should undergo an echocardiographic evaluation. Renal abnormalities should be assessed by abdominal US. Neonatal hypoglycemia can be associated with Beckwith–Weideman syndrome. Blood samples for genetic evaluation should be obtained as well. No pressure should be placed on the omphalocele sac in an effort to reduce its contents because this maneuver may increase the risk of rupture of the sac or may interfere with abdominal venous return. Prophylactic broad-spectrum antibiotics should be administered in case of rupture. The subsequent treatment and outcome is determined by the size of the omphalocele. In general terms, small to medium sized defects have a significantly better prognosis than extremely large defects in which the liver is present. In these cases, not only is the management of the abdominal wall defect a significant challenge, but these patients often have concomitant pulmonary insufficiency that can lead to significant morbidity and mortality. If possible, and if the pulmonary status will permit it, a primary repair of the omphalocele should be undertaken. In preparing infants with omphalocele for transport, risks arising from associated anomalies should be specifically addressed. Infants with an omphalocele do not have as significant fluid and temperature losses as those with gastroschisis, but these losses are still higher than those with an intact abdominal wall. The sac itself can be covered with saline-soaked gauze and an impervious dressing to minimize these losses. An NG tube should be inserted and placed to suction.

Surgical Management

There is currently no completely accepted technique to treat giant omphaloceles and two methods are used the most: staged closure and delayed closure.

Immediate Primary Closure Treatment options in infants with omphalocele depend on the size of the defect, the baby's gestational age, and the presence of associated anomalies. Defects that are less than 1. 5 cm in diameter are referred to as a hernia of the cord and are repaired shortly after birth if there are no major associated anomalies. The defects that are larger but still easy to close as they have minimal associated loss of abdominal domain also can be closed in the neonatal period. Primary closure consists of excision of the sac and closure of the fascia and skin over the abdominal contents. It is not unusual for an omphalomesenteric duct remnant to be associated with a small omphalocele. The intra-abdominal pressure can become elevated during reduction and repair, leading to abdominal compartment syndrome. Therefore, in larger defects, some surgeons will measure bladder pressure and have mesh available if primary closure is not feasible.

Staged Neonatal Closure In many cases, the loss of domain in the peritoneal cavity prevents primary closure without an undue increase in intra-abdominal pressure. Multiple methods have been proposed to obtain primary abdominal wall closure in these babies. Staged closure in the neonates may involve different techniques like serial inversion of the amnionic sac, excision of the sac and replacement with mesh and closed. Amnion inversion allows gradual reduction of the sac followed by sac excision and primary or mesh closure [173, 174].

Scarification Treatment In case the neonate has cardiac or respiratory problems or too large defect, the surgeon thinks that this cannot be corrected by a surgical repair, Nonoperative techniques is adopted that uses an agent for allowing an eschar grow over the intact amnion sac. Over the time, there is epithelialization of eschar, leaving a ventral hernia. The ventral hernia repair is performed using a variety of techniques: primary fascial closure, autologous repair with component separation, or mesh repair.

Large Ruptured Cmphalocele Is one of the most Ruptured Omphalocele challenging pediatric surgical conditions to manage. At birth, there is the urgent need to cover the exposed viscera like a gastroschisis (Fig. **4.55**). However, the abdominal wall configuration and the defect itself are usually not amenable for placing a spring-loaded silo. In addition, as opposed to gastroschisis, there is a much more substantial loss of intra-abdominal domain that makes gradual reduction of the viscera very difficult. The goal is to cover the exposed abdominal viscera, which can be challenging. One small series had good outcomes and result in survival despite high incidences of abnormalities like intestinal fistulas, sepsis, and pulmonary hypoplasia. In most cases, a silo will have to be fashioned by suturing to the abdominal wall and skin together. Despite the creation of a silo, the reduction is usually still not possible, and some surgeons have advocated the use of biologic mesh to create a bed for skin to grow over and be grafted. At that point, the delayed closure of the ventral hernia may be contemplated. Respiratory issues such as pulmonary hypoplasia may complicate the management.

Postoperative Course

After any type of neonatal repair, most patients will require mechanical ventilation for several days. Feeding may commence when bowel activity resumes. Antibiotics are administered postoperatively for only 24–48 hours unless there are concerns for a wound infection. If a ventral hernia develops, repair may be deferred for 1 year or later to allow stabilization and a natural increase in abdominal domain. The method used for closure (primary *vs* staged with delayed primary closure or mesh) has not been shown to affect length of hospitalization, likely because the patient numbers are very small and because patient selection plays a role [175]. Pulmonary hypoplasia and hypertension are associated with omphalocele, especially the large or giant varieties. Although the etiology of this complication is unclear, it may be related to disrupted thoracic development due to the abdominal wall defect, which leads to pulmonary hypoplasia.

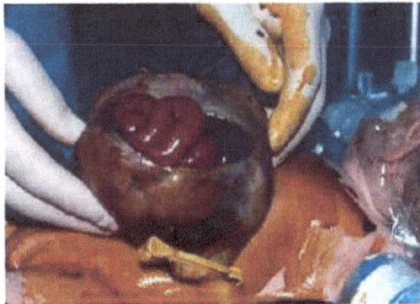

Fig. (4.55). This neonate was born with an omphalocele that ruptured during delivery. Thus, immediate management was needed. The sac was removed, and a silo was created.

Long-term Outcomes

For omphalocele patients are also closely dependent on the associated anomalies and conditions. Several long-term medical problems can develop in patients with large omphaloceles (Fig. **4.54**). These include gastroesophageal reflux disease (GERD), pulmonary insufficiency, recurrent lung infections or asthma, and feeding difficulty with failure to thrive [176]. The respiratory insufficiency associated with giant omphaloceles may be secondary to abnormal thoracic development, with a narrow thorax and small lung area leading to pulmonary hypoplasia. Also, it may be associated with poor intrauterine diaphragmatic motion and altered chest wall development. Prolonged respiratory difficulties can occur in up to 20% of infants with giant omphaloceles, leading to increased time of mechanical ventilation and the need for supplemental oxygen during the neonatal period. Some neonates may require a tracheostomy.

Umbilical Hernia

Umbilical hernia is a common disorder in children and is frequently evaluated and treated by pediatric and general surgeons. Unlike other hernias of childhood, a fascial defect is present at birth but may resolve without the need for an operation. There are multiple factors that affect the incidence or prevalence of umbilical hernia in the general population. These may include age, race, gestational age, and coexisting disorders. In the United States, umbilical hernias are present in 15–25% of newborns or approximately 800,000 children annually [177, 178].

Anatomy

After birth, closure of the umbilical ring is the result of complex interactions with the lateral body wall folding in a medial direction, fusion of the rectus abdominis muscles into the linea alba, and umbilical orifice contraction that is aided by elastic fibers from the obliterated umbilical arteries. Fibrous proliferation of the surrounding lateral connective tissue plates and mechanical stress from rectus muscle tension also may help with natural closure. Failure of these closure processes results in an umbilical hernia. The hernia sac is peritoneum and is usually very adherent to the dermis of the umbilical skin. The range of fascial defect's diameter is from several millimeters to 5 cm or more. Its size does not depend upon the extent of skin protrusion. Sometimes it may show large proboscis-like alarming protrusions (Fig. **4.56**) merely with small defects. The assessment of the actual fascial defect by palpation is important to know whether operative or nonoperative treatment is appropriate.

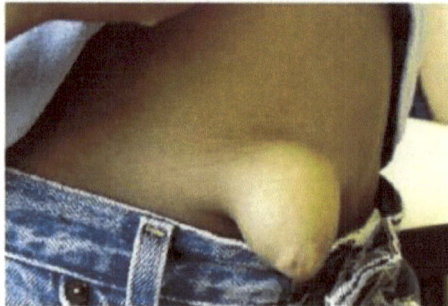

Fig. (4.56). This 5-year-old child showing a large proboscis-like umbilical hernia.

Treatment

For many years, it has been elaborated that there is spontaneous closure in cases of umbilical hernia in infants until ages of 4-5 years. Measures like Pressure dressings and other devices have not effect in its closure or reduction, neither these measures enhance the closure process. Instead they may result in skin irritation and breakdown. A number of studies have demonstrated spontaneous resolution rates of >90% of hernias by 1 year of age the primary danger associated with observation is the possibility of incarceration or strangulation. Studies have shown these complications to be quite rare, with an incidence less than 1%. Patients bearing small fascial defects ranging from 0. 5–1. 5 cm in diameter are more prone to incarceration.

CONSENT FOR PUBLICATION

Not applicable.

CONFLICT OF INTEREST

The author declares no conflict of interest, financial or otherwise.

ACKNOWLEDGEMENTS

Declared none.

REFERENCES

[1]   Pedersen R N, Garne E, Loane M, Korsholm L, Husby S. Infantile hypertrophic pyloric stenosis: a comparative study of incidence and other epidemiological characteristics in seven European regions. J Matern Fetal Neonatal Med 2008; 21(9): 599-604.
        [http://dx.doi.org/10. 1080/14767050802214824] [PMID: 18828050]

[2]   Sommerfield T, Chalmers J, Youngson G, Heeley C, Fleming M, Thomson G. The changing epidemiology of infantile hypertrophic pyloric stenosis in Scotland. Arch Dis Child 2008; 93(12): 1007-11.
        [http://dx.doi.org/10. 1136/adc. 2007. 128090] [PMID: 18285388]

[3]   Persson S, Ekbom A, Granath F, Nordenskjöld A. Parallel incidences of sudden infant death syndrome and infantile hypertrophic pyloric stenosis: a common cause? Pediatrics 2001; 108(4): E70.
        [http://dx.doi.org/10. 1542/peds. 108. 4. e70] [PMID: 11581478]

[4]   Schechter R, Torfs C P, Bateson T F. The epidemiology of infantile hypertrophic pyloric stenosis. Paediatr Perinat Epidemiol 1997; 11(4): 407-27.
        [http://dx.doi.org/10. 1046/j. 1365-3016. 1997. d01-32. x] [PMID: 9373863]

[5]   Honein M A, Paulozzi L J, Himelright I M, *et al.* Infantile hypertrophic pyloric stenosis after pertussis prophylaxis with erythromcyin: a case review and cohort study. Lancet 1999; 354(9196): 2101-5.
        [http://dx.doi.org/10. 1016/S0140-6736(99)10073-4] [PMID: 10609814]

[6]   Mitchell L E, Risch N. The genetics of infantile hypertrophic pyloric stenosis. A reanalysis. Am J Dis Child 1993; 147(11): 1203-11.
        [http://dx.doi.org/10. 1001/archpedi. 1993. 02160350077012] [PMID: 8237916]

[7]   Rasmussen L, Green A, Hansen L P. The epidemiology of infantile hypertrophic pyloric stenosis in a Danish population, 1950-84. Int J Epidemiol 1989; 18(2): 413-7.
        [http://dx.doi.org/10. 1093/ije/18. 2. 413] [PMID: 2767855]

[8]   Spitz L, Zail S S. Serum gastrin levels in congenital hypertrophic pyloric stenosis. J Pediatr Surg 1976; 11(1): 33-5.
       [http://dx.doi.org/10. 1016/0022-3468(76)90166-4] [PMID: 1245992]

[9]   Vanderwinden J M, Mailleux P, Schiffmann S N, Vanderhaeghen J J, De Laet M H. Nitric oxide synthase activity in infantile hypertrophic pyloric stenosis. N Engl J Med 1992; 327(8): 511-5.
       [http://dx.doi.org/10. 1056/NEJM199208203270802] [PMID: 1378938]

[10]   White M C, Langer J C, Don S, DeBaun M R. Sensitivity and cost minimization analysis of radiology *versus* olive palpation for the diagnosis of hypertrophic pyloric stenosis. J Pediatr Surg 1998; 33(6): 913-7.
       [http://dx.doi.org/10. 1016/S0022-3468(98)90673-X] [PMID: 9660228]

[11]   Breaux C W Jr, Georgeson K E, Royal S A, Curnow A J. Changing patterns in the diagnosis of hypertrophic pyloric stenosis. Pediatrics 1988; 81(2): 213-7.
       [PMID: 3277156]

[12]   Keller H, Waldmann D, Greiner P. Comparison of preoperative sonography with intraoperative findings in congenital hypertrophic pyloric stenosis. J Pediatr Surg 1987; 22(10): 950-2.
       [http://dx.doi.org/10. 1016/S0022-3468(87)80598-5] [PMID: 3316593]

[13]   Lamki N, Athey P A, Round M E, Watson A B Jr, Pfleger M J. Hypertrophic pyloric stenosis in the neonate--diagnostic criteria revisited. Can Assoc Radiol J 1993; 44(1): 21-4.
       [PMID: 8425150]

[14]   Malcom G E III, Raio C C, Del Rios M, Blaivas M, Tsung J W. Feasibility of emergency physician diagnosis of hypertrophic pyloric stenosis using point-of-care ultrasound: a multi-center case series. J Emerg Med 2009; 37(3): 283-6.
       [http://dx.doi.org/10. 1016/j. jemermed. 2007. 11. 053] [PMID: 18572347]

[15]   Boneti C, McVay M R, Kokoska E R, Jackson R J, Smith S D. Ultrasound as a diagnostic tool used by surgeons in pyloric stenosis. J Pediatr Surg 2008; 43(1): 87-91.
       [http://dx.doi.org/10. 1016/j. jpedsurg. 2007. 09. 027] [PMID: 18206462]

[16]   Meissner P E, Engelmann G, Troeger J, Linderkamp O, Nuetzenadel W. Conservative treatment of infantile hypertrophic pyloric stenosis with intravenous atropine sulfate does not replace pyloromyotomy. Pediatr Surg Int 2006; 22(12): 1021-4.
       [http://dx.doi.org/10. 1007/s00383-006-1751-3] [PMID: 17021743]

[17]   Kawahara H, Takama Y, Yoshida H, *et al.* Medical treatment of infantile hypertrophic pyloric stenosis: should we always slice the "olive"? J Pediatr Surg 2005; 40(12): 1848-51.
       [http://dx.doi.org/10. 1016/j. jpedsurg. 2005. 08. 025] [PMID: 16338303]

[18]   Kawahara H, Imura K, Nishikawa M, Yagi M, Kubota A. Intravenous atropine treatment in infantile hypertrophic pyloric stenosis. Arch Dis Child 2002; 87(1): 71-4.
       [http://dx.doi.org/10. 1136/adc. 87. 1. 71] [PMID: 12089130]

[19]   Ogawa Y, Higashimoto Y, Nishijima E, *et al.* Successful endoscopic balloon dilatation for hypertrophic pyloric stenosis. J Pediatr Surg 1996; 31(12): 1712-4.
       [http://dx.doi.org/10. 1016/S0022-3468(96)90059-7] [PMID: 8986998]

[20]   Yusuf T E, Brugge W R. Endoscopic therapy of benign pyloric stenosis and gastric outlet obstruction. Curr Opin Gastroenterol 2006; 22(5): 570-3.
       [http://dx.doi.org/10. 1097/01. mog. 0000239874. 13867. 41] [PMID: 16891891]

[21]   Wu S-F, Lin H-Y, Huang F-K, *et al.* Efficacy of medical treatment for infantile hypertrophic pyloric stenosis: a meta-analysis. Pediatr Neonatol 2016; 57(6): 515-21.
       [http://dx.doi.org/10. 1016/j. pedneo. 2016. 02. 005] [PMID: 27215474]

[22]   Dalton B G, Gonzalez K W, Boda S R, Thomas P G, Sherman A K, St Peter S D. Optimizing fluid resuscitation in hypertrophic pyloric stenosis. J Pediatr Surg 2016; 51(8): 1279-82.
       [http://dx.doi.org/10. 1016/j. jpedsurg. 2016. 01. 013] [PMID: 26876090]

[23] Adibe O O, Nichol P F, Lim F Y, Mattei P. Ad libitum feeds after laparoscopic pyloromyotomy: a retrospective comparison with a standardized feeding regimen in 227 infants. J Laparoendosc Adv Surg Tech A 2007; 17(2): 235-7.
[http://dx.doi.org/10. 1089/lap. 2006. 0143] [PMID: 17484656]

[24] Lee S L, Sydorak R M, Lau S T. Air insufflation of the stomach f ing laparoscopic pyloromyotomy may not detect perforation. J Pediatr Surg 2009; 44: 1631-7.

[25] Georgeson K E, Corbin T J, Griffen J W, Breaux C W Jr. An analysis of feeding regimens after pyloromyotomy for hypertrophic pyloric stenosis. J Pediatr Surg 1993; 28(11): 1478-80.
[http://dx.doi.org/10. 1016/0022-3468(93)90435-N] [PMID: 8301463]

[26] Sullivan K J, Chan E, Vincent J, Iqbal M, Wayne C, Nasr A. Feeding post-pyloromyotomy: a meta-analysis. Pediatrics 2016; 137(1): e20152550.
[http://dx.doi.org/10. 1542/peds. 2015-2550] [PMID: 26719292]

[27] Markel T A, Scott M R, Stokes S M, Ladd A P. A randomized trial to assess advancement of enteral feedings following surgery for hypertrophic pyloric stenosis. J Pediatr Surg 2017; 52(4): 534-9.
[http://dx.doi.org/10. 1016/j. jpedsurg. 2016. 09. 069] [PMID: 27829521]

[28] St Peter S D, Tsao K, Sharp S W, Holcomb G W III, Ostlie D J. Predictors of emesis and time to goal intake after pyloromyotomy: analysis from a prospective trial. J Pediatr Surg 2008; 43(11): 2038-41.
[http://dx.doi.org/10. 1016/j. jpedsurg. 2008. 04. 008] [PMID: 18970937]

[29] Kimura K, Loening-Baucke V. Bilious vomiting in the newborn: rapid diagnosis of intestinal obstruction. Am Fam Physician 2000; 61(9): 2791-8.
[PMID: 10821158]

[30] Mustafawi A R, Hassan M E. Congenital duodenal obstruction in children: a decade's experience. Eur J Pediatr Surg 2008; 18(2): 93-7.
[http://dx.doi.org/10. 1055/s-2008-1038478] [PMID: 18437652]

[31] Stiefel D, Stallmach T, Sacher P. Acute appendicitis in neonates: complication or morbus sui generis? Pediatr Surg Int 1998; 14(1-2): 122-3.
[http://dx.doi.org/10. 1007/s003830050457] [PMID: 9880719]

[32] Coughlin J P, Gauderer M W, Stern R C, Doershuk C F, Izant R J Jr, Zollinger R M Jr. The spectrum of appendiceal disease in cystic fibrosis. J Pediatr Surg 1990; 25(8): 835-9.
[http://dx.doi.org/10. 1016/0022-3468(90)90186-D] [PMID: 2205712]

[33] Kwan K Y, Nager A L. Diagnosing pediatric appendicitis: usefulness of laboratory markers. Am J Emerg Med 2010; 28(9): 1009-15.
[http://dx.doi.org/10. 1016/j. ajem. 2009. 06. 004] [PMID: 20825931]

[34] Choi D, Park H, Lee Y R, *et al.* The most useful findings for diagnosing acute appendicitis on contrast-enhanced helical CT. Acta Radiol 2003; 44(6): 574-82.
[http://dx.doi.org/10. 1080/02841850312331287819] [PMID: 14616200]

[35] Cappendijk V C, Hazebroek F W. The impact of diagnostic delay on the course of acute appendicitis. Arch Dis Child 2000; 83(1): 64-6.
[http://dx.doi.org/10. 1136/adc. 83. 1. 64] [PMID: 10869003]

[36] Results of the North American trial of piperacillin/tazobactam compared with clindamycin and gentamicin in the treatment of severe intra-abdominal infections. Eur J Surg Suppl 1994; 573(573): 61-6.
[PMID: 7524798]

[37] Styrud J, Eriksson S, Nilsson I, *et al.* Appendectomy *versus* antibiotic treatment in acute appendicitis. a prospective multicenter randomized controlled trial. World J Surg 2006; 30(6): 1033-7.
[http://dx.doi.org/10. 1007/s00268-005-0304-6] [PMID: 16736333]

[38] Raveenthiran V. Knowledge of ancient Hindu surgeons on Hirschsprung disease: evidence from

Sushruta Samhita of circa 1200-600 BC. J Pediatr Surg 2011; 46(11): 2204-8.
[http://dx.doi.org/10. 1016/j. jpedsurg. 2011. 07. 007] [PMID: 22075360]

[39]   Smith G H H, Cass D. Infantile Hirschsprung's disease—is barium enema useful? Pediatr Surg Int
       1991; 6: 318-21.
       [http://dx.doi.org/10. 1007/BF00178647]

[40]   Georgeson K E, Fuenfer M M, Hardin W D. Primary laparoscopic pull-through for Hirschsprung's
       disease in infants and children. J Pediatr Surg 1995; 30(7): 1017-21.
       [http://dx.doi.org/10. 1016/0022-3468(95)90333-X] [PMID: 7472924]

[41]   Marty T L, Matlak M E, Hendrickson M, Black R E, Johnson D G. Unexpected death from
       enterocolitis after surgery for Hirschsprung's disease. Pediatrics 1995; 96(1 Pt 1): 118-21.
       [PMID: 7596698]

[42]   Huppertz H I, Soriano-Gabarró M, Grimprel E, *et al.* Intussusception among young children in
       Europe. Pediatr Infect Dis J 2006; 25(1) (Suppl.): S22-9.
       [http://dx.doi.org/10. 1097/01. inf. 0000197713. 32880. 46] [PMID: 16397426]

[43]   Stringer M D, Pablot S M, Brereton R J. Paediatric intussusception. Br J Surg 1992; 79(9): 867-76.
       [http://dx.doi.org/10. 1002/bjs. 1800790906] [PMID: 1422744]

[44]   Weihmiller S N, Buonomo C, Bachur R. Risk stratification of children being evaluated for
       intussusception. Pediatrics 2011; 127(2): e296-303.
       [http://dx.doi.org/10. 1542/peds. 2010-2432] [PMID: 21242220]

[45]   Daneman A, Navarro O. Intussusception. Part 1: a review of diagnostic approaches. Pediatr Radiol
       2003; 33(2): 79-85.
       [http://dx.doi.org/10. 1007/s00247-002-0832-2] [PMID: 12557062]

[46]   Mirza B. Recurrent intussusception: management options. APSP J Case Rep 2011; 2(1): 9.
       [PMID: 22953276]

[47]   Bai Y Z, Chen H, Wang W L. A special type of postoperative intussusception: ileoileal intussusception
       after surgical reduction of ileocolic intussusception in infants and children. J Pediatr Surg 2009; 44(4):
       755-8.
       [http://dx.doi.org/10. 1016/j. jpedsurg. 2008. 08. 011] [PMID: 19361636]

[48]   Kluth D, Jaeschke-Melli S, Fiegel H. The embryology of gut rotation. Semin Pediatr Surg 2003; 12(4):
       275-9.
       [http://dx.doi.org/10. 1053/j. sempedsurg. 2003. 08. 009] [PMID: 14655167]

[49]   Stewart D R, Colodny A L, Daggett W C. Malrotation of the bowel in infants and children: a 15 year
       review. Surgery 1976; 79(6): 716-20.
       [PMID: 1273757]

[50]   Brenner E C. Congenital defects of the anus and rectum. Surg Gynecol Obstet 1915; 20: 579-88.

[51]   Levitt M A, Peña A. Anorectal Malformations http://www. OJRD. com/content/2/1/33

[52]   Stoll C, Alembik Y, Dott B, Roth M P. Associated malformations in patients with anorectal anomalies.
       Eur J Med Genet 2007; 50(4): 281-90.
       [http://dx.doi.org/10. 1016/j. ejmg. 2007. 04. 002] [PMID: 17572165]

[53]   Levitt M A, Kant A, Peña A. The morbidity of constipation in patients with anorectal malformations. J
       Pediatr Surg 2010; 45(6): 1228-33.
       [http://dx.doi.org/10. 1016/j. jpedsurg. 2010. 02. 096] [PMID: 20620325]

[54]   Nio M, Ohi R, Miyano T, Saeki M, Shiraki K, Tanaka K. Five- and 10-year survival rates after surgery
       for biliary atresia: a report from the Japanese Biliary Atresia Registry. J Pediatr Surg 2003; 38(7): 997-
       1000.
       [http://dx.doi.org/10. 1016/S0022-3468(03)00178-7] [PMID: 12861525]

[55]   Chandra R S. Biliary atresia and other structural anomalies in the congenital polysplenia syndrome. J

Pediatr 1974; 85(5): 649-55.
[http://dx.doi.org/10. 1016/S0022-3476(74)80508-1] [PMID: 4472512]

[56]   Davenport M, Savage M, Mowat A P, Howard E R. Biliary atresia splenic malformation syndrome: an etiologic and prognostic subgroup. Surgery 1993; 113(6): 662-8.
[PMID: 8506525]

[57]   Tan C E, Driver M, Howard E R, Moscoso G J. Extrahepatic biliary atresia: a first-trimester event? Clues from light microscopy and immunohistochemistry. J Pediatr Surg 1994; 29(6): 808-14.
[http://dx.doi.org/10. 1016/0022-3468(94)90377-8] [PMID: 7521396]

[58]   Tyler K L, Sokol R J, Oberhaus S M, *et al.* Detection of reovirus RNA in hepatobiliary tissues from patients with extrahepatic biliary atresia and choledochal cysts. Hepatology 1998; 27(6): 1475-82.
[http://dx.doi.org/10. 1002/hep. 510270603] [PMID: 9620316]

[59]   Chiba T. Japanese biliary atresia Registry. In: Ohi R, Ed. biliary atresia. Tokyo: Icom Associates 1991.

[60]   Chiba T. Japanese biliary atresia Registry. In: Ohi R, Ed. biliary atresia. Tokyo: Icom Associates 1991.

[61]   Balistreri W F. Neonatal cholestasis. J Pediatr 1985; 106(2): 171-84.
[http://dx.doi.org/10. 1016/S0022-3476(85)80282-1] [PMID: 3881579]

[62]   Ukarapol N, Wongsawasdi L, Ong-Chai S, Riddhiputra P, Kongtawelert P. Hyaluronic acid: additional biochemical marker in the diagnosis of biliary atresia. Pediatr Int 2007; 49(5): 608-11.
[http://dx.doi.org/10. 1111/j. 1442-200X. 2007. 02423. x] [PMID: 17875085]

[63]   Javitt N B, Keating J P, Grand R J, Harris R C. Serum bile acid patterns in neonatal hepatitis and extrahepatic biliary atresia. J Pediatr 1977; 90(5): 736-9.
[http://dx.doi.org/10. 1016/S0022-3476(77)81238-9] [PMID: 856962]

[64]   Abramson S J, Berdon W E, Altman R P, Amodio J B, Levy J. Biliary atresia and noncardiac polysplenic syndrome: US and surgical considerations. Radiology 1987; 163(2): 377-9.
[http://dx.doi.org/10. 1148/radiology. 163. 2. 3550880] [PMID: 3550880]

[65]   Zhou L, Shan Q, Tian W, Wang Z, Liang J, Xie X. Ultrasound for the diagnosis ofbiliary atresia: a meta-analysis. AJR Am J Roentgenol 2016; 206(5): W73-82.
[http://dx.doi.org/10. 2214/AJR. 15. 15336] [PMID: 27010179]

[66]   Boughanim M, Benachi A, Dreux S, Delahaye S, Muller F. Nonvisualization of the fetal gallbladder by second-trimester ultrasound scan: strategy of clinical management based on four examples. Prenat Diagn 2008; 28(1): 46-8.
[http://dx.doi.org/10. 1002/pd. 1912] [PMID: 18186137]

[67]   Kasai M. Treatment of biliary atresia with special reference to hepatic porto-enterostomy and its modifications. Prog Pediatr Surg 1974; 6: 5-52.
[PMID: 4596366]

[68]   Andrews W S, Pau C M, Chase H P, Foley L C, Lilly J R. Fat soluble vitamin deficiency in biliary atresia. J Pediatr Surg 1981; 16(3): 284-90.
[http://dx.doi.org/10. 1016/S0022-3468(81)80681-1] [PMID: 7252728]

[69]   Hernanz-Schulman M, Ambrosino M M, Freeman P C, Quinn C B. Common bile duct in children: sonographic dimensions. Radiology 1995; 195(1): 193-5.
[http://dx.doi.org/10. 1148/radiology. 195. 1. 7892467] [PMID: 7892467]

[70]   Davenport M, Stringer M D, Howard E R. Biliary amylase and congenital choledochal dilatation. J Pediatr Surg 1995; 30(3): 474-7.
[http://dx.doi.org/10. 1016/0022-3468(95)90059-4] [PMID: 7539079]

[71]   Jeong I H, Jung Y S, Kim H, *et al.* Amylase level in extrahepatic bile duct in adult patients with choledochal cyst plus anomalous pancreatico-biliary ductal union. World J Gastroenterol 2005; 11(13): 1965-70.
[http://dx.doi.org/10. 3748/wjg. v11. i13. 1965] [PMID: 15800987]

[72]   Todani T, Watanabe Y, Narusue M, Tabuchi K, Okajima K. Congenital bile duct cysts: Classification, operative procedures, and review of thirty-seven cases including cancer arising from choledochal cyst. Am J Surg 1977; 134(2): 263-9.
[http://dx.doi.org/10. 1016/0002-9610(77)90359-2] [PMID: 889044]

[73]   Miyano T, Yamataka A, Li L. Congenital biliary dilatation. Semin Pediatr Surg 2000; 9(4): 187-95.
[http://dx.doi.org/10. 1053/spsu. 2000. 18843] [PMID: 11112836]

[74]   Alonso-Lej F, Rever W B Jr, Pessagno D J. Congenital choledochal cyst, with a report of 2, and an analysis of 94, cases. Surg GynecolObstet Int Abstr Surg 1959; 108(1): 1-30.
[PMID: 13625059]

[75]   Jang J Y, Yoon C H, Kim K M. Endoscopic retrograde cholangiopancreatography in pancreatic and biliary tract disease in Korean children. World J Gastroenterol 2010; 16(4): 490-5.
[http://dx.doi.org/10. 3748/wjg. v16. i4. 490] [PMID: 20101777]

[76]   Park D H, Kim M H, Lee S K, *et al.* Can MRCP replace the diagnostic role of ERCP for patients with choledochal cysts? Gastrointest Endosc 2005; 62(3): 360-6.
[http://dx.doi.org/10. 1016/j. gie. 2005. 04. 026] [PMID: 16111952]

[77]   Yamataka A, Ohshiro K, Okada Y, *et al.* Complications after cyst excision with hepaticoenterostomy for choledochal cysts and their surgical management in children *versus* adults. J Pediatr Surg 1997; 32(7): 1097-102.
[http://dx.doi.org/10. 1016/S0022-3468(97)90407-3] [PMID: 9247242]

[78]   Whitington P F, Black D D. Cholelithiasis in premature infants treated with parenteral nutrition and furosemide. J Pediatr 1980; 97(4): 647-9.
[http://dx.doi.org/10. 1016/S0022-3476(80)80033-3] [PMID: 6775066]

[79]   total parentral nutrition (TPN) and gallbladder diseases in neonates. Sonographic assessment J ultrasound Med 1987; 6: 243.

[80]   kasai M, Suzuki S: A new operation for "non-correctable" biliary atresia: hepatic portoenterostomy. Shujyutsu 1959; 13: 733.

[81]   Kamisawa T, Takuma K, Egawa N, Tsuruta K, Sasaki T. A new embryological theory of the pancreatic duct system. Dig Surg 2010; 27(2): 132-6.
[http://dx.doi.org/10. 1159/000286906] [PMID: 20551658]

[82]   Okahara M, Mori H, Kiyosue H, Yamada Y, Sagara Y, Matsumoto S. Arterial supply to the pancreas; variations and cross-sectional anatomy. Abdom Imaging 2010; 35(2): 134-42.
[http://dx.doi.org/10. 1007/s00261-009-9581-0] [PMID: 19777288]

[83]   Otto A K, Neal M D, Slivka A N, Kane T D. An appraisal of endoscopic retrograde cholangiopancreatography (ERCP) for pancreaticobiliary disease in children: our institutional experience in 231 cases. Surg Endosc 2011; 25(8): 2536-40.
[http://dx.doi.org/10. 1007/s00464-011-1582-8] [PMID: 21359895]

[84]   Park A J, Latif S U, Ahmad M U, *et al.* A comparison of presentation and management trends in acute pancreatitis between infants/toddlers and older children. J Pediatr Gastroenterol Nutr 2010; 51(2): 167-70.
[http://dx.doi.org/10. 1097/MPG. 0b013e3181cea545] [PMID: 20479687]

[85]   Morinville V D, Husain S Z, Bai H, *et al.* Definitions of pediatric pancreatitis and survey of present clinical practices. J Pediatr Gastroenterol Nutr 2012; 55(3): 261-5.
[http://dx.doi.org/10. 1097/MPG. 0b013e31824f1516] [PMID: 22357117]

[86]   Bai H X, Lowe M E, Husain S Z. What have we learned about acute pancreatitis in children? J Pediatr Gastroenterol Nutr 2011; 52(3): 262-70.
[http://dx.doi.org/10. 1097/MPG. 0b013e3182061d75] [PMID: 21336157]

[87]   Herman R, Guire K E, Burd R S, Mooney D P, Ehlrich P F. Utility of amylase and lipase as predictors

of grade of injury or outcomes in pediatric patients with pancreatic trauma. J Pediatr Surg 2011; 46(5): 923-6.
[http://dx.doi.org/10. 1016/j. jpedsurg. 2011. 02. 033] [PMID: 21616253]

[88]   Iglesias-Garcia J, Domínguez-Muñoz J E, Castiñeira-Alvariño M, Luaces-Regueira M, Lariño-Noia J. Quantitative elastography associated with endoscopic ultrasound for the diagnosis of chronic pancreatitis. Endoscopy 2013; 45(10): 781-8.
[http://dx.doi.org/10. 1055/s-0033-1344614] [PMID: 24019131]

[89]   Bollen T L, Singh V K, Maurer R, *et al.* A comparative evaluation of radiologic and clinical scoring systems in the early prediction of severity in acute pancreatitis. Am J Gastroenterol 2012; 107(4): 612-9.
[http://dx.doi.org/10. 1038/ajg. 2011. 438] [PMID: 22186977]

[90]   Al-Omran M, Albalawi Z H, Tashkandi M F, Al-Ansary L A. Enteral *versus* parenteral nutrition for acute pancreatitis. Cochrane Database Syst Rev 2010; (1): : CD002837.
[http://dx.doi.org/10. 1002/14651858. CD002837. pub2] [PMID: 20091534]

[91]   Tenner S, Baillie J, DeWitt J, Vege S S. American College of Gastroenterology guideline: management of acute pancreatitis. Am J Gastroenterol 2013; 108(9): 1400-1415, 1416.
[http://dx.doi.org/10. 1038/ajg. 2013. 218] [PMID: 23896955]

[92]   Li J, Wang R, Tang C. Somatostatin and octreotide on the treatment of acute pancreatitis - basic and clinical studies for three decades. Curr Pharm Des 2011; 17(16): 1594-601.
[http://dx.doi.org/10. 2174/138161211796196936] [PMID: 21548873]

[93]   Lévy P, Domínguez-Muñoz E, Imrie C, Löhr M, Maisonneuve P. Epidemiology of chronic pancreatitis: burden of the disease and consequences. United European Gastroenterol J 2014; 2(5): 345-54.
[http://dx.doi.org/10. 1177/2050640614548208] [PMID: 25360312]

[94]   Schneider L, Müller E, Hinz U, Grenacher L, Büchler M W, Werner J. Pancreas divisum: a differentiated surgical approach in symptomatic patients. World J Surg 2011; 35(6): 1360-6.
[http://dx.doi.org/10. 1007/s00268-011-1076-9] [PMID: 21472371]

[95]   Moran A, Brunzell C, Cohen R C, *et al.* Clinical care guidelines for cystic fibrosis-related diabetes: a position statement of the American Diabetes Association and a clinical practice guideline of the Cystic Fibrosis Foundation, endorsed by the Pediatric Endocrine Society. Diabetes Care 2010; 33(12): 2697-708.
[http://dx.doi.org/10. 2337/dc10-1768] [PMID: 21115772]

[96]   Neff L P, Mishra G, Fortunato J E, Laudadio J, Petty J K. Microlithiasis, endoscopic ultrasound, and children: not just little gallstones in little adults. J Pediatr Surg 2011; 46(3): 462-6.
[http://dx.doi.org/10. 1016/j. jpedsurg. 2010. 09. 007] [PMID: 21376193]

[97]   Beltrand J, Caquard M, Arnoux J B, *et al.* Glucose metabolism in 105 children and adolescents after pancreatectomy for congenital hyperinsulinism. Diabetes Care 2012; 35(2): 198-203.
[http://dx.doi.org/10. 2337/dc11-1296] [PMID: 22190679]

[98]   Jazrawi S F, Barth B A, Sreenarasimhaiah J. Efficacy of endoscopic ultrasound-guided drainage of pancreatic pseudocysts in a pediatric population. Dig Dis Sci 2011; 56(3): 902-8.
[http://dx.doi.org/10. 1007/s10620-010-1350-y] [PMID: 20676768]

[99]   Kandula L, Whitcomb D C, Lowe M E. Genetic issues in pediatric pancreatitis. Curr Gastroenterol Rep 2006; 8(3): 248-53.
[http://dx.doi.org/10. 1007/s11894-006-0083-8] [PMID: 16764792]

[100] Majumder S, Chari S T. Chronic pancreatitis. Lancet 2016; 387(10031): 1957-66.
[http://dx.doi.org/10. 1016/S0140-6736(16)00097-0] [PMID: 26948434]

[101] Mathur A, Gorden P, Libutti S K. Insulinoma. Surg Clin North Am 2009; 89(5): 1105-21.
[http://dx.doi.org/10. 1016/j. suc. 2009. 06. 009] [PMID: 19836487]

[102] Grant C S. Insulinoma. Surg Oncol Clin N Am 1998; 7(4): 819-44.
[http://dx.doi.org/10. 1016/S1055-3207(18)30247-3] [PMID: 9735136]

[103] Soloni P, Cecchetto G, Dall'igna P, Carli M, Toffolutti T, Bisogno G. Management of unresectable solid papillary cystic tumor of the pancreas. A case report and literature review. J Pediatr Surg 2010; 45(5): e1-6.
[http://dx.doi.org/10. 1016/j. jpedsurg. 2010. 02. 045] [PMID: 20438906]

[104] Campanile M, Nicolas A, LeBel S, Delarue A, Guys J M, de Lagausie P. Frantz's tumor: is mutilating surgery always justified in young patients? Surg Oncol 2011; 20(2): 121-5.
[http://dx.doi.org/10. 1016/j. suronc. 2009. 12. 003] [PMID: 20106656]

[105] Nossal G J, Austin C M, Pye J, Mitchell J. Antigens in immunity. XII. Antigen trapping in the spleen. Int Arch Allergy Appl Immunol 1966; 29(4): 368-83.
[http://dx.doi.org/10. 1159/000229718] [PMID: 5934923]

[106] Pai S Y, Reinherz E L. Immune response. 2015.

[107] Karakousis G C, Fraker D L. The spleen. Greenfield's Surgery: Scientific Principles and Practice. 6th ed., Philadelphia, PA: Wolters Kluwer 2016.

[108] Greig J D, Sweet E M, Drainer I K. Splenic torsion in a wandering spleen, presenting as an acute abdominal mass. J Pediatr Surg 1994; 29(4): 571-2.
[http://dx.doi.org/10. 1016/0022-3468(94)90096-5] [PMID: 8014820]

[109] Schmidt S P, Andrews H G, White J J. The splenic snood: an improved approach for the management of the wandering spleen. J Pediatr Surg 1992; 27(8): 1043-4.
[http://dx.doi.org/10. 1016/0022-3468(92)90555-L] [PMID: 1403532]

[110] Allen K B, Andrews G. Pediatric wandering spleen--the case for splenopexy: review of 35 reported cases in the literature. J Pediatr Surg 1989; 24(5): 432-5.
[http://dx.doi.org/10. 1016/S0022-3468(89)80395-1] [PMID: 2661792]

[111] Palanivelu C, Rangarajan M, Senthilkumar R, Parthasarathi R, Kavalakat A J. Laparoscopic mesh splenopexy (sandwich technique) for wandering spleen. JSLS 2007; 11(2): 246-51.
[PMID: 17761090]

[112] Halpert B, Gyorkey F. Accessory spleen in the tail of the pancreas. AMA Arch Pathol 1957; 64(3): 266-9.
[PMID: 13457581]

[113] Crawford D L P P, Moore J T. Hypertrophied splenic remnants in hereditary spherocytosis. Contemp Surg 1998; 53: 103-4.

[114] Putschar W G, Manion W C. Splenicgonadal fusion. Am J Pathol 1956; 32(1): 15-33.
[PMID: 13275562]

[115] Rathaus V, Zissin R, Goldberg E. Spontaneous rupture of an epidermoid cyst of spleen: preoperative ultrasonographic diagnosis. J Clin Ultrasound 1991; 19(4): 235-7.
[http://dx.doi.org/10. 1002/jcu. 1870190410] [PMID: 1646230]

[116] Accinni A, Bertocchini A, Madafferi S, Natali G, Inserra A. Ultrasound-guided percutaneous sclerosis of congenital splenic cysts using ethyl alcohol 96% and minocycline hydrochloride 10%: A pediatric series. J Pediatr Surg 2016; 51(9): 1480-4.
[http://dx.doi.org/10. 1016/j. jpedsurg. 2016. 05. 005] [PMID: 27320839]

[117] Morgenstern L. Nonparasitic splenic cysts: pathogenesis, classification, and treatment. J Am Coll Surg 2002; 194(3): 306-14.
[http://dx.doi.org/10. 1016/S1072-7515(01)01178-4] [PMID: 11893134]

[118] Young N S, Brown K E. Parvovirus B19. N Engl J Med 2004; 350(6): 586-97.
[http://dx.doi.org/10. 1056/NEJMra030840] [PMID: 14762186]

[119] Rescorla F J, West K W, Engum S A, Grosfeld J L. Laparoscopic splenic procedures in children: experience in 231 children. Ann Surg 2007; 246(4): 683-7.
[http://dx.doi.org/10. 1097/SLA. 0b013e318155abb9] [PMID: 17893505]

[120] Davis P W, Williams D A, Shamberger R C. Immune thrombocytopenia: surgical therapy and predictors of response. J Pediatr Surg 1991; 26(4): 407-12.
[http://dx.doi.org/10. 1016/0022-3468(91)90987-5] [PMID: 2056400]

[121] Fonkalsrud E W, Philippart M, Feig S. Ninety-five percent splenectomy for massive splenomegaly: a new surgical approach. J Pediatr Surg 1990; 25(2): 267-9.
[http://dx.doi.org/10. 1016/0022-3468(90)90437-E] [PMID: 2303995]

[122] Farah R A, Rogers Z R, Thompson W R, Hicks B A, Guzzetta P C, Buchanan G R. Comparison of laparoscopic and open splenectomy in children with hematologic disorders. J Pediatr 1997; 131(1 Pt 1): 41-6.
[http://dx.doi.org/10. 1016/S0022-3476(97)70122-7] [PMID: 9255190]

[123] Gigot J F, Jamar F, Ferrant A, *et al*. Inadequate detection of accessory spleens and splenosis with laparoscopic splenectomy. A shortcoming of the laparoscopic approach in hematologic diseases. Surg Endosc 1998; 12(2): 101-6.
[http://dx.doi.org/10. 1007/s004649900607] [PMID: 9479721]

[124] Gelmini R, Romano F, Quaranta N, *et al*. Sutureless and stapleless laparoscopic splenectomy using radiofrequency: LigaSure device. Surg Endosc 2006; 20(6): 991-4.
[http://dx.doi.org/10. 1007/s00464-005-0470-5] [PMID: 16738999]

[125] Romano F, Gelmini R, Caprotti R, *et al*. Laparoscopic splenectomy: ligasure *versus* EndoGIA: a comparative study. J Laparoendosc Adv Surg Tech A 2007; 17(6): 763-7.
[http://dx.doi.org/10. 1089/lap. 2007. 0005] [PMID: 18158806]

[126] Lai P B, Leung K L, Ho W S, Yiu R Y, Leung B C, Lau W Y. The use of liposucker for spleen retrieval after laparoscopic splenectomy. Surg Laparosc Endosc Percutan Tech 2000; 10(1): 39-40.
[http://dx.doi.org/10. 1097/00129689-200002000-00009] [PMID: 10872525]

[127] Golkar F C, Ross S B, Sperry S, *et al*. Patients' perceptions of laparoendoscopic single-site surgery: the cosmetic effect. Am J Surg 2012; 204(5): 751-61.
[http://dx.doi.org/10. 1016/j. amjsurg. 2011. 07. 026] [PMID: 23140831]

[128] Fan Y, Wu S D, Kong J, Su Y, Tian Y, Yu H. Feasibility and safety of single-incision laparoscopic splenectomy: a systematic review. J Surg Res 2014; 186(1): 354-62.
[http://dx.doi.org/10. 1016/j. jss. 2013. 09. 010] [PMID: 24135373]

[129] Delaitre B, Maignien B. [Splenectomy by the laparoscopic approach. Report of a case]. Presse Med 1991; 20(44): 2263.
[PMID: 1838167]

[130] Szold A, Kamat M, Nadu A, Eldor A. Laparoscopic accessory splenectomy for recurrent idiopathic thrombocytopenic purpura and hemolytic anemia. Surg Endosc 2000; 14(8): 761-3.
[http://dx.doi.org/10. 1007/s004640000209] [PMID: 10954825]

[131] Minkes R K, Lagzdins M, Langer J C. Laparoscopic *versus* open splenectomy in children. J Pediatr Surg 2000; 35(5): 699-701.
[http://dx.doi.org/10. 1053/jpsu. 2000. 6010] [PMID: 10813328]

[132] Winslow E R, Brunt L M. Perioperative outcomes of laparoscopic *versus* open splenectomy: a meta-analysis with an emphasis on complications. Surgery 2003; 134(4): 647-53.
[http://dx.doi.org/10. 1016/S0039-6060(03)00312-X] [PMID: 14605626]

[133] Eber S W, Langendörfer C M, Ditzig M, *et al*. Frequency of very late fatal sepsis after splenectomy for hereditary spherocytosis: impact of insufficient antibody response to pneumococcal infection. Ann Hematol 1999; 78(11): 524-8.
[http://dx.doi.org/10. 1007/s002770050550] [PMID: 10602897]

[134] Baird P A, MacDonald E C. An epidemiologic study of congenital malformations of the anterior abdominal wall in more than half a million consecutive live births. Am J Hum Genet 1981; 33(3): 470-8.
[PMID: 6454342]

[135] Mortellaro V E, St Peter S D, Fike F B, Islam S. Review of the evidence on the closure of abdominal wall defects. Pediatr Surg Int 2011; 27(4): 391-7.
[http://dx.doi.org/10. 1007/s00383-010-2803-2] [PMID: 21161242]

[136] Lap C C M M, Brizot M L, Pistorius L R, *et al.* Outcome of isolated gastroschisis; an international study, systematic review and meta-analysis. Early Hum Dev 2016; 103: 209-18.
[http://dx.doi.org/10. 1016/j. earlhumdev. 2016. 10. 002] [PMID: 27825040]

[137] Lausman A Y, Langer J C, Tai M, *et al.* Gastroschisis: what is the average gestational age of spontaneous delivery? J Pediatr Surg 2007; 42(11): 1816-21.
[http://dx.doi.org/10. 1016/j. jpedsurg. 2007. 07. 005] [PMID: 18022429]

[138] Feldkamp M L, Carmichael S L, Shaw G M, Panichello J D, Moore C A, Botto L D. Maternal nutrition and gastroschisis: findings from the National Birth Defects Prevention Study. Am J Obstet Gynecol 2011; 204(5): 404. e1-404. e10.
[http://dx.doi.org/10. 1016/j. ajog. 2010. 12. 053] [PMID: 21396620]

[139] Browne M L, Hoyt A T, Feldkamp M L, *et al.* Maternal caffeine intake and risk of selected birth defects in the National Birth Defects Prevention Study. Birth Defects Res A Clin Mol Teratol 2011; 91(2): 93-101.
[http://dx.doi.org/10. 1002/bdra. 20752] [PMID: 21254365]

[140] Frolov P, Alali J, Klein M D. Clinical risk factors for gastroschisis and omphalocele in humans: a review of the literature. Pediatr Surg Int 2010; 26(12): 1135-48.
[http://dx.doi.org/10. 1007/s00383-010-2701-7] [PMID: 20809116]

[141] Stoll C, Alembik Y, Dott B, Roth M P. Risk factors in congenital abdominal wall defects (omphalocele and gastroschisi): a study in a series of 265,858 consecutive births. Ann Genet 2001; 44(4): 201-8.
[http://dx.doi.org/10. 1016/S0003-3995(01)01094-2] [PMID: 11755106]

[142] Islam S. Clinical care outcomes in abdominal wall defects. Curr Opin Pediatr 2008; 20(3): 305-10.
[http://dx.doi.org/10. 1097/MOP. 0b013e3282ffdc1e] [PMID: 18475100]

[143] D'Antonio F, Virgone C, Rizzo G, *et al.* Prenatal risk factors and outcomes in gastroschisis: a meta-analysis. Pediatrics 2015; 136: E159-69.

[144] Page R, Ferraro Z M, Moretti F, Fung K F. Gastroschisis: antenatal sonographic predictors of adverse neonatal outcome. J Pregnancy 2014; 2014: 239406-13.
[http://dx.doi.org/10. 1155/2014/239406] [PMID: 25587450]

[145] Overcash R T, DeUgarte D A, Stephenson M L, *et al.* Factors associated with gastroschisis outcomes. Obstet Gynecol 2014; 124(3): 551-7.
[http://dx.doi.org/10. 1097/AOG. 0000000000000425] [PMID: 25162255]

[146] Geslin D, Clermidi P, Gatibelza M-E, *et al.* What prenatal ultrasound features are predictable of complex or vanishing gastroschisis? A retrospective study. Prenat Diagn 2017; 37(2): 168-75.
[http://dx.doi.org/10. 1002/pd. 4984] [PMID: 27981591]

[147] Cağlar M, Hakgüder G, Ateş O, *et al.* Amniotic fluid ferritin as a marker of intestinal damage in gastroschisis: a time course experimental study. J Pediatr Surg 2007; 42(10): 1710-5.
[http://dx.doi.org/10. 1016/j. jpedsurg. 2007. 05. 027] [PMID: 17923200]

[148] Fasching G, Haeusler M, Mayr J, Schimpl G, Haas J, Puerstner P. Can levels of interleukins and matrix metalloproteinases in the amniotic fluid predict postnatal bowel function in fetuses with gastroschisis? J Pediatr Surg 2005; 40(12): 1887-91.
[http://dx.doi.org/10. 1016/j. jpedsurg. 2005. 08. 032] [PMID: 16338312]

[149] Sbragia L, Schmidt A F, Moraes S, *et al.* Inflammatory response in a rat model of gastroschisis is associated with an increase of NF-kappaB. Braz J Med Biol Res 2010; 43(2): 160-5.
[http://dx.doi.org/10. 1590/S0100-879X2010005000005] [PMID: 20098844]

[150] Kale A, Kale E, Akdeniz N, Canoruc N. Elevated amniotic fluid amino acid levels in fetuses with gastroschisis. Braz J Med Biol Res 2006; 39(8): 1021-5.
[http://dx.doi.org/10. 1590/S0100-879X2006000800004] [PMID: 16906276]

[151] Zani-Ruttenstock E, Zani A, Paul A, Diaz-Cano S, Ade-Ajayi N. Interstitial cells of Cajal are decreased in patients with gastroschisis associated intestinal dysmotility. J Pediatr Surg 2015; 50(5): 750-4.
[http://dx.doi.org/10. 1016/j. jpedsurg. 2015. 02. 029] [PMID: 25783375]

[152] Langer J C, Longaker M T, Crombleholme T M, *et al.* Etiology of intestinal damage in gastroschisis. I: Effects of amniotic fluid exposure and bowel constriction in a fetal lamb model. J Pediatr Surg 1989; 24(10): 992-7.
[http://dx.doi.org/10. 1016/S0022-3468(89)80200-3] [PMID: 2530329]

[153] Snyder C L, St Peter S D. Trends in mode of delivery for gastroschisis infants. Am J Perinatol 2005; 22(7): 391-6.
[http://dx.doi.org/10. 1055/s-2005-872591] [PMID: 16215928]

[154] Jansen L A, Safavi A, Lin Y, MacNab Y C, Skarsgard E D. Preclosure fluid resuscitation influences outcome in gastroschisis. Am J Perinatol 2012; 29(4): 307-12.
[http://dx.doi.org/10. 1055/s-0031-1295639] [PMID: 22094919]

[155] Corona-Rivera J R, Nieto-García R, López-Marure E, *et al.* Associated congenital anomalies in infants with isolated gastroschisis: A single-institutional experience. Am J Med Genet A 2016; 170A(2): 316-21.
[http://dx.doi.org/10. 1002/ajmg. a. 37433] [PMID: 26464049]

[156] Arnold M A, Chang D C, Nabaweesi R, *et al.* Risk stratification of 4344 patients with gastroschisis into simple and complex categories. J Pediatr Surg 2007; 42(9): 1520-5.
[http://dx.doi.org/10. 1016/j. jpedsurg. 2007. 04. 032] [PMID: 17848242]

[157] Abdullah F, Arnold M A, Nabaweesi R, *et al.* Gastroschisis in the United States 1988-2003: analysis and risk categorization of 4344 patients. J Perinatol 2007; 27(1): 50-5.
[http://dx.doi.org/10. 1038/sj. jp. 7211616] [PMID: 17036030]

[158] Molik K A, Gingalewski C A, West K W, *et al.* Gastroschisis: a plea for risk categorization. J Pediatr Surg 2001; 36(1): 51-5.
[http://dx.doi.org/10. 1053/jpsu. 2001. 20004] [PMID: 11150437]

[159] Youssef F, Laberge J-M, Puligandla P, Emil S. Determinants of outcomes in patients with simple gastroschisis. J Pediatr Surg 2017; 52(5): 710-4.
[http://dx.doi.org/10. 1016/j. jpedsurg. 2017. 01. 019] [PMID: 28188037]

[160] Youssef F, Cheong L H A, Emil S. Gastroschisis outcomes in North America: a comparison of Canada and the United States. J Pediatr Surg 2016; 51(6): 891-5.
[http://dx.doi.org/10. 1016/j. jpedsurg. 2016. 02. 046] [PMID: 27004440]

[161] Emil S, Canvasser N, Chen T, Friedrich E, Su W. Contemporary 2-year outcomes of complex gastroschisis. J Pediatr Surg 2012; 47(8): 1521-8.
[http://dx.doi.org/10. 1016/j. jpedsurg. 2011. 12. 023] [PMID: 22901911]

[162] Saleem I, St. Peter S D, Qureshi F, *et al.* The Impact of Complex Gastroschisis on Morbidity and Survival. AAP National Conference & Exhibition.

[163] Aldrink J H, Caniano D A, Nwomeh B C. Variability in gastroschisis management: a survey of North American pediatric surgery training programs. J Surg Res 2012; 176(1): 159-63.
[http://dx.doi.org/10. 1016/j. jss. 2011. 05. 012] [PMID: 21737095]

[164]　Gonzalez D O, Cooper J N, St Peter S D, *et al.* Variability in outcomes after gastroschisis closure across U. S. children's hospitals. J Pediatr Surg 2017. Epub ahead of print [PMID: 28483165]

[165]　Houben C, Davenport M, Ade-Ajayi N, Flack N, Patel S. Closing gastroschisis: diagnosis, management, and outcomes. J Pediatr Surg 2009; 44(2): 343-7.
[http://dx.doi.org/10. 1016/j. jpedsurg. 2008. 10. 084] [PMID: 19231531]

[166]　Lepigeon K, Van Mieghem T, Vasseur Maurer S, Giannoni E, Baud D. Gastroschisis--what should be told to parents? Prenat Diagn 2014; 34(4): 316-26.
[http://dx.doi.org/10. 1002/pd. 4305] [PMID: 24375446]

[167]　Bergholz R, Boettcher M, Reinshagen K, Wenke K. Complex gastroschisis is a different entity to simple gastroschisis affecting morbidity and mortality-a systematic review and meta-analysis. J Pediatr Surg 2014; 49(10): 1527-32.
[http://dx.doi.org/10. 1016/j. jpedsurg. 2014. 08. 001] [PMID: 25280661]

[168]　Brantberg A, Blaas H-G K, Haugen S E, Eik-Nes S H. Characteristics and outcome of 90 cases of fetal omphalocele. Ultrasound Obstet Gynecol 2005; 26(5): 527-37.
[http://dx.doi.org/10. 1002/uog. 1978] [PMID: 16184512]

[169]　Sadler T W. The embryologic origin of ventral body wall defects. Semin Pediatr Surg 2010; 19(3): 209-14.
[http://dx.doi.org/10. 1053/j. sempedsurg. 2010. 03. 006] [PMID: 20610194]

[170]　Solerte L. Three-dimensional multiplanar ultrasound in a limb-body wall complex fetus: clinical evidence for counseling. J Matern Fetal Neonatal Med 2006; 19(2): 109-12.
[http://dx.doi.org/10. 1080/14767050400028840] [PMID: 16581607]

[171]　Tassin M, Descriaud C, Elie C, *et al.* Omphalocele in the first trimester: prediction of perinatal outcome. Prenat Diagn 2013; 33(5): 497-501.
[http://dx.doi.org/10. 1002/pd. 4102] [PMID: 23529817]

[172]　Cohen-Overbeek T E, Tong W H, Hatzmann T R, *et al.* Omphalocele: comparison of outcome following prenatal or postnatal diagnosis. Ultrasound Obstet Gynecol 2010; 36(6): 687-92.
[http://dx.doi.org/10. 1002/uog. 7698] [PMID: 20509138]

[173]　Yokomori K, Ohkura M, Kitano Y, Hori T, Nakajo T. Advantages and pitfalls of amnion inversion repair for the treatment of large unruptured omphalocele: results of 22 cases. J Pediatr Surg 1992; 27(7): 882-4.
[http://dx.doi.org/10. 1016/0022-3468(92)90391-J] [PMID: 1640338]

[174]　de Lorimier A A, Adzick N S, Harrison M R. Amnion inversion in the treatment of giant omphalocele. J Pediatr Surg 1991; 26(7): 804-7.
[http://dx.doi.org/10. 1016/0022-3468(91)90143-H] [PMID: 1832715]

[175]　Islam S. Advances in surgery for abdominal wall defects: gastroschisis and omphalocele. Clin Perinatol 2012; 39(2): 375-86.
[http://dx.doi.org/10. 1016/j. clp. 2012. 04. 008] [PMID: 22682386]

[176]　Biard J M, Wilson R D, Johnson M P, *et al.* Prenatally diagnosed giant omphaloceles: short- and long-term outcomes. Prenat Diagn 2004; 24(6): 434-9.
[http://dx.doi.org/10. 1002/pd. 894] [PMID: 15229842]

[177]　Arias E. United States Life Tables, 2011. Natl Vital Stat Rep 2015; 64(11): 1-63.
[PMID: 26460931]

[178]　Keshtgar A S, Griffiths M. Incarceration of umbilical hernia in children: is the trend increasing? Eur J Pediatr Surg 2003; 13(1): 40-3.
[http://dx.doi.org/10. 1055/s-2003-38299] [PMID: 12664414]

CHAPTER 5

Undescended Testis (Cryptorchidism)

Assalah T. Gumer[1] and **Sultan M. Ghanim**[2,*]

[1] 6th Grade Medical College, Faculty of Medicine, University of Kufa, Iraq

[2] ME Unit, Medical College, Faculty of Medicine, University of Kufa, Iraq

Abstract: This chapter will discuss common genital tract diseases in pediatric age group. These include undescended testis, testicular neoplasm, ovarian cyst, and ovarian neoplasm, and ambiguous genitalia. Undescended testis incidence is 30% in pre-term and 3% in full-term infants and it is associated with an increased risk of infertility and malignancy. Testicular neoplasm has different types; the most common type is yolk sac tumor. Ovarian cysts are quite common in childhood and adolescence age groups. Lastly, we will discuss ambiguous genitalia, which should address as a medical emergency condition during evaluation.

Keywords: Genital Diseases, Neoplasms, Pediatrics.

GENITALIA

This is a condition in which one testis or both testes fail to descend into the scrotum before birth. The Undescended testis is associated with histological and morphologic changes as early as months of age, atrophy of Leydig cells, decrease in tubular diameter, and impaired spermatogenesis can occur by 2 years of age. Incidence 30% of preterm infants, 3% of full-term infants. The testicle may reside in the retro perineum, in the internal inguinal ring, in the inguinal canal, or even at the external ring. Retractile testis is a normally descended testis that retracts into the inguinal canal but can be brought down into the scrotal sac during the examination It is thought to result from a hyper reflexive cremasteric muscle contraction and does not require operative intervention (Fig. **5.1**).

* **Corresponding author Sultan M. Ghanim:** ME Unit, Medical College, Faculty of Medicine, University of Kufa, Iraq; Tel: +9647816669997; E-mail: sultanmalsaadi@uokufa.edu.iq

Sultan M. Ghanim, Najah R. Hadi and Nada Al-Haris (Eds.)

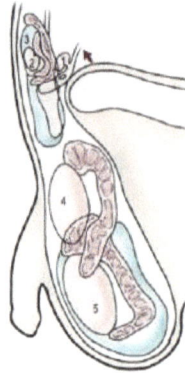

Fig. (5.1). Testicular descent shown in males: 1, 90 mm crown–rump length (CRL) (12–24 weeks of gestational age); 2, 125 mm CRL (15–17 weeks) [3], 230 mm CRL (24–26 weeks); 4, 280 mm CRL (28–30 weeks); 5, at term.

DIAGNOSIS

There is widespread confusion in primary care owing to the historical variability in defining what constitutes a UDT, thus requiring a careful evaluation of history of the patient and a physical examination. The supine and frog-legged sitting position are the key positions in which patients are examined in warm rooms. The examination of the scrotum is conducted for hypoplasia and the presence of testis. Solitary testis showing compensatory hypertrophy may represent the Monorchia. The fingers are used to palpate and feel. By moving fingers, the area starting from the iliac crest up to the inguinal canal is felt until the scrotum is reached. With the help of a hand, the location of the testis is evaluated, and subcutaneous structures toward the scrotum are pushed inside. The scrotum is not touched before the location of the testis as this may activate the cremasteric reflex, leading to the retraction of the testis. The walking of fingers may be done by using a lubricating gel or soap to avoid friction. Gentle pressure is applied in the mid-abdominal line to push the testis into the inguinal canal. A cross-legged sitting or squatting position is important for the identification of the testis. The accurate physical examination of a ticklish or obese boy is often challenging. Due to challenges during the physical examination, up to 20% of non-palpable testes are considered palpated when the diagnosis is being conducted during anesthesia in the operating room [1, 2]. During diagnosis, the retractile testes and low UDTs are pushed by hand into the scrotum, and the retractile testes remain there until displaced by a cremasteric reflex, whereas the low UDT retracts back up to its abnormal location once released. Most of the time, the ipsilateral hemiscrotum is often underdeveloped with a UDT and fully developed with a retractile testis. When any testis is not palpable, one must differentiate anorchia, androgen insensitivity syndrome, or a chromosomal abnormality from bilateral non-palpable UDT.

Moreover, a rare (but potentially life-threatening condition) should also be considered. A phenotypically male newborn with bilateral non-palpable gonads, even in the presence of an otherwise normal-appearing penis, could represent a masculinized 46, XX baby with congenital adrenal hyperplasia (CAH). If the diagnosis is delayed, the salt-wasting form of CAH can lead to severe electrolyte imbalance and cardiovascular compromise. In such cases, karyotyping is warranted. To avoid unnecessary surgical exploration in a 46XY patient with anorchia, studies to determine the presence of viable testicular tissue should include serum MIF, inhibit B, follicle-stimulating hormone (FSH), luteinizing hormone (LH), and testosterone [3]. If the child is <9–12 months of age, serum MIS and inhibit B should be undetectable in the absence of viable testes. The elevation of FSH level above the mean indicates in a boy having age less than 9 years; it suggests the presence of anorchia for sure. If Human chorionic gonadotropin (HCG) stimulation elevates testosterone level with normal LH and FSH levels, functioning testicular tissue could be the possible cause and the patient needs to undergo further investigation. However, under normal testosterone levels, nonfunctional testicular tissue may be diagnosed with further investigation. However, it is impossible to distinguish between normal non-palpable testes and functioning testicular remnants in Human chorionic gonadotropin (HCG) stimulation [4]. Imaging studies are rarely helpful in determining the presence or location of a UDT and may delay timely referral for surgical treatment [5]. Therefore, their routine use is not recommended. The literature has revealed in the research conducted that an expert surgeon can better diagnose and locate the UDT than some imaging techniques like ultrasonography (US), computed tomography (CT), or magnetic resonance imaging (MRI). These imaging techniques are less sensitive in detecting soft tissue masses <1 cm than an expert examiner or surgeon [6]. Usually, in bilateral non-palpable testes, MRI with gadolinium is more helpful in detecting the abdominal testes as MRI gives a a bright appearance to the testicular tissue [7, 8]. However, these cases can be better evaluated with serum hormones and markers. MRI tends to add little to the diagnosis while incurring costs and exposure to contrasts agent and anesthesia. Although, the accuracy of US is low despite being easy to perform. It adds to the expenditure on the part of patient and has the sensitivity of 45% and specificity of 78%, respectively. In brief, Imaging does not help diagnose testicular absence. It is critical to not "miss" an intra-abdominal testicle. If an imaging test existed, that could definitively prove that the testicle was absent (as opposed to Undescended), this would be a valuable tool. Currently, however, no such imaging study exists.

FERTILITY

Bilateral testes biopsies at the time of orchidopexy helped in revealing that histologically abnormal UDT and, to a lesser degree, its contralateral descended mate may be the causes of infertility [10, 11]. Patients having UDT in their history on analysis show subnormal semen. Since fertility is associated with the position of UDT, abdominal or canalicular testes in men resulted in infertility as compared with the men having inguinal testes (83.3% *vs* . 90%) [13, 14]. Despite these findings, both men with a previous history of unilateral UDT showed an infertility rate of (~10%) equivalent to that of the normal population [14 - 16]. Men having bilateral UDT if diagnosed and treated early exhibited paternity rates of 50–65%. We may deduce that these men have six times more chances of being infertile than the normal population of men [17, 18].

Mechanisms of infertility in UDT are directly associated with some cells and structures. These include the Sertoli and Leydig cells, as well as Wolffian duct abnormalities (vasal and epididymal). Already insufficient sperms are stopped by these abnormalities, and their transport is limited. The testicular temperature in a UDT becomes high, and this results in the immaturity of the Sertoli cells in monkeys [19]. Histopathology results exhibit that lack of Leydig cell proliferation and delay in the transformation of gonocytes to dark adult spermatogonia is caused by the blunted normal testosterone surge at 60–90 days postnatal. In the rat model, early orchiopexy for UDT resulted in the preservation of germ cell number and spermatogenesis compared to the germ cell apoptosis in untreated rats [21]. The delayed orchidopexy up to 3 years compared to the normal 9 months resulting in less testicular growth in boys [22]. A clinical trial was conducted in young boys related to Neoadjuvant LH-releasing hormone (LHRH), and this showed that orchidopexy increases the fertility index (spermatogonia/tubule) if the boys are treated. Another clinical trial on Neoadjuvant Gonadotropin-releasing hormone therapy revealed that fertility is improved, although this therapy gave better results if administered before 24 months [24].

RISK OF MALIGNANCY

UDT is linked with malignancy and may increase the risk of malignancy by two to eightfold (25)(26). This risk appears to vary with the gonad's location: The risk is far less (only 1%) in the case of inguinal and while it is slightly riskier (up to 5%) in the case of abdominal testes [27, 28]. The malignancies may be seminomas or non-seminomas, depending upon some features. Malignancies that initiate in testes and remain located in the abdomen are frequently seminomas (74%) [29, 30]. While cancers that are developed after successful orchidopexy, regardless of the original location, are frequently non-seminomatous germ cell tumors without taking location into account, and these usually constitute 63% of the malignancies [31, 32]. A significant percentage of men (10%) having testicular cancer may have a history of UDT [33].

The changes in the micro and macro environment of the UDT seem to be connected with the increased risk of malignancy; this is stated by two competing theories known as "position theory" and "testicular digenesis" theory. A study was conducted in 2007 on 16,983 Swedish men. They underwent orchidopexy before attaining the age of 13 and 2.23 of such patients showed the risk of developing cancer at later stages of their lives [34]. Those patients who were operated on at or after attaining the age of 13 showed a bit higher risk of developing cancer in the future. The percentage of that risk was 5.40 as compared with normal men. Another study revealed that patients who underwent orchidopexy before 10 years of age have a six times less risk of developing malignancies than those who underwent orchidopexy after more than 10 years [35]. These associations between ages of orchidopexy with a decrease in cancer risk need further verification yet provide compelling evidence for early surgical intervention. Moreover, by placing the gonad in an accessible location, orchidopexy facilitates subsequent testicular examination and can potentially help with early cancer detection.

The alternate "common cause" or "testicular digenesis" theory hypothesizes that hormonal or genetic causes could possibly trigger the malignancy. This may influence both Cryptorchidism and testicular cancer [36]. In 15-20% of the patients suffering from UDT, the testicular tumor may initiate in the normally descended contralateral testis. Thus these testes are more prone to risk [37].

The incidence of carcinoma *in situ* (CIS) is usually diagnosed in patients suffering from Cryptorchidism compared to non-affected at the post-pubertal stage. The ratio of CIS in men with Cryptorchidism is 2–4%. Early 5 years of the patients' life witness the invasion of germ cell tumors in 50% of the cases, as soon as the CIS progresses. Although the history of a young child who is CIS diagnosed at the time of orchiopexy is not obvious. Such patients undergo frequent biopsies after puberty; it is unclear if this intervention leads to benefits in cancer prevention [39].

Treatment

Males with bilateral Undescended testicles are often infertile. The testis is subjected to a higher temperature, resulting in decreased spermatogenesis, if unilateral palpable testis in the inguinal canal, standard dartos pouch orchidopexy is performed in 6 months to 1 year of age. Undescended testis is not palpable in the inguinal canal, a diagnostic laparoscopy is useful if the testicular vessels are seen exiting the internal ring, an open inguinal orchidopexy is performed If intra-abdominal testis two-stage Fowler-Stephens orchidopexy can be considered testicular vessels are ligated as a first stage tallow collateral circulation to develop for 6 months before orchidopexy is performed as a second stage of the procedure. If both testes are nonpalpable, a human chorionic Gonadotropin (hCG) stimulation test is carried out to confirm the presence of functioning testis. If a functioning testes are present, diagnostic laparoscopy is performed to identify the testes and to determine surgical therapy (Fig. **5.2**).

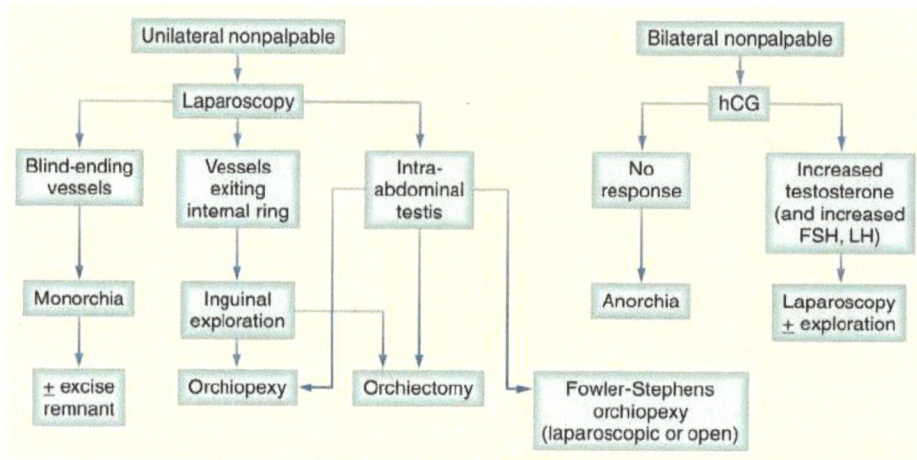

Fig. (5.2). Algorithm for the management of nonpalpable undescended testes. (Adapted from Lee KL, Shortleaf LD: Undescended testis and testicular tumors In Ashcraft KW, Holcomb GW, Holcomb GW III, *et al* , editors: Pediatric surgery, ed 4, Philadelphia, 2005, Elsevier Saunders, pp 706–716.

Indications for Operation

If physical examination findings consistent with Cryptorchidism, there is a future risk of testicular cancer. Orchidopexy positions the test is where it can be easily examined, however, it does not -minimize the risk of developing cancer. Potential future increased risk of infertility or subfertility with undescended testis psychosocial factor to allow normal self-image.

Hormonal Treatment

The use of hormonal therapy in treating UDT is yet to be established. Buserelin is an LHRH agonist being used in Europe frequently to treat UDT (40), but its success is more prominent in cases with the testis at or distal to the external inguinal ring [41, 42]. Some research has recommended the HCG therapy in bilateral UDT to restore a normal endocrine milieu and enhance germ cell maturation [43]. Some trials that have combined Buserelin and HCG therapy have shown success results upto 60% while orchidopexy was conducted in 40% of the cases. The USFDA has not yet allowed the use of Buserelin. In addition, clinical trials using LHRH in Neoadjuvant fashion in young boys undergoing orchidopexy have indicated an improvement in fertility [23]. The 2014 AUA update on

Cryptorchidism does not recommend the use of hormonal therapy to induce testicular descent [9]. Providers have largely embraced these guidelines, and thus routine use of hormonal therapy for UDT in North America is now rare.

Possible Complications

Wound infection, Bleeding, Testicular ascent, and Testicular atrophy.

Testicular neoplasm

Testicular cancer is not very common in children, and its prevalence is only 1-2% of all pediatric solid tumors. Usually, the incidences of pediatric testicular tumors appear between ages 12 and 24 months in neonates; another peak is followed during puberty. Before the age of puberty, boys exhibit a very high percentage of benigntesticular lesions than post-pubertal and adult males [47, 56].

Management of testicular tumors in prepubertal boys thus differs rather dramatically from postpubertal males, as testis-sparing procedures (*i.e.*, partial orchiectomy) are favored in the former. Conversely, in postpubertal patients and adults' curative treatment tends to favor a radical orchiectomy. Malignant, germ cell cancers tend to respond well to chemotherapy, and the need for retroperitoneal lymph node dissection (RPLND) is relatively rare [48]. In previous reports, germ cell tumors were thought to comprise 65–85% of pediatric testicular tumors. This was largely based on tumor registries that reported >60% yolk sac tumors (YST) and approximately 20% teratoma, Table **5.1**.

Table 5.1. Primary testes tumor types in 395 boys under 12 years of age.

Tumor type	Frequency %
Yolk sac	62
Teratoma	23
Stromal(unspecified)	4
Epidermoid cyst	3
Juvenile granulose cell	3
Sertoli cell	3
Leyding cell	1
Gonadoblastoma	1

Current literature reports indicate teratoma and Epidermoid cysts are the most common neoplasms in prepubertal children [28, 49]. Data also now support the rationale for testis-sparing surgery in prepubertal patients with negative serum markers (particularly α-fetoprotein [AFP], which is almost universally elevated in patients with YSTs) (Fig. **5.3**) [46]. There are several patient populations that have an increased risk for neoplasms. In particular, males with gonadal digenesis, hypovirilization, and disorders of sexual development have an increased incidence of gonadal tumors, particularly Gonadoblastoma.

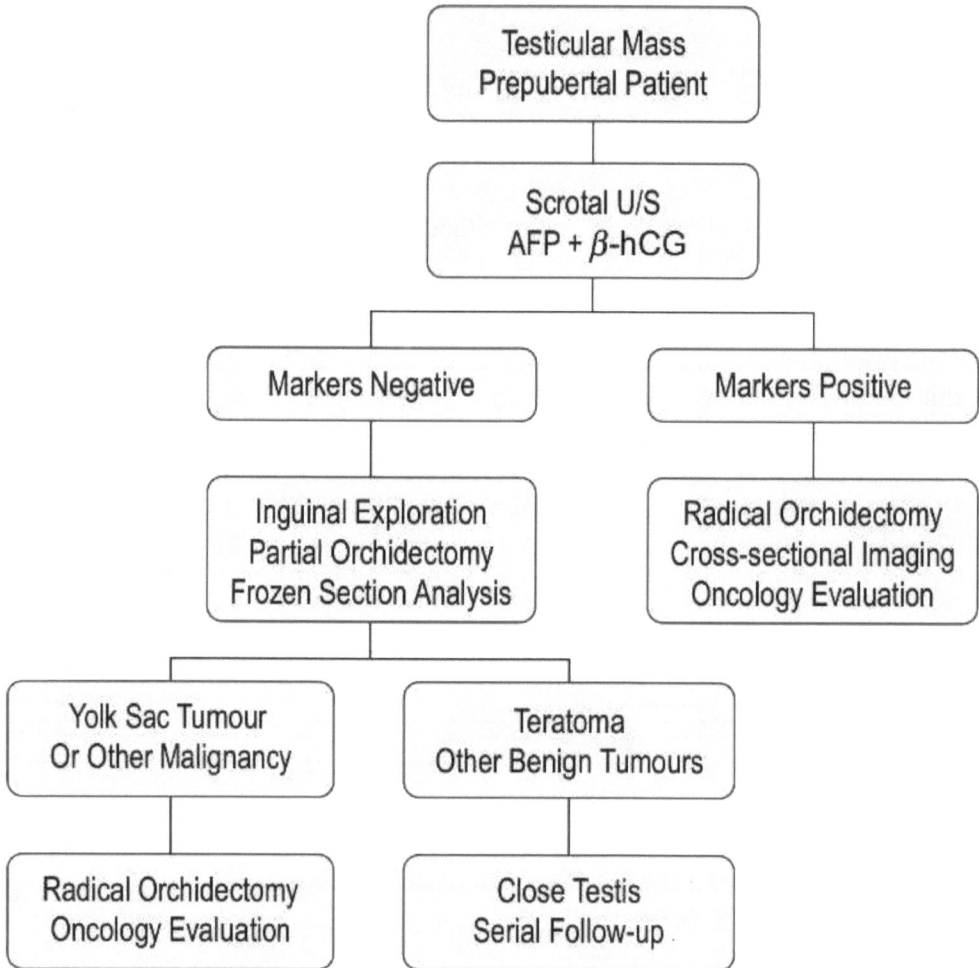

Fig. (5.3). This algorithm depicts the management of the prepubertal male with a testicular mass that is suspicious for cancer.

PRESENTATION AND DIAGNOSIS

A painless scrotal mass is a testicular tumor, (Fig. **5.4**). The enlarged scrotum is a feature that must not be ignored. Sometimes, a tumor arising in a UDT may cause torsion associated with acute abdominal pain. Malignancy typically is non-tender, does not transilluminate, and is associated with normal urinalysis. An associated hydrocele in 15–20% of patients may impede adequate testicular examination [46]. Hormonally active tumors can cause precocious puberty. A color Doppler US and serum tumor markers (AFP, β hCG, and lactate dehydrogenase [LDH]) should be obtained to make an initial assessment for a testicular mass. US is nearly 100% sensitive for detecting a testicular tumor; anechoic cystic lesions usually suggest benign disease [48]. Internal calcifications and a mass with "onion-skin" alternating hypo-and hyperechoic lesions suggest an epidermoid cyst or teratoma [51]. These findings obtained as a part of the initial evaluation are important in doing pre-operative planning for a testis sparing operation. Serum tumor marker levels help in diagnosis and are also take into account in the follow-up of testicular malignancy.

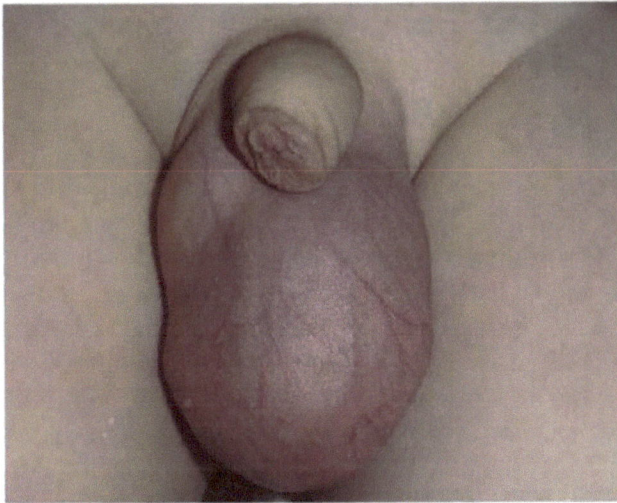

Fig. (5.4). This 3-year-old child presented with a painless scrotal mass and elevated AFP. He underwent a radical orchiectomy for a yolk sac tumor.

AFP or Alpha-Fetoprotein is a glycoprotein. Various benign and malignant diseases, including YSTs of the testis, show an elevation in its levels. The half-life of AFP is approximately 5.5 days, and the normal adult levels (<10 ng/mL) are not achieved until around 10 months of age [52]. β-hCG is a glycoprotein produced by some seminomas and mixed germ cell tumors, as well as choriocarcinoma. The half-life of β-hCG is 24 hours and cannot be detected in significant amounts in boys (<5 IU/ L). Once the high-risk testicular cancer is diagnosed, Histologically a CT scan is done for evaluation of metastatic disease and planning for RPLND, but it may carry a 15–20% false-negative rate [53].

MRI also has been used and may ultimately replace CT in children for diagnosis and follow-up due to the high ionizing radiation of CT and risk of future malignancy [54]. Prepubertal testis tumors are staged using the Children's Oncology Group staging system Table **5.2**.

Table 5.2. Children's Oncology Group Staging System for Testicular Cancer.

Stage	Features
I	Limited to testes Completely resected by high inguinal orchiectomy No clinical, radiographic, or histological evidence of disease beyond the testes. Patients with normal or unknown tumour markers at diagnosis must have a negative ipsilateral retroperitoneal node sampling to confirm stage 1 disease
II	Trans-scrotal biopsy or orchiectomy Microscopic disease in scrotum or high in spermatic cord (<5 cm from proximal end) Failure of tumour markers to normalize or decrease with an appropriate half-life
III	Retroperitoneal lymph node involvement No visceral or extra-abdominal involvement
IV	Distant metastases

CARCINOMA *IN SITU*

Carcinoma *in situ* (CIS) is considered a a premalignant lesion of the testis. Cancer that is developed in at least 50% of the testes may develop the CIS [38], usually in patients with UDT and DSD, as both the conditions are associated with higher chances of testicular cancer than that in the general population [55]. Testicular microlithiasis (Fig. **5.5**) may be associated with an increased risk of CIS as well as testicular germ cell tumors [56 - 58]. The presence of microlithiasis in testis is not conclusively considered premalignant. Rather, it appears to be a marker of an increased risk of cancer, which may be increasingly important in infertile men with atrophic testes or those with known testicular cancer and microlithiasis in the contralateral gonad [26, 59]. Endocrinological alterations in patients undergoing puberty may cause CIS, although its history in such patients before puberty is not obvious. When a testicular biopsy is performed at the time of orchidopexy, CIS is seen in 0.36–0.45% of cases [60, 61]. 2- 4% of the men with a history of UDT are more prone to CIS. An annual testicular examination and the testicular US may help in managing the CIS if identified in testis before puberty. After puberty, a biopsy of the contralateral testis and unilateral orchiectomy could be the possible treatment. If CIS is diagnosed in the remaining testes, radiation treatment is receommended [62]. The fertility implications of this treatment option can be significant, and the decision has to be taken in the context of cancer risk against the need for hormone supplementation and infertility.

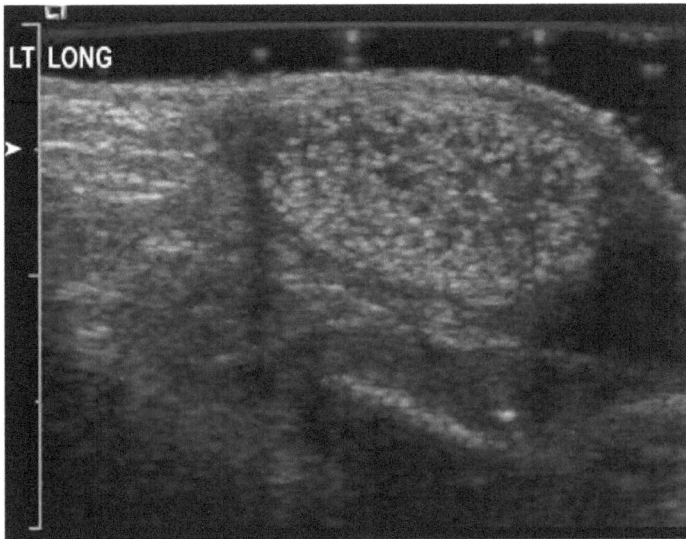

Fig. (5.5). This ultrasound image depicts diffuse microlithiasis in this testis that may be associated with an increased risk of carcinoma *in situ* and/ or germ cell tumors.

GERM CELL TUMORS

Yolk Sac Tumors

Endodermal sinus tumors, embryonal adenocarcinoma, orchioblastomas, or Teillum tumors are also termed as YSTs, which usually appear in the initial two years of life. These may appear as firm yellow/white bodies. Under the microscope, they are characterized by Schiller–Duval bodies (Fig. **5.6**) and stain positive for AFP [64, 65]. Contrary to the behavior of embryonal carcinoma in adults, YST (which is histologically similar) in children has a more indolent course and spread hematogenously. Approximately 95% of YSTs are confined to the testis, and metastases to the retroperitoneum are uncommon (5%) [47]. The lungs are the most common site of distant metastasis, and retroperitoneal metastases are seen only 5% of the time [48]. 99% of the cases exhibit the 5-year survival for YST. The radical inguinal orchiectomy is the standard diagnostic and therapeutic procedure adopted in YST, and this alone is usually curative in children. To redcuce the risk of metastases, the clamping of spermatic cord is done as soon it enters the inguinal canal. Abdominopelvic CT and chest radiography (CXR), histological examination of the radical orchiectomy specimen, and determination of serum tumor markers are some of the pre-requisites for Staging of YST.

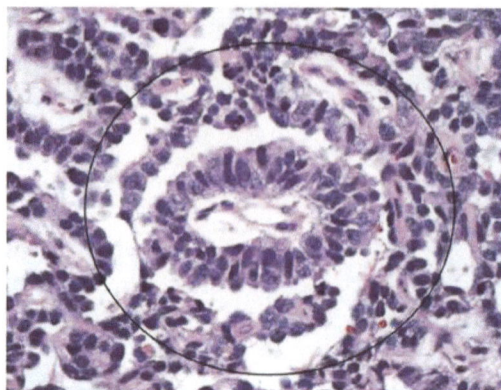

Fig. (5.6). Yolk sac tumors are firm and yellow/white in appearance. Under the microscope, they are characterized by Schiller–Duval bodies and stain positive for α-fetoprotein. The Schiller–Duval body is the structure in the circle. It is composed of a central papillary structure within a cystic space lined by malignant cells.

Stage I tumors can be treated by radical inguinal orchiectomy [66] as these are limited to the testes. Measurement of tumor markers every month and CXRs every 2 months, Abdominopelvic CT or MRI after every 3 months in the first year and every 6 months for the next year is done to treat and diagnose this. However, this practice may be overly aggressive in a child whose tumor markers remain normal. If there is no recurrence till two years, the follow-up is postponed for 6 month or a year [64].

Traditionally, RPLND was recommended for boys with unknown or normal markers at diagnosis to confirm stage I disease. Although confirmatory RPLND may still be considered, it is used less often because stage I YST has a high likelihood of stage I presentation (85%), has a propensity for hematogenously spread to the lungs RPLND has a high complication rate in children. The risk of recurrence is approximately 20% and almost always can be salvaged with chemotherapy [48].

Stage II disease includes those tumors with residual disease in the scrotum or high proximal inguinal cord, node involvement on imaging, or that showing increase in the tumor markers after orchiectomy. Tumors diagnosed and treated with trans-scrotal biopsy should be considered stage II because trans-scrotal violation alters their normal lymphatic drainage. Lymphatic drainage of the testis occurs through the retroperitoneal nodes, while the Lymphatic drainage of the scrotum occurs into the inguinal nodes. Combination chemotherapy with cisplatin, etoposide, and bleomycin (PEB) is recommended for all patients with stage II disease. Due to significant ototoxicity and nephrotoxicity with cisplatin, the UK Children's

Cancer Study Group substituted carboplatin for cisplatin and was able to maintain a 100% event-free survival at 5 years [67]. After chemotherapy, the cases of persistent retroperitoneal mass or elevated AFP are very rare. In such cases, an RPLND is usually considered.

Stage III disease: Imaging studies witnessed the enlarged retroperitoneal spread (lymph node >4cm) during this stage. Biopsy is used to confirm suspected nodal metastases, such as lymph nodes >1–2 cm on CT. Metastases beyond the retroperitoneum or to any viscera define stage IV disease. For both stage III and stage IV disease, chemotherapy followed by RPLND is suggested as a possible treatment. The overall survival approaches 100% [47].

Teratoma

Teratoma account for over 40% of testicular tumors in prepubertal children, Histologically, ectoderm, endoderm, and mesoderm, which are layers of embryonic tissue, constitute teratoma. Grossly, they can contain differentiated tissue such as cartilage, muscle, bone, fat, and a cystic component. A benign course is followed by teratoma before puberty, and testis-sparing surgery could be the possible treatment, (Fig. **5.7**) [67, 68]. A study revealed the effectiveness of the testis-sparing approach. There were no signs of tumor recurrence even after a long-term mean follow-up of 7 years in the ipsilateral or contralateral gonad [69]. Also, no radiographic follow-up is recommended for prepubertal patients who undergo partial orchiectomy [48]. However, if one accepts the dysplasia theory, whether benign or malignant, the unilateral testicular tumor could pose an increased risk for the contralateral testis.

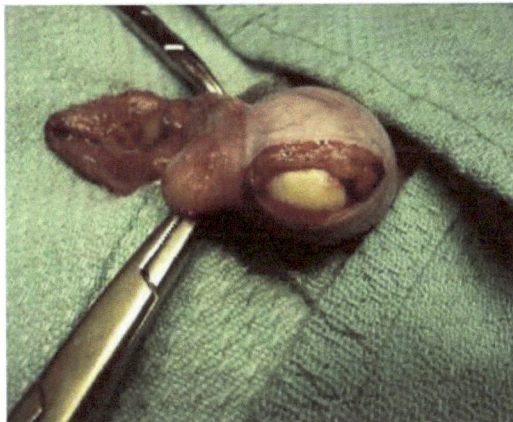

Fig. (5.7). A 4-year-old child was found to have a painless testicular mass. Serum markers were negative. At operation, this well-demarcated tumor was encountered that was amenable to a testis-sparing operation. Frozen analysis was consistent with a benign tumor (teratoma).

On the other hand, radical inguinal orchiectomy is suggested at or after puberty as teratoma usually follows a malignant post-pubertal course. The enucleated tumor should always be sent for frozen section examination. If immature elements or pubertal changes are seen (*i.e.*, spermatogenesis on the normal somniferous tubules surrounding the margin), radical orchiectomy is the possible cure suggested by the literature [70]. Elevated AFP or focus of YST may indicate potential recurrence.

Epidermoid cysts comprise about 15% of pediatric testis tumors, and asmonodermal teratoma follow a benign course. As such, a testis-sparing approach can be taken [48].

Mixed Germ Cell Tumor

20% of pediatric/adolescent germ cell tumors are mixed with germ cell tumors almost exclusively in post-pubertal patients. Hepatocarcinoma can be seen in an operatively corrected UDT. It is associated with the presence of YST, embryonal carcinoma, choriocarcinoma, and seminomas [71], and 80% of the cases exhibited it presence in the testis only. The value of RPLND in children has been challenged over the years, and management in children/ adolescents tends to follow management guidelines established for adult patients in which these neoplasms are more common [72].

Seminomas

Seminomas are rare in children but are the most common tumor in an uncorrected abdominal UDT. Radical orchiectomy and retroperitoneal radiation could cure the Seminomas, following guidelines for adult patients [73].

Gonadal stromal tumor

Leydig Cell Tumors

This is a non-germ cell tumor (NGCTs), and its incidence is often reported in boys of 5-9 years of age [48, 74]. Its incidence is associated with the appearance of three signs, including a unilateral testicular mass (90–93%), precocious puberty, and elevated 17-ketosteroid levels; these signs are called its clinical triad. The production of testosterone and occasionally other androgens may result in signs of precocious puberty and gynecomastia in 20% of the patients [75]. Precocious puberty may also be caused by pituitary lesions, Leydig cell hyperplasia, and CAH. The evaluations may include pituitary/adrenal axis by assaying for 17-ketosteroids, FSH, LH, and dexamethasone suppression test. Reinke crystals on histological examination are pathognomonic for this tumor and can be found in 35–40% of all patients, (Fig. **5.8**) [76]. Testis-sparing nucleation is also considered when diagnosed preoperatively, as Leydig cell tumors may follow a benign course [77].

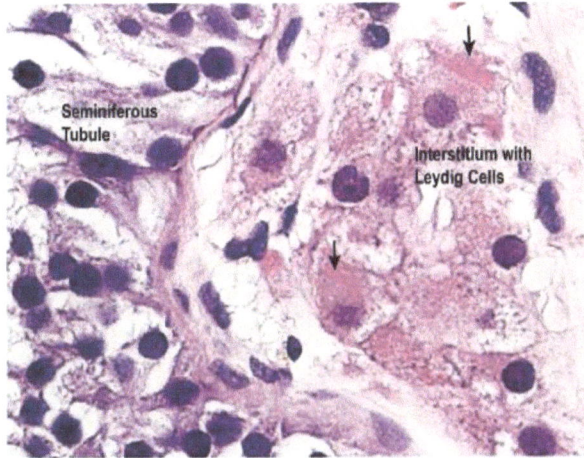

Fig. (5.8). On histologic examination, Reinke crystals (arrows) are pathognomonic for a Leydig cell tumor and are found in up to 40% of these tumors [80, 81].

The Granulose Cell Tumor

This tumor also follows a benign course, and testis-sparing surgery again could be the possible cure. Neonates undergoing this tumor exhibit the symptoms like scrotal swelling, normal age-adjusted AFP levels, and a complex, cystic, multi-septated, hypoechoic mass on the testicular US [78].

The Sertoli Cell Tumor

This tumor is a rare form of NGCT. A small percentage of patients have gynecomastia, though these tumors are typically not as hormonally active as Leydig cell tumors [79]. In children under five years, this tumor follows the benign course, and testis-sparing surgery could be the possible cure. Older children, however, should have a metastatic evaluation with imaging [48].

Gonadoblastoma is a form of NGCT usually associated with a DSD and typically occurring in digenetic gonads. The patients are generally 46XY phenotypic females with complete androgen insensitivity syndrome (CAIS) and intraabdominal testes undergoing virilization at puberty. One-third of patients exhibit bilateral gonadal lesions. There is a small risk of malignant degeneration in 10% of the patients. Historically early gonadectomy was recommended, especially in a female children (Table **5.3**).

Table 5.3. Neoplasms in female children and adolescent.

Tumor Neoplasm	Appearance	Marker	Other Information
Teratoma (dermoid)	Irregular, cystic and solid	None	Most common germ cell tumor 6-8% malignant and immature, may be associated with other germ cell tumors
Dysgerminoma	Thick, white, opaque: cytological reactivity with ALP	None	Inspect other ovary 15-20% bilateral, 95% cure (stage I) Chemotherapy is only required in case of advanced disease
Endodermal sinus tumor Also known as (yolk sac tumor)	Solid and cystic Schiller-Duval bodies	AFP	Primarily unilateral Surgery and chemotherapy is the cure 15% survival rate after stage I
Embryonal carcinoma	Smooth with area of haemorrhage and necrosis Schiller-Duval bodies	β-hCG	mixed germ cell tumor 60% endocrinological active (precocious puberty) Surgery and chemotherapy with a (50% survival stage I)
Choriocarcinoma	Syncytiotrophoblasts and cyto trophoblasts	β-hCG	Rare primary tumor in children surgery and chemotherapy is the cure
Mixed germ cell tumor	Predominantly solid or cystic depending on the composition	AFP	Composed of Dysgerminoma and endodermal sinus tumor
Sex cord-stromal tumor	Granulose-theca or sertoli-Leyding cells	None	Prevalent in younger patients Isosexual precocious puberty
Juvenile granulosa –theca cell tumour	Very vascular	None	Malignancy related to the percentage of granulosa cells Pure thecomas benign Surgery for stage I Surgery and chemotherapy for advanced disease Variable malignant potential
Sertoli-leyding cell tumors (arrhenoblastoma) Epithelial tumours Serous cystadenoma Mucinous cystadenoma Serous or mucinous cystadenocarcinoma	Predominantly cystic Predominantly cystic with septations		Commonly large size have borderline variants Low malignant potential From coelomic epithelium Rare in children and adolescent

Tumor Neoplasm	Appearance	Marker	Other Information
Miscellaneous tumours Polyembryoma Gonadoblastoma Mesothelioma Metastatic disease	Tissues resemble embryos with all three germ cell types (amniotic cavity, yolk sac, placental primordia)		Predominantly dysgenetic gonads

Currently, however, there is significant debate about the timing and need for gonadectomy. Some surgeons advocate for the preservation of the gonads until adolescence, as puberty can be aided by the peripheral conversion of androgens to estrogens. Others, including many affected patients, are electing to preserve their intra-abdominal gonads indefinitely [82]. Patients with mixed gonadal dysgenesis raised as males should have their streak gonads and UDTs removed, though some suggest that scrotal testes can be preserved because they are less prone to malignancy and can be surveyed more easily.

Ovarian Cysts and Tumour

Ovarian cysts are commonly seen at all ages on pelvic imaging. Most will resolve spontaneously. They can be managed expectantly without surgical management. Most of the ovarian neoplasms that require operation are benign, with the most common neoplasms being mature teratomas and mucinous and serous cystadenomas. Malignant tumors of the ovary are uncommon in the adolescent population, with the malignancy rate slightly higher in childhood than in adolescence [83].

OVARIAN CYSTS IN THE NEONATE

Prenatally diagnosed intra-abdominal cyst, Simple cysts, and Complex cystic masses in neonates be associated with utero or neonatal torsion, with an extremely rare risk of malignancy [84].

Management

observation for all asymptomatic neonatal ovarian cysts regardless of size as most will involutes within the first year of life (spare up to 50% of neonates an operative procedure) [85, 86]. Operative intervention may be necessary if the symptoms include persistent masses, torsion, hemorrhage, mass effect, the recurrence of a cyst after aspiration, the development of acute abdominal symptoms, or other associated signs\symptoms. The ideal surgical approach is laparoscopic and would involve an ovarian sparing surgery (OSS) which should be used for all cysts regardless of size, complexity, or presence of antenatal or postnatal torsion. If aspiration is the chosen method of treatment, a minimally invasive technique is also preferred, this provides the advantage of confirmation of the diagnosis of an ovarian cyst.

OVARIAN CYSTS IN CHILDREN

In children, small cysts exhibiting follicular development and atresia are very common. A large, persistent complex mass with solid components is often associated with diagnosing an ovarian tumour like cystic teratoma or stromal tumour. These ovarian cysts may result in symptoms like early breast development or vaginal bleeding. When cysts are noted to be associated with pubertal changes, an endocrine evaluation is needed. When bilateral ovarian masses are noted in conjunction with pubertal changes, special consideration should be given to the diagnoses of Dysgerminoma or hypothyroidism. Dysgerminoma requires an evaluation with karyotyping and operative removal. The ovarian cysts seen with hypothyroidism will resolve with thyroid replacement without surgical intervention. The size, the presence of symptoms, and cyst composition are the factors determining the management of ovarian cysts in children. The exploration is needed for ovarian masses that are symptomatic or associated with worrisome radiologic signs. If there are no signs of malignancy, ovarian tissue is conserved to a possible extent.

OVARIAN CYSTS IN ADOLESCENTS

This is a very common disorder in adolescence showing ovulatory dysfunction, associated with rupture, pain, hemorrhage, or a mass in the pelvis. These may appear incidentally at the time of conducting other tests. The signs and symptoms like endometriosis, pelvic inflammatory disease disorders of the fallopian tube, congenital uterine anomalies, or disorders of pregnancy are associated with OVARIAN CYSTS in adolescence.

(Fig. **5.9**) Bilateral enlarged multicystic ovaries were found in an 8-year-old with precocious puberty due to hypothyroidism. The pretreatment ultrasound of the right ovary (A) shows a large multicystic ovary. (B) Following thyroid replacement therapy, there has been a resolution in the size of the ovary.

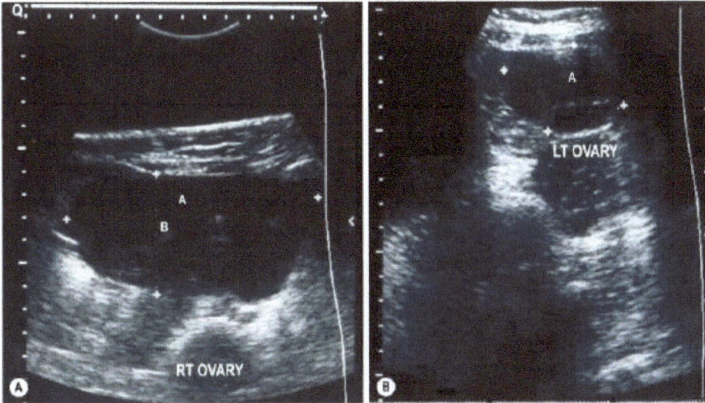

Fig. (5.9). This algorithm is useful for conducting a preoperative evaluation regarding the eligibility of the patient for surgery.

Evaluation

The evaluation is based on the full history, menstrual function and sexual activity, pregnancy, or any signs of a sexually transmitted infection. US is the initial imaging test of choice for evaluation of the ovary completion of urinary screening for (pregnancy, gonorrhea, chlamydia). The management of ovarian cysts with a low rate of malignancy, the high rate of functional cysts or benign tumors in adolescents is done by a conservative approach. Observation is the initial therapy in such cases.

Ambiguous Genitalia

Embryology

Sixth fetal week is the time when the differentiation in the sex could possibly be made. Before the Sixth fetal week, every fetus has Wolffian (male) and müllerian (female) ducts, and this differentiation is influenced by the SRY, which is the sex determining region of the Y chromosome. The shorter arm of the Y chromosome is the place where this is present at the distal end. The SRY influences the genetic changes that lead to the differentiation of gonads in the mammalian urogenital ridge. The Sertoli cells of the seminiferous tubules release Secretion of Müllerian-inhibiting substance (MIS), leading to the retrogression of müllerian ducts and other associated structures like the anlage of the uterus, Fallopian tubes, and the upper vagina takes place, indicating towards the male sex. If there is no production of MIS in the absence of SRY in the Y chromosome, the müllerian duct and its derivatives start developing, indicating towards female phenotype. Sometimes mutations or deletions alter the functioning of SRY, giving rise to the abnormalities. In case of any problem or abnormality, the variants of the intersex syndrome are as following:

a. True hermaphroditism: showing both ovarian and testicular gonadal tissue

b. Male pseudohermaphroditism: testicles only as in males

c. Female pseudohermaphroditism: ovarian tissue only as in females

d. Mixed gonadal dysgenesis: usually underdeveloped or imperfectly formed gonads.

Female Pseudohermaphroditism

The most common cause of pseudohermaphroditism in females is congenital adrenal hyperplasia. These children have a 46XX karyotype but have been exposed to excessive androgens in utero. Common enzyme deficiencies include 21- hydroxylase,11-hydroxylase, and 3β-hydroxysteroid dehydrogenase.

These deficiencies result in the overproduction of intermediary steroid hormones, which results in masculinization of the external genitalia of the XX fetus. These patients are unable to synthesize cortisol. In 90%of cases, deficiency of 21-hydroxylase causes adrenocorticotropic hormone (ACTH) to stimulate the secretion of excessive quantities of adrenal androgen, which masculinizes the developing female (Fig. **5.10**). These infants are prone to salt loss and require cortisol replacement. Those with mineralocorticoid deficiency also require fludrocortisone replacement.

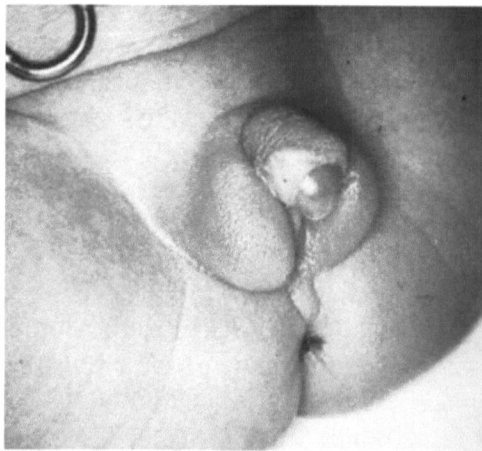

Fig. (5.10). An adrenogenital syndrome is represented by enlarged clitoris and labioscrotal folds in a baby.

Management

In patients with intersex variants or abnormalities, genetic background and family history needs to be evaluated. The study of anatomic structures by physical examination (US) could possibly indicate the reason for abnormality. Some biochemical factors in serum and urine could possibly lead to defects in enzymes. The other technique used is laparoscopy for gonadal biopsy.

Treatment

Correction of electrolyte and volume losses in cases of congenital adrenal hyperplasia and replacement of hormone deficiency are the possible solutions. Surgical assignment of gender should never be determined at the first operation. Although historically female gender had been assigned, there is abundant and convincing evidence that are raising a genotypic male as a female has devastating consequences, not only anatomically but also psychosocially. This is particularly relevant given the role of pre-and postnatal hormones on gender imprinting and identity. In general terms surgical reconstruction should be performed after a full genetic workup and with the involvement of pediatric endocrinologists (pediatric plastic surgeons) and ethicists with expertise in gender issues. Discussion with the family also plays an important role. This approach will reduce the anxiety associated with these disorders and help to ensure the normal physical and emotional development of these patients.

Evaluation of the Newborn with Ambiguous Genitalia

It is very disturbing for the family if ambiguous genitalia is diagnosed in newborns. It is treated as a medical emergency. Usually, genital ambiguity is obvious; still, the tests conducted and the finding of hospitals like the nonpalpable testis and DSD evaluation is extremely important. Despite the absence of classic ambiguity, a high degree of DSD conditions may be found in such patients [87]. Table **5.4** indicates some abnormal physical examinations that may warrant consideration for DSD.

Table 5.4. Physical examination for DSD.

Apparent Female	Unsure	Apparent Male
Clitoral hypertrophy Fused labia Palpable gonad	Ambiguous genitalia	Impalpable testes Severe hypospadias Hypospadias and cryptorchidism

The family history may include maternal hormone exposure, previous fetal death, or a history of genital ambiguity. The examination may consist of the physiology of genitalia. Palpable gonads are one of the important steps in evaluation. It represents a testis or ovotestis and rules out 46, XX DSD, in which only ovaries are present, or PGD, in which only only exists streak gonads are present. The palpability of both gonads may indicate 46, XY DSD. The palpability of one gonad generally implies MGD or ovotesticular DSD. Phallic stretched length, clitoral size, and the position of the urogenital sinus is important while making an evaluation. Palpable uterus may be revealed while conducting a rectal examination. The assessment for the stigmata of Turner syndrome associated with MGD and PGD is also done while making an evaluation. An elevated ACTH production in CAH may also by noted by the bronzing of the areola or scrotum. A karyotype or fluorescent *in situ* hybridization to identify X and Y chromosomes is also a part of initial metabolic evaluation. 17-OH progesterone levels should be obtained after 3 or 4 days; in the meantime, spurious elevations resulting from the stress related to birth usually subsides. The monitoring of electrolyte levels to assess the salt-wasting with CAH is also done. 5α-reductase deficiency is evaluated by checking Testosterone and DHT levels [88]. An elevated LH level and a low MIS level suggest testis dysgenesis or absence. ACTH or hCG stimulation tests, although being controversial, can be performed.

Genetic evaluation for DSDs has always involved a karyotype. Historically, due to cost and the relative difficulty in sequencing, previous diagnostic evaluations have relied heavily on biochemical and phenotypic features. However, for patients with 46, XY DSD or 46, XX who have the ovotesticular or testicular disease, diagnosis may be difficult using such approaches. With the advent of next-generation sequencing, more widespread genetic testing for DSD has gained momentum. Currently, more than 80 genes either play a role in sexual development or have led to DSD development [89]. An in-depth review of some of the more common genes involved in DSD is available [90]. A recent review of studies from 2015 and 2016 using more nontargeted genetic testing approaches found that 35% of patients with 46, XY received a genetic diagnosis [91]. This increased genetic diagnostic rate allows for better clarification of a phenotypically diverse populations. The Society of Endocrinology in the United Kingdom has developed an algorithm for genetic testing that includes karyotype followed by microarray, followed either by single-gene testing or panel testing, finally followed by whole-exome or whole-genome sequencing if no diagnosis is found with initial testing [92]. Although these tests improve the molecular diagnostic rate, their effect on treatment for patients with DSDs is less clear, and we will likely continue to learn more as larger groups of patients are evaluated. The pelvic US is of the early imaging studies that indicate the presence of a uterus or a gonad. In the US, the differentiation of a testis, ovotestis, or ovary is not possible. The confluence of a vagina and urethra and its relation to the urethral sphincter (Fig. **5.11** and **5.12**) is evaluated by a genitogram. Gonal biopsy is done for diagnostic purposes. Metabolic evaluation is important for the assessment of levels of CAH. The endoscopy has no role in diagnosis, still, it is conducted to characterize the internal duct structure and the level of confluence of the urogenital sinus. Endoscopy also plays an important role in planning reconstructive procedures [93]. This gender-assignment team includes a pediatric urologist/surgeon, endocrinologist, geneticist, neonatologist, psychologist, and social worker. Such teams do the evaluation of all newborns with ambiguous genitalia. The team compiles valuable information revealed by all the tests conducted, and this information is presented before the parents in a conference. The gender assessment team works on the goals like preservation of sexual function and any reproductive potential with the least number of operations appropriate gender appearance with stable gender identity and psychosocial well-being of the newborn [94].

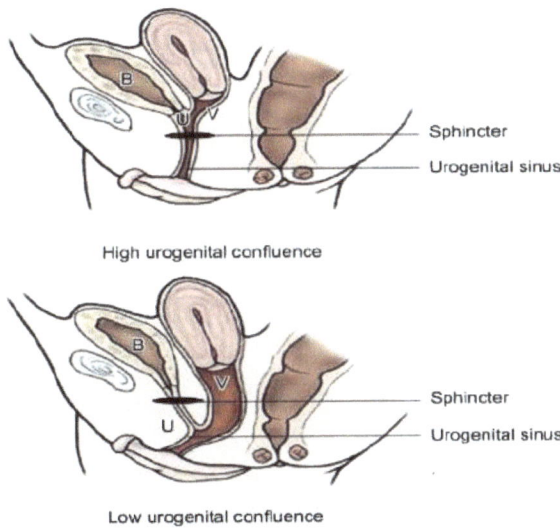

High urogenital confluence

Low urogenital confluence

Fig 5.11. High *versus* low urogenital confluence.

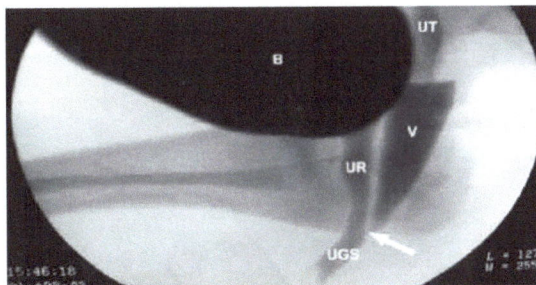

Fig. (5.12). Genitogram showing the lower confluence.

CONCLUSION

Sexual development already starts in childhood, when toddlers start to explore their body and interact with other children by inducing games such as "doctor" and "patient", building up their sexual identity. An impaired body image, as well as impaired self-esteem, problems with incontinence, dependence on parental help, and other psychosocial factors may interfere with normal sexual development during childhood and adolescence. These factors might be the reason that a significant number of adult patients with an anorectal malformation (ARM) is dissatisfied with their partnership and sexuality or report some forms of sexual dysfunction. In agreement with the wish for specialized training in sexuality and sexual issues of the majority of pediatric surgeons in many reviews studies, it has been recently exclaimed that there is an urgent need for an up-to-date sexual health education not only for present-day physicians, but also for medical students and patients to improve sexual health care.

CONSENT FOR PUBLICATION

Not Applicable.

CONFLICT OF INTEREST

The author declares no conflict of interest, financial or otherwise.

ACKNOWLEDGEMENTS

Declared none.

REFERENCES

[1]   Docimo SG. The results of surgical therapy for cryptorchidism: a literature review and analysis. J Urol 1995; 154(3): 1148-52.
        [http://dx.doi.org/10.1016/S0022-5347(01)67015-0] [PMID: 7637073]

[2]   Kirsch AJ, Escala J, Duckett JW, *et al.* Surgical management of the nonpalpable testis: the Children's Hospital of Philadelphia experience. J Urol 1998; 159(4): 1340-3.
        [http://dx.doi.org/10.1016/S0022-5347(01)63613-9] [PMID: 9507881]

[3]   Teo AQ, Khan AR, Williams MPL, Carroll D, Hughes IA. Is surgical exploration necessary in bilateral anorchia? J Pediatr Urol 2013; 9(1): e78-81.
        [http://dx.doi.org/10.1016/j.jpurol.2012.09.006] [PMID: 23079081]

[4]   Jarow JP, Berkovitz GD, Migeon CJ, Gearhart JP, Walsh PC. Elevation of serum gonadotropins establishes the diagnosis of anorchism in prepubertal boys with bilateral cryptorchidism. J Urol 1986; 136(1 Pt 2): 277-9.
        [http://dx.doi.org/10.1016/S0022-5347(17)44840-3] [PMID: 2873261]

[5]   Kanaroglou N, To T, Zhu J, *et al.* Inappropriate use of ultrasound in management of pediatric cryptochidism. Pediatrics 2015; 136(3): 479-86.
        [http://dx.doi.org/10.1542/peds.2015-0222] [PMID: 26260719]

[6]   Esposito C, Cardona R, Centonze A, *et al.* Impact of laparoscopy on the management of an unusual case of nonpalpable testis in an adult patient. Surg Endosc 2003; 17(8): 1324.
[http://dx.doi.org/10.1007/s00464-002-4283-5] [PMID: 12739128]

[7]   De Filippo RE, Barthold JS, González R. The application of magnetic resonance imaging for the preoperative localization of nonpalpable testis in obese children: an alternative to laparoscopy. J Urol 2000; 164(1): 154-5.
[http://dx.doi.org/10.1016/S0022-5347(05)67484-8] [PMID: 10840451]

[8]   Landa HM, Gylys-Morin V, Mattrey RF, Krous HF, Kaplan GW, Packer MG. Magnetic resonance imaging of the cryptorchid testis. Eur J Pediatr 1987; 146 (Suppl. 2): S16-7.
[http://dx.doi.org/10.1007/BF00452861] [PMID: 2891511]

[9]   Kolon TF, Herndon CDA, Baker LA, *et al.* Evaluation and treatment of cryptorchidism: AUA guideline. J Urol 2014; 192(2): 337-45.
[http://dx.doi.org/10.1016/j.juro.2014.05.005] [PMID: 24857650]

[10]   Huff DS, Hadziselimovic F, Snyder HM III, Blythe B, Ducket JW. Histologic maldevelopment of unilaterally cryptorchid testes and their descended partners. Eur J Pediatr 1993; 152 (Suppl. 2): S11-4.
[http://dx.doi.org/10.1007/BF02125425] [PMID: 8101802]

[11]   Rusnack SL, Wu H-Y, Huff DS, *et al.* Testis histopathology in boys with cryptorchidism correlates with future fertility potential. J Urol 2003; 169(2): 659-62.
[http://dx.doi.org/10.1016/S0022-5347(05)63986-9] [PMID: 12544338]

[12]   Puri P, O'Donnell B. Semen analysis of patients who had orchidopexy at or after seven years of age. Lancet 1988; 2(8619): 1051-2.
[http://dx.doi.org/10.1016/S0140-6736(88)90067-0] [PMID: 2903280]

[13]   Lee PA, Coughlin MT, Bellinger MF. Paternity and hormone levels after unilateral cryptorchidism: association with pretreatment testicular location. J Urol 2000; 164(5): 1697-701.
[http://dx.doi.org/10.1016/S0022-5347(05)67087-5] [PMID: 11025752]

[14]   Lee PA. Fertility in cryptorchidism. Does treatment make a difference? Endocrinol Metab Clin North Am 1993; 22(3): 479-90.
[http://dx.doi.org/10.1016/S0889-8529(18)30146-4] [PMID: 7902276]

[15]   Chilvers C, Dudley NE, Gough MH, Jackson MB, Pike MC. Undescended testis: the effect of treatment on subsequent risk of subfertility and malignancy. J Pediatr Surg 1986; 21(8): 691-6.
[http://dx.doi.org/10.1016/S0022-3468(86)80389-X] [PMID: 2875145]

[16]   Lee PA, Coughlin MT. The single testis: paternity after presentation as unilateral cryptorchidism. J Urol 2002; 168(4 Pt 2): 1680-2.
[http://dx.doi.org/10.1097/00005392-200210020-00005] [PMID: 12352333]

[17]   Lee PA, Coughlin MT. Fertility after bilateral cryptorchidism. Evaluation by paternity, hormone, and semen data. Horm Res 2001; 55(1): 28-32.
[PMID: 11423739]

[18]   Lee PA, O'Leary LA, Songer NJ, Coughlin MT, Bellinger MF, LaPorte RE. Paternity after bilateral cryptorchidism. A controlled study. Arch Pediatr Adolesc Med 1997; 151(3): 260-3.
[http://dx.doi.org/10.1001/archpedi.1997.02170400046008] [PMID: 9080933]

[19]   Singh R, Hamada AJ, Bukavina L, Agarwal A. Physical deformities relevant to male infertility. Nat Rev Urol 2012; 9(3): 156-74.
[http://dx.doi.org/10.1038/nrurol.2012.11] [PMID: 22349654]

[20]   Hadziselimović F, Thommen L, Girard J, Herzog B. The significance of postnatal gonadotropin surge for testicular development in normal and cryptorchid testes. J Urol 1986; 136(1 Pt 2): 274-6.
[http://dx.doi.org/10.1016/S0022-5347(17)44839-7] [PMID: 2873260]

[21]   Mizuno K, Hayashi Y, Kojima Y, Kurokawa S, Sasaki S, Kohri K. Early orchiopexy improves

subsequent testicular development and spermatogenesis in the experimental cryptorchid rat model. J Urol 2008; 179(3): 1195-9.
[http://dx.doi.org/10.1016/j.juro.2007.10.029] [PMID: 18206164]

[22] Kollin C, Karpe B, Hesser U, Granholm T, Ritzén EM. Surgical treatment of unilaterally undescended testes: testicular growth after randomization to orchiopexy at age 9 months or 3 years. J Urol 2007; 178(4 Pt 2): 1589-93.
[http://dx.doi.org/10.1016/j.juro.2007.03.173] [PMID: 17707045]

[23] Jaganathan K, Ahmed S, Henderson A, Rané A. Current management strategies for testicular microlithiasis. Nat Clin Pract Urol 2007; 4(9): 492-7.
[http://dx.doi.org/10.1038/ncpuro0856] [PMID: 17823602]

[24] Schwentner C, Oswald J, Kreczy A, *et al.* Neoadjuvant gonadotropin-releasing hormone therapy before surgery may improve the fertility index in undescended testes: a prospective randomized trial. J Urol 2005; 173(3): 974-7.
[http://dx.doi.org/10.1097/01.ju.0000153562.07287.77] [PMID: 15711353]

[25] Pohl H. The Location and Fate of the Cryptorchid and Impalpable Testes Dialogues in Pediatric Urology. Pearl River, NY: William J. Miller Associates 1997; pp. 3-4.

[26] Herrinton LJ, Zhao W, Husson G. Management of cryptorchism and risk of testicular cancer. Am J Epidemiol 2003; 157(7): 602-5.
[http://dx.doi.org/10.1093/aje/kwg012] [PMID: 12672679]

[27] Li FP, Fraumeni JF. Testicular cancers in children: epidemiologic characteristics. J Natl Cancer Inst 1972; 48(6): 1575-81.
[PMID: 5066470]

[28] Ross JH, Rybicki L, Kay R. Clinical behavior and a contemporary management algorithm for prepubertal testis tumors: a summary of the Prepubertal Testis Tumor Registry. J Urol 2002; 168(4 Pt 2): 1675-8.
[http://dx.doi.org/10.1097/00005392-200210020-00004] [PMID: 12352332]

[29] Wood HM, Elder JS. Cryptorchidism and testicular cancer: separating fact from fiction. J Urol 2009; 181(2): 452-61.
[http://dx.doi.org/10.1016/j.juro.2008.10.074] [PMID: 19084853]

[30] Raja MA, Oliver RT, Badenoch D, Blandy JP. Orchidopexy and transformation of seminoma to non-seminoma. Lancet 1992; 339(8798): 930.
[http://dx.doi.org/10.1016/0140-6736(92)90967-8] [PMID: 1348319]

[31] Halme A, Kellokumpu-Lehtinen P, Lehtonen T, Teppo L. Morphology of testicular germ cell tumours in treated and untreated cryptorchidism. Br J Urol 1989; 64(1): 78-83.
[http://dx.doi.org/10.1111/j.1464-410X.1989.tb05527.x] [PMID: 2569902]

[32] Jones BJ, Thornhill JA, O'Donnell B, *et al.* Influence of prior orchiopexy on stage and prognosis of testicular cancer. Eur Urol 1991; 19(3): 201-3.
[http://dx.doi.org/10.1159/000473619] [PMID: 1677333]

[33] Pike MC, Chilvers C, Peckham MJ. Effect of age at orchidopexy on risk of testicular cancer. Lancet 1986; 1(8492): 1246-8.
[http://dx.doi.org/10.1016/S0140-6736(86)91389-9] [PMID: 2872394]

[34] Pettersson A, Richiardi L, Nordenskjold A, Kaijser M, Akre O. Age at surgery for undescended testis and risk of testicular cancer. N Engl J Med 2007; 356(18): 1835-41.
[http://dx.doi.org/10.1056/NEJMoa067588] [PMID: 17476009]

[35] Walsh TJ, Dall'Era MA, Croughan MS, Carroll PR, Turek PJ. Prepubertal orchiopexy for cryptorchidism may be associated with lower risk of testicular cancer. J Urol 2007; 178(4 Pt 1): 1440-6.
[http://dx.doi.org/10.1016/j.juro.2007.05.166] [PMID: 17706709]

[36]   Asklund C, Jørgensen N, Kold Jensen T, *et al.* Biology and e ology of testicular dysgenesis syndrome. BJU Int 2004; 93(3): 6-11.

[37]   Akre O, Pettersson A, Richiardi L. Risk of contralateral testicular cancer among men with unilaterally undescended testis: a meta analysis. Int J Cancer 2009; 124(3): 687-9.
[http://dx.doi.org/10.1002/ijc.23936] [PMID: 18973229]

[38]   Dieckmann KP, Skakkebaek NE. Carcinoma *in situ* of the testis: review of biological and clinical features. Int J Cancer 1999; 83(6): 815-22.
[http://dx.doi.org/10.1002/(SICI)1097-0215(19991210)83:6<815::AID-IJC21>3.0.CO;2-Z]   [PMID: 10597201]

[39]   Giwercman A, Müller J, Skakkeboek NE. Cryptorchidism and testicular neoplasia. Horm Res 1988; 30(4-5): 157-63.
[http://dx.doi.org/10.1159/000181053] [PMID: 2907892]

[40]   Bica DT, Hadziselimovic F. Buserelin treatment of cryptorchidism: a randomized, double-blind, placebo-controlled study. J Urol 1992; 148(2 Pt 2): 617-21.
[http://dx.doi.org/10.1016/S0022-5347(17)36670-3] [PMID: 1353540]

[41]   Hadziselimović F, Huff D, Duckett J, *et al.* Long-term effect of luteinizing hormone-releasing hormone analogue (buserelin) on cryptorchid testes. J Urol 1987; 138(4 Pt 2): 1043-5.
[http://dx.doi.org/10.1016/S0022-5347(17)43495-1] [PMID: 2888905]

[42]   Lala R, Matarazzo P, Chiabotto P, *et al.* Early hormonal and surgical treatment of cryptorchidism. J Urol 1997; 157(5): 1898-901.
[http://dx.doi.org/10.1016/S0022-5347(01)64897-3] [PMID: 9112559]

[43]   Lala R, Matarazzo P, Chiabotto P, de Sanctis C, Canavese F, Hadziselimovic F. Combined therapy with LHRH and HCG in cryptorchid infants. Eur J Pediatr 1993; 152 (Suppl. 2): S31-3.
[http://dx.doi.org/10.1007/BF02125433] [PMID: 8101810]

[44]   Giannopoulos MF, Vlachakis IG, Charissis GC. 13 Years' experience with the combined hormonal therapy of cryptorchidism. Horm Res 2001; 55(1): 33-7.
[PMID: 11423740]

[45]   Waldschmidt J, Doede T, Vygen I. The results of 9 years of experience with a combined treatment with LH-RH and HCG for cryptorchidism. Eur J Pediatr 1993; 152 (Suppl. 2): S34-6.
[http://dx.doi.org/10.1007/BF02125434] [PMID: 8101811]

[46]   Pohl HG, Shukla AR, Metcalf PD, *et al.* Prepubertal testis tumors: actual prevalence rate of histological types. J Urol 2004; 172(6 Pt 1): 2370-2.
[http://dx.doi.org/10.1097/01.ju.0000144402.13556.74] [PMID: 15538270]

[47]   Wu HY, Snyder HM III. Pediatric urologic oncology: bladder, prostate, testis. Urol Clin North Am 2004; 31(3): 619-27.
[http://dx.doi.org/10.1016/j.ucl.2004.04.004] [PMID: 15313070]

[48]   Agarwal PK, Palmer JS. Testicular and paratesticular neoplasms in prepubertal males. J Urol 2006; 176(3): 875-81.
[http://dx.doi.org/10.1016/j.juro.2006.04.021] [PMID: 16890643]

[49]   Walsh TJ, Grady RW, Porter MP, Lin DW, Weiss NS. Incidence of testicular germ cell cancers in U.S. children: SEER program experience 1973 to 2000. Urology 2006; 68(2): 402-5.
[http://dx.doi.org/10.1016/j.urology.2006.02.045] [PMID: 16904461]

[50]   Pohl HG, Shukla AR, Metcalf PD, *et al.* Prepubertal testis tumors: actual prevalence rate of histological types. J Urol 2004; 172(6 Pt 1): 2370-2.
[http://dx.doi.org/10.1097/01.ju.0000144402.13556.74] [PMID: 15538270]

[51]   Langer JE, Ramchandani P, Siegelman ES, Banner MP. Epidermoid cysts of the testicle: sonographic and MR imaging features. AJR Am J Roentgenol 1999; 173(5): 1295-9.

[http://dx.doi.org/10.2214/ajr.173.5.10541108] [PMID: 10541108]

[52]   Ohama K, Nagase H, Ogino K, *et al.* Alpha-fetoprotein (AFP) levels in normal children. Eur J Pediatr Surg 1997; 7(5): 267-9.
[http://dx.doi.org/10.1055/s-2008-1071168] [PMID: 9402482]

[53]   Pizzocaro G, Zanoni F, Salvioni R, Milani A, Piva L, Pilotti S. Difficulties of a surveillance study omitting retroperitoneal lymphadenectomy in clinical stage I nonseminomatous germ cell tumors of the testis. J Urol 1987; 138(6): 1393-6.
[http://dx.doi.org/10.1016/S0022-5347(17)43652-4] [PMID: 2824862]

[54]   Cho J-H, Chang J-C, Park B-H, Lee JG, Son CH. Sonographic and MR imaging findings of testicular epidermoid cysts. AJR Am J Roentgenol 2002; 178(3): 743-8.
[http://dx.doi.org/10.2214/ajr.178.3.1780743] [PMID: 11856711]

[55]   Wallace TM, Levin HS. Mixed gonadal dysgenesis. A review of 15 patients reporting single cases of malignant intratubular germ cell neoplasia of the testis, endometrial adenocarcinoma, and a complex vascular anomaly. Arch Pathol Lab Med 1990; 114(7): 679-88.
[PMID: 2163601]

[56]   Trout AT, Chow J, McNamara ER, *et al.* Association between t lar microlithiasia and testicular neoplasia: large multicenter study in a pediatric population. Radiology 2017; 285(2): 576-83.
[http://dx.doi.org/10.1148/radiol.2017162625] [PMID: 28715257]

[57]   Heller HT, Oliff MC, Doubilet PM, O'Leary MP, Benson CB. Testicular microlithiasis: prevalence and association with primary testicular neoplasm. J Clin Ultrasound 2014; 42(7): 423-6.
[http://dx.doi.org/10.1002/jcu.22144] [PMID: 24585495]

[58]   Cooper ML, Kaefer M, Fan R, Rink RC, Jennings SG, Karmazyn B. Testicular microlithiasis in children and associated testicular cancer. Radiology 2014; 270(3): 857-63.
[http://dx.doi.org/10.1148/radiol.13130394] [PMID: 24475810]

[59]   van Casteren NJ, Looijenga LHJ, Dohle GR. Testicular microlithiasis and carcinoma *in situ* overview and proposed clinical guideline. Int J Androl 2009; 32(4): 279-87.
[http://dx.doi.org/10.1111/j.1365-2605.2008.00937.x] [PMID: 19207616]

[60]   Hadziselimović F, Hecker E, Herzog B. The value of testicular biopsy in cryptorchidism. Urol Res 1984; 12(3): 171-4.
[http://dx.doi.org/10.1007/BF00255917] [PMID: 6148798]

[61]   Cortes D, Thorup JM, Visfeldt J. Cryptorchidism: aspects of fertility and neoplasms. A study including data of 1,335 consecutive boys who underwent testicular biopsy simultaneously with surgery for cryptorchidism. Horm Res 2001; 55(1): 21-7.
[PMID: 11423738]

[62]   Heidenreich A, Moul JW. Contralateral testicular biopsy procedure in patients with unilateral testis cancer: is it indicated? Semin Urol Oncol 2002; 20(4): 234-8.
[http://dx.doi.org/10.1053/suro.2002.36980] [PMID: 12489055]

[63]   Kay R. Prepubertal Testicular Tumor Registry. J Urol 1993; 150(2 Pt 2): 671-4.
[http://dx.doi.org/10.1016/S0022-5347(17)35581-7] [PMID: 8392120]

[64]   Wu HY, Snyder HM. Advances in Pediatric Urologic Oncology. AUA Update Series XXII 2003.

[65]   Wold LE, Kramer SA, Farrow GM. Testicular yolk sac and embryonal carcinomas in pediatric patients: comparative immunohistochemical and clinicopathologic study. Am J Clin Pathol 1984; 81(4): 427-35.
[http://dx.doi.org/10.1093/ajcp/81.4.427] [PMID: 6367423]

[66]   Hayes-Lattin B, Nichols CR. Testicular cancer: a prototypic tumor of young adults. Semin Oncol 2009; 36(5): 432-8.
[http://dx.doi.org/10.1053/j.seminoncol.2009.07.006] [PMID: 19835738]

[67] Mann JR, Raafat F, Robinson K, *et al.* The United Kingdom Children's Cancer Study Group's second germ cell tumor study: carboplatin, etoposide, and bleomycin are effective treatment for children with malignant extracranial germ cell tumors, with acceptable toxicity. J Clin Oncol 2000; 18(22): 3809-18.
[http://dx.doi.org/10.1200/JCO.2000.18.22.3809] [PMID: 11078494]

[68] Rushton HG, Belman AB, Sesterhenn I, Patterson K, Mostofi FK. Testicular sparing surgery for prepubertal teratoma of the testis: a clinical and pathological study. J Urol 1990; 144(3): 726-30.
[http://dx.doi.org/10.1016/S0022-5347(17)39567-8] [PMID: 2388338]

[69] Shukla AR, Woodard C, Carr MC, *et al.* Experience with testis sparing surgery for testicular teratoma. J Urol 2004; 171(1): 161-3.
[http://dx.doi.org/10.1097/01.ju.0000101185.90327.b4] [PMID: 14665867]

[70] Marina NM, Cushing B, Giller R, *et al.* Complete surgical excision is effective treatment for children with immature teratomas with or without malignant elements: A Pediatric Oncology Group/Children's Cancer Group Intergroup Study. J Clin Oncol 1999; 17(7): 2137-43.
[http://dx.doi.org/10.1200/JCO.1999.17.7.2137] [PMID: 10561269]

[71] Mann JR, Gray ES, Thornton C, *et al.* Mature and immature extracranial teratomas in children: the UK Children's Cancer Study Group Experience. J Clin Oncol 2008; 26(21): 3590-7.
[http://dx.doi.org/10.1200/JCO.2008.16.0622] [PMID: 18541896]

[72] Batata MA, Whitmore WF Jr, Chu FC, *et al.* Cryptorchidism and testicular cancer. J Urol 1980; 124(3): 382-7.
[http://dx.doi.org/10.1016/S0022-5347(17)55458-0] [PMID: 6107388]

[73] Motzer RJ, Jonasch E, Agarwal N, *et al.* Testicular cancer. Version 2.2015. J Natl Compr Canc Netw 2015; 13(6): 772-99.
[http://dx.doi.org/10.6004/jnccn.2015.0092] [PMID: 26085393]

[74] Perry C, Servadio C. Seminoma in childhood. J Urol 1980; 124(6): 932-3.
[http://dx.doi.org/10.1016/S0022-5347(17)55740-7] [PMID: 6108374]

[75] Coppes MJ, Rackley R, Kay R. Primary testicular and paratesticular tumors of childhood. Med Pediatr Oncol 1994; 22(5): 329-40.
[http://dx.doi.org/10.1002/mpo.2950220506] [PMID: 8127257]

[76] Cheville JC, Sebo TJ, Lager DJ, Bostwick DG, Farrow GM. Leydig cell tumor of the testis: a clinicopathologic, DNA content, and MIB-1 comparison of nonmetastasizing and metastasizing tumors. Am J Surg Pathol 1998; 22(11): 1361-7.
[http://dx.doi.org/10.1097/00000478-199811000-00006] [PMID: 9808128]

[77] Jain M, Aiyer HM, Bajaj P, Dhar S. Intracytoplasmic and intranuclear Reinke's crystals in a testicular Leydig-cell tumor diagnosed by fine-needle aspiration cytology: a case report with review of the literature. Diagn Cytopathol 2001; 25(3): 162-4.
[http://dx.doi.org/10.1002/dc.2029] [PMID: 11536438]

[78] Henderson CG, Ahmed AA, Sesterhenn I, Belman AB, Rushton HG. Enucleation for prepubertal leydig cell tumor. J Urol 2006; 176(2): 703-5.
[http://dx.doi.org/10.1016/j.juro.2006.03.083] [PMID: 16813923]

[79] Shukla AR, Huff DS, Canning DA, *et al.* Juvenile granulosa cell tumor of the testis: contemporary clinical management and pathological diagnosis. J Urol 2004; 171(5): 1900-2.
[http://dx.doi.org/10.1097/01.ju.0000120223.29924.3b] [PMID: 15076304]

[80] Gabrilove JL, Freiberg EK, Leiter E, Nicolis GL. Feminizing and non-feminizing Sertoli cell tumors. J Urol 1980; 124(6): 757-67.
[http://dx.doi.org/10.1016/S0022-5347(17)55652-9] [PMID: 7003168]

[81] Gourlay WA, Johnson HW, Pantzar JT, McGillivray B, Crawford R, Nielsen WR. Gonadal tumors in disorders of sexual differentiation. Urology 1994; 43(4): 537-40.
[http://dx.doi.org/10.1016/0090-4295(94)90251-8] [PMID: 8154078]

[82]   Olsen MM, Caldamone AA, Jackson CL, Zinn A. Gonadoblastoma in infancy: indications for early gonadectomy in 46XY gonadal dysgenesis. J Pediatr Surg 1988; 23(3): 270-1.
[http://dx.doi.org/10.1016/S0022-3468(88)80738-3] [PMID: 3357146]

[83]   Cools M, Wolffenbuttel KP, Drop SLS, Oosterhuis JW, Looijenga LH. Gonadal development and tumor formation at the crossroads of male and female sex determination. Sex Dev 2011; 5(4): 167-80.
[http://dx.doi.org/10.1159/000329477] [PMID: 21791949]

[84]   Oltmann SC, Garcia N, Barber R, Huang R, Hicks B, Fischer A. Can we preoperatively risk stratify ovarian masses for malignancy? J Pediatr Surg 2010; 45(1): 130-4.
[http://dx.doi.org/10.1016/j.jpedsurg.2009.10.022] [PMID: 20105592]

[85]   Cho MJ, Kim DY, Kim SC. Ovarian cyst aspiration in the neonate: m mally invasive surgery. J Pediatr Adolesc Gynecol 2015; 28(5): 348-53.
[http://dx.doi.org/10.1016/j.jpag.2014.10.003] [PMID: 26148782]

[86]   Monnery-Noché ME, Auber F, Jouannic JM, *et al*. Fetal and neonatal ovarian cysts: is surgery indicated? Prenat Diagn 2008; 28(1): 15-20.
[http://dx.doi.org/10.1002/pd.1915] [PMID: 18186135]

[87]   Papic JC, Billmire DF, Rescorla FJ, Finnell SM, Leys CM. Management of neonatal ovarian cysts and its effect on ovarian preservation. J Pediatr Surg 2014; 49(6): 990-3.
[http://dx.doi.org/10.1016/j.jpedsurg.2014.01.040] [PMID: 24888849]

[88]   Kaefer M, Diamond D, Hendren WH, *et al*. The incidence of intersexuality in children with cryptorchidism and hypospadias: stratification based on gonadal palpability and meatal position. J Urol 1999; 162(3 Pt 2): 1003-6.
[http://dx.doi.org/10.1097/00005392-199909000-00010] [PMID: 10458421]

[89]   Huseman DA. The Genitalia Intersex. 4th ed., In: Gillenwater JY, Grayhack JT, Howards SS, Mitchell ME, eds. In: Gillenwater JY, Grayhack JT, Howards SS, Mitchell ME, Eds. Philadelphia: Lippincott Williams & Wilkins 2002.

[90]   Kim JH, Kang E, Heo SH, *et al*. Diagnostic yield of targeted gene panel sequencing to identify the genetic etiology of disorders of sex development. Mol Cell Endocrinol 2017; 444: 19-25.
[http://dx.doi.org/10.1016/j.mce.2017.01.037] [PMID: 28130116]

[91]   Ahmed SF, Bashamboo A, Lucas-Herald A, McElreavey K. Understanding the genetic aetiology in patients with XY DSD. Br Med Bull 2013; 106: 67-89.
[http://dx.doi.org/10.1093/bmb/ldt008] [PMID: 23529942]

[92]   Kremen J, Chan YM, Swartz JM. Recent findings on the genetics of disorders of sex development. Curr Opin Urol 2017; 27(1): 1-6.
[http://dx.doi.org/10.1097/MOU.0000000000000353] [PMID: 27798415]

[93]   Ahmed SF, Achermann JC, Arlt W, *et al*. Society for Endocrinology UK guidance on the initial evaluation of an infant or an adolescent with a suspected disorder of sex development (Revised 2015). Clin Endocrinol (Oxf) 2016; 84(5): 771-88.
[http://dx.doi.org/10.1111/cen.12857] [PMID: 26270788]

[94]   Diamond DA. Sexual differentiation: normal and abnormal. In: Walsh PC, Retik AB, Vaughn ED, Jr, Wein AJ, Eds. Campbell's Urology. 8th ed. Philadelphia: WB Saunders 2002; pp. 2395-427.

[95]   Meyer-Bahlburg HF. Gender assignment and reassignment in intersexuality: controversies, data, and guidelines for research. Adv Exp Med Biol 2002; 511: 199-223.
[http://dx.doi.org/10.1007/978-1-4615-0621-8_12] [PMID: 12575763]

CHAPTER 6

Pediatric Malignancy

Noor Al-Huda I. Khalaf[1], **Hiba A. Mirza**[1] and **Sultan M. Ghanim**[2,*]

[1] *6th Grade Medical College, Faculty of Medicine, University of Kufa, Iraq*

[2] *ME Unit, Medical College, Faculty of Medicine, University of Kufa, Iraq*

Abstract: Cancer is the second leading cause of death in children after trauma and accounts for approximately 11% of all pediatric deaths in the United States. In the western countries, leukemia, central nervous system (CNS) tumors, lymphomas, neuroblastomas and nephroblastomas account for most pediatric malignancies. Neuroblastoma and nephroblastoma are among the more common solid abdominal tumors. The prognoses for these cancers have improved after numerous multicentre trials. The following description will be restricted to the most commonly encountered tumors in children.

Keywords: Malignancy, Pediatric, Surgery.

RENAL TUMORS

Classification of Renal Tumors

Wilms tumor (favorable, unfavorable)
Renal cell carcinoma
Renal tumors associated with TFE3 or TFEB translocations
Clear cell sarcoma
Malignant rhabdoid tumor of the kidney
Renal cell sarcoma
Renal adenocarcinoma
Ossifying renal tumor of infancy
Renal medullary carcinoma
Renal neurogenic tumor
Renal teratoma Metanephric tumor (adenoma, stromal tumor, adenofibroma)
Mesoblastic nephroma
Angiolipoma
Cystic nephroma or partially cystic nephroma
Diffuse hyperblastic perilobar nephroblastomatosis
Nephrogenic rest

* **Corresponding author Sultan M. Ghanim:** ME Unit, Medical College, Faculty of Medicine, University of Kufa, Iraq; Tel: +9647816669997; E-mail: sultanmalsaadi@uokufa.edu.iq

Sultan M. Ghanim, Najah R. Hadi and Nada Al-Haris (Eds.)

Wilms Tumor

Renal tumor arising from pluripotent embryonic renal precursor cells, most are diagnosed between 1 and 5 years with the peak incidence at age 3. Tumors tend to occur earlier in malethan female. WT incidence decreases over the age of 10 and is less common under 6 months of age. Bilateral Wilms tumors (BWT) occur in 4–13% of patients [1, 2].

Metastasis of Nephroblastoma

In 5% of cases, the nephroblastoma is bilateral. Metastasis mostly occurs in regional lymph nodes and lungs. Typically; blastema is present in the tumor, consisting of clusters of cells with hyperchromatic ovoid nuclei. Within the blastema, different structures can be observed, including rosettes, tubules, and pseudo-glomerular structures (Fig. **6.1**) [3].

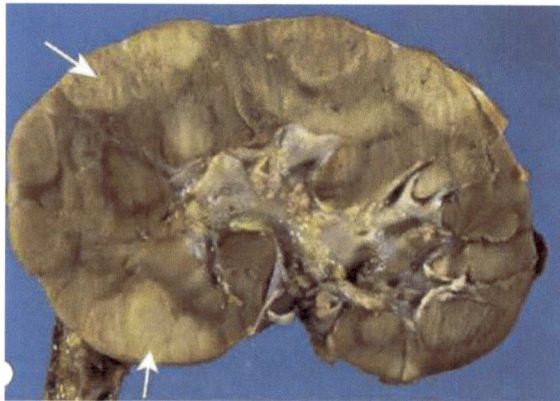

Fig. (6.1). A resected kidney with a similar pattern of DHPLN reveals extensive involvement of the periphery of the cortex by severely hypertrophied nephrogenic rests (arrows). Resection of such kidneys should be avoided because, in most cases, the hypertrophy will resolve and the kidney will have excellent preservation of its function.

Causes of Nephroblastoma

The most often cited genetic anomalies in Wilms tumor involve chromosomal loci 11p13 (WT1) and 11p15 (WT2). Other factors influencing tumor development are the loss of heterozygosity and genomic imprinting (Fig. **6.2**). Nephrogenesis in the normal kidney is usually complete by 34 to 36 weeks' gestation. The presence of nephrogenic rests (NRs; persistent metanephric tissue in the kidney after the 36th week of gestation) has been associated with the occurrence of WT [5]. NR are considered precursor lesions to WT. However, only a small number develop clonal transformation resulting in the development of WT. The presence of multiple or diffuse NRs is termed nephroblastomatosis [6].

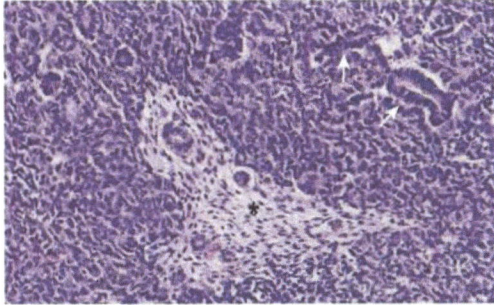

Fig. (6.2). The classic "triphasic" histologic pattern (blastemal, epithelial, and mesenchymal derivatives) of a Wilms tumor is seen on this H&E slide. There is a predominance of small undifferentiated blastemal cells in the image that surround a few neoplastic ducts and tubular epithelial structures (solid arrows). In the center is an island (asterisk) of spindle-shaped fibroblastic mesenchymal cells that surround a few tubules. The neoplastic cells in the image lack the requisite features of an anaplastic variant.

Associated with Multiple Genetic Syndromes (10% of all WT Cases)

1. Beckwith–Wiedemann syndrome (visceromegaly, macroglossia, omphalocele, hyperinsulinemic hypoglycemia).
2. WAGR syndrome (WT with aniridia, genitourinary malformations, and mental retardation).
3. Denys–Drash syndrome (nephropathy, renal failure, male pseudoher-maphroditism, and WT).
4. Sporadic aniridia.
5. Isolated hemihypertrophy.
6. Genital anomalies.
7. Simpson-Golabi-Behmel syndrome (General overgrowth in height and weight with characteristic facial features) [7, 8].

The differential diagnosis for a malignant abdominal mass in a child includes:

- WT
- Neuroblastoma
- Hepatoblastoma
- Rhabdomyosarcoma
- lymphoma

Clinical Presentation of Wilms' Tumor

Symptoms;

- History of asymptomatic painless abdominal mass 85% of cases (discovered by a parent while bathing or dressing the child)

- Hematuria (33%)
- Fever
- Weight loss
- Nausea or vomiting
- Lethargy and fatigue

Signs;

- Abdominal mass painless palpable firm fixed most do not cross the midline. At friable tumor caution when palpitating abdomen tumor may rupture.
- Hypertension in 20%; Hypertension occurs as a result of either renin secretion by tumor cells or compression of the renal vasculature by the tumor.
- Pallor.
- Varicocele or inguinal hernia.
- Abdominal vein distended.
- Potential stigmata of genetic syndrome [9].

Diagnosis of Wilms' Tumor

• Ct Scan of the Chest and Abdomen

Characterize the mass, identify the presence of metastases, provide information on the opposite kidney and indicate the presence of nephrogenic rests, which are precursor lesions to Wilms' tumor (Figs. **6.3** and **6.4**).

• Abdominal US

Screening study for an abdominal mass to determine its site of origin and assess for possible intravascular or ureteral extension [10]

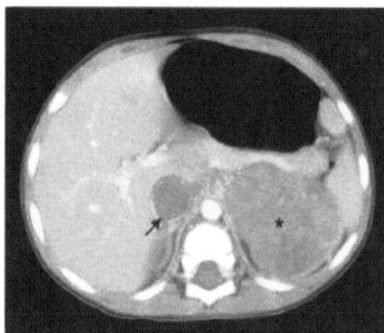

Fig. (6.3). A transverse cut of a CT scan demonstrating a left Wilms tumor (asterisk) that extends into the inferior vena cava (arrow).

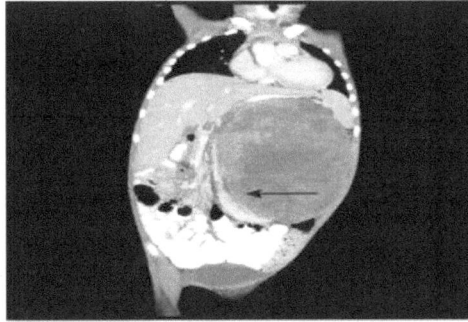

Fig. (6.4). CT scan of a 4-year-old boy found on routine physical examination demonstrating a very large left renal tumor and the classic "claw sign" of a Wilms tumor that occurs with extension of the thin lip of renal parenchyma (arrow) over the tumor.

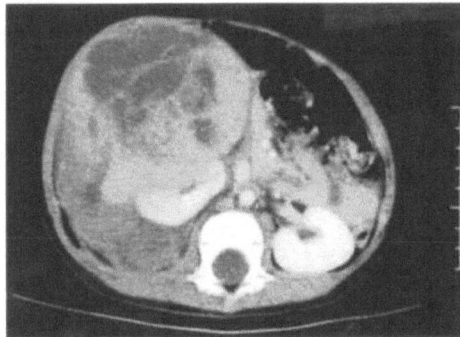

Fig. (6.5). CT scan of a 3-year-old boy who presented with a history of abdominal pain, fever, and a right flank mass. The tumor is very large, with extension outside the renal capsule into the retroperitoneal tissues posterior to the kidney. Despite its size, this lesion was able to be completely resected. Lymph nodes and specimen margins were negative for tumor. This tumor was therefore stage II, and the infant was able to avoid both anthracycline therapy and abdominal irradiation because of the complete resection.

Staging of Wilms Tumor According to the National Wilms Tumor Study Group (NWT) [11]

Table 6.1. Staging Criteria COG STAGING SYSTEM.

Stage	Criteria
I	The tumor is limited to the kidney and has been completely resected. The tumor was not ruptured, nor was biopsy performed prior to removal No penetration of the renal capsule or involvement of renal sinus vessels
II	The tumor extends beyond the capsule of the kidney but was completely resected with no evidence of tumor at or beyond the margins of resection There is penetration of the renal capsule or invasion of the renal sinus vessels

Stage	Criteria
III	. Gross or microscopic residual tumor remains postoperatively, including in operable tumor, positive surgical margins, tumor spillage, regional lymph node metastases, positive peritoneal cytology, or transected tumor thrombus. The tumor was ruptured or biopsied prior to removal.
IV	IIIIV Hematogenous metastases or lymph node metastases are present outside the abdomen (*e.g.*, lung, liver, bone, brain).
V	Bilateral renal involvement is present at diagnosis, and each side may be considered to have a "local" stage.

Treatment

Radical resection (nephroureterectomy) of affected kidney with evaluation for staging, followed by chemotherapy (low stages) and radiation (higher stages). The goal of surgery is complete removal of the tumor. It is crucial to avoid tumor rupture or injury to contiguous organs [14].

Preoperative Chemotherapy

1-Extension of tumor thrombus into the IVC that extends to the level of the hepatic veins, and tumor that extends above the level of the hepatic veins
2-Tumor involves contiguous structures
3-Bilateral tumors
4-Tumor in a solitary kidney
5-Pulmonary compromise due to extensive pulmonary metastases [12, 13].

Prognosis is very good. The 5-year survival rate is 80%; for stage I patients, it is even higher at 90%.

Prognostic factors: Tumor size, Grade of the tumor as anaplasia confers an unfavorable prognosis, older age is associated with poorer prognosis. And Lymph node involvement is associated with poorer prognosis [15].

Follow-Up

For follow-up surveillance, abdominal sonography is a suitable method as it avoids further exposure to radiation. During treatment, it is important to be aware of the possible presence of sinusoidal obstruction syndrome (formerly called veno- occlusive disease) affecting the small hepatic veins. It is a common side effect of the cytostatic drug actinomycin D, which represents the key substance in chemotherapy for wilms [16].

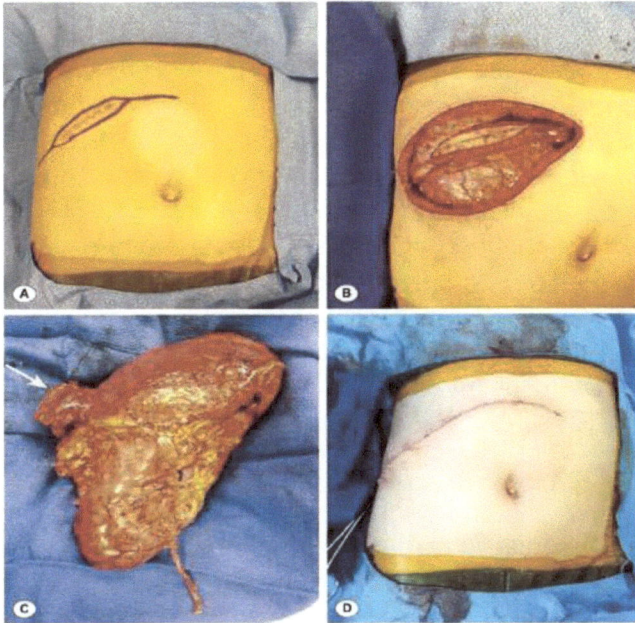

Fig. (6.6). This young child presented with a very large right-sided Wilms tumor that measured more than 15 cm in greatest diameter. An open biopsy was initially performed due to the concern about tumor spill with attempted resection. At the second operation, the previous incision has been outlined in (A). It is important to remove the previous incision down to the tumor to prevent seeding the second incision with tumor. In (B) the previous incision and tract remains attached to the underlying kidney. In (C) the resected specimen is seen. Note the initial incision and tract (arrow) are attached to the specimen. In (D) the incision following the second operation has been closed.

Neonatal Wilms Tumor

Rare and include benign and malignant tumors. It accounts for greater than 50% of the renal tumors. After 3 months of age, it accounts for less than 10%. Renal tumors in children less than 7 months of age found that 63.4% were WT. Eighty-two per cent of these were stage I/II. In contrast, RTK presented with advanced disease (53% stage III/IV). Outcomes paralleled older children with excellent results for neonates with WT (5-year OS of 93.4%) and poor outcome for RTK (5-year OS of 16.4%) [1, 17].

Extrarenal Wilms Tumor

An extrarenal site of primary WT is uncommon. These extrarenal tumors be have identically to tumor arising within the kidney and should be treated both locally and systematically base on the same criteria, common sites of occurrence of extrarenal WT include the retroperitoneum, inguinal canal, scrotum, and vagina. Less common sites are the uterus, cervix, ovary, and the presacral space [19, 20].

Renal Cell Carcinoma

Children with RCC are generally older than those with WT. The mean age at presentation with RCC was 14 years. Clinical stage at the time of diagnosis and complete tumor resection were meaningful prognostic factors. Radical nephrectomy and regional lymphadenectomy have been the primary modality for cure, and children with distant spread have a grave prognosis. Overall survival was much worse than for WT, with a five-year survival of only 30%. Survival was 60% in children with complete resection of the primary tumor and zero in those with only partial resection. Survival was also stage dependent: 92.5% for stage I 84.5% for stage II, 72.7%for stage III, and12.7%for stage IV. RCC is remarkably resistant to chemotherapy, preventing cure in most children with metastatic disease [21].

Neuroblastoma

Third most common pediatric malignancy, small blue round cell tumor (SBRCT) an Embryonal tumor originating from primitive neural crest cells. Neuroblastomas belong to a group of tumors classified as the small round blue cell" tumors (Fig. **6.7**). Others in this category include Ewing's sarcoma, non-Hodgkin's lymphoma, primitive neuroectodermal tumors (PNETs) and undifferentiated soft tissue sarcomas such as rhabdomyosarcoma, these +ve for neuron specific enolase. Patients have advanced disease at the time of presentation unlike Wilms' tumor.

Neuroblastoma may cross the midline, but Wilm'stumours do so only rarely [22].

Anatomical Site

Adrenal gland (50% cases)

Paraaortic abdominal paraspinal ganglia—25%

Posterior mediastinum —20%

Neck— 1%

Pelvis— 4% (organ of zuckerkandel) [23]

Incidence

90% of cases: < 5 year

97% are diagnosed by 10 years

Median age at diagnosis: 22 months

15% cancer-related deaths in children

Neuroblastoma is a heterogeneous disease. Tumors can spontaneously regress or mature, or display a very aggressive, malignant phenotype. The cause is unknown, but association with: Hirschsprung disease, Neurofibromatosis, Beckwith-Wiedemann syndromecongenital central hypoventilation syndrome (Ondine curse) and pheochromocytoma [24]. Metastatic extension occurs in lymphatic and hematogenous patterns. Only rarely does neuroblastoma metastasize to lung or brain, spinal cord, heart and these are usually manifestations of end-stage disease. The clinical presentation depends on the site of the primary and the presence of metastases.

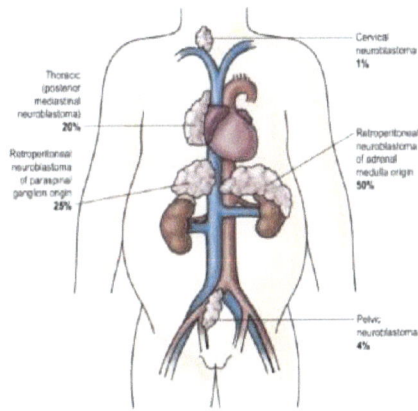

Fig. (6.7). Primary sites for neuroblastoma is depicted in this anatomic drawing (Reprinted from Davidoff AM. Neuroblastoma, in: Oldham KT, Colombani PM, Foglia RP, *et al*, editors, Principles and Practice of Pediatric Surgery. Philadelphia: Lippincott Williams & Wilkins; 2005).

Presentation

Symptomatic Abdominal Mass Constitutional symptoms (Lethargy, Weakness, Irritability, Weight-loss, pain).

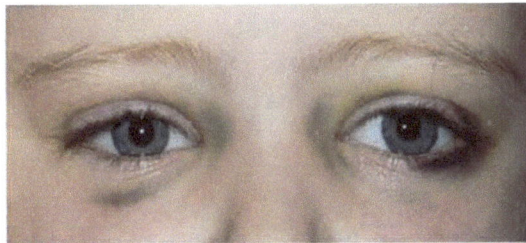

Fig. (6.8). Clinical evidence of metastatic neuroblastoma. "Raccoon eyes," characteristic of metastatic neuroblastoma in the posterior orbital venous plexus, are seen in a child with stage 4 disease.

Signs

- Asymptomatic abdominal mass (palpable in 50% of cases)
- Respiratory distress or dysphagia (mediastinal tumors)
- Altered defecation or urination (pelvic or paraspinal tumors)
- Altered gait (paraspinaltumors)
- Horner's syndrome (upper chest or neck tumors)
- HTN (20%–35%)
- Opsomyoclonus (Kinsbourne syndrome/dancing eyes and dancing feet)
- Secretory diarrhea; excessive secretion of catecholamine or vasoactive intestinal peptide by the tumor.

More than 40% of patients have metastatic disease at diagnosis.

- Limp (Hutchinson syndrome)
- Hepatomegaly (Pepper syndrome)
- Raccoon eyes (retroorbital venous plexus spread) (Fig. **6.8**)
- Distant lymph node enlargement
- Palpable non tender subcutaneous bluish nodules (infants with stage IVS tumors) [25, 26]

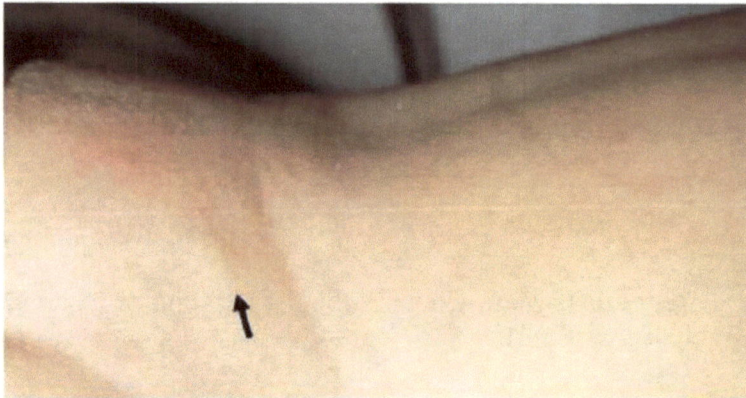

Fig. (6.9). "Blueberry muffin" spot (arrow) in the skin, characteristic of metastatic neuroblastoma, is seen in the suprapubic region of an infant with a 4S neuroblastoma (Courtesy Stephen Shochat, MD, St, Jude Children's Research Hospital, and Memphis, TN).

Histopathological Classification

Shimada and colleagues first developed an age linked classification system of neuroblastic tumors based on tumor morphology in which neuroblastomas were divided into two prognostic subgroups, favorable histology and unfavorable histology, Additional factors that contribute to the prognostic distinction include the MKI, which is defined as the number of tumor cells in mitosis or karyorrhexis per 5000 neuroblastic cells (*i.e.*, low MKI, <100 cells; intermediate, 100–200 cells; high > 200 cells), and the patient's age (<1.5 years, 1.55 years, >5 years). The INPC is based mainly on morphologic changes associated with the maturational sequence of neuroblastic tumors. The INPC classifies neuroblastic tumors into three morphologic categories (Fig. **6.9**):

- neuroblastoma
- ganglioneuroblastoma
- ganglioneuroma

Add independent prognostic information beyond the prognostic contribution of age. This particularly important in patients with MYCN non amplified tumors who are older than 18 months and have stage 3 disease, or 12 to 18 months of age and have stage 4 disease, or have 4S disease. Ganglioneuroblastomas contain cells that are transitioning toward differentiation but are not completely differentiated / mature. Also, <50% of the total volume is made up of neuroblastic cells. Divided into 'intermixed' and 'nodular' subtypes (worse prognosis), depending on the distribution of the neuroblastic cells. Neuroblastomas are, by definition, Schwannianstroma poor (<50% of the tumor tissue) and can be sub typed as undifferentiated, poorly differentiated, or differentiating. Undifferentiated requires supplemental diagnostic methods such as immune histochemistry, electron microscopy, orcytogenetics. Moreover, neuropil is not present. In poorly differentiated, <5% of tumor cells have features of differentiation, and neuropil is present. Differentiating tumors demonstrate >5% of tumor cells differentiating toward ganglion cells [27, 28].

Laboratory finding

Elevated urinary catecholamines (24hr estimation): Vanillylmandelic acid (VMA) and Homovanillic acid (HVA**),** is of clinical value in diagnosing neuroblastoma and determining the response to therapy. And markers of tumor progression or relapse and serve as a surrogate prognostic indicator. Elevated levels of serum catecholamines: (dopamine, norepinephrine). CBC with differential: signs of marrow infiltration. Lactate Dehydrogenase; lack of specificity, great prognostic significance, high serum levels reflect high proliferative activity or a large tumor burden, LDH level higher than 1500 IU/L appears to be associated with a poor prognosis. Monitor disease activity or the response to therapy, Ferritin elevation, serumferritin (>150ng/mL) reflect a large tumor burdenor rapid tumor progression, indicates a poor prognosis. Levels often return to normal during clinical remission. N-myc oncogene and DNA ploidy; myc oncogene associated with neuroblastoma [29].

Radiology Findings

MRI scan of primary tumor examine extent of disease. CT of chest, abdomen, pelvis stage disease and Bone scan look for metastasis (Fig. **6.10**).

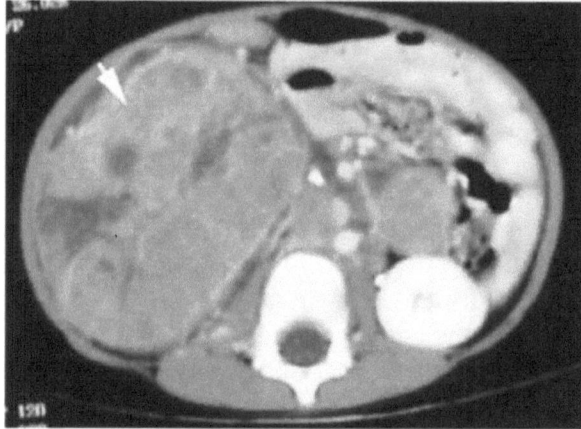

Fig. (6.10). Abdominal neuroblastoma arising from the right retroperitoneum (arrow).

Metaiodobenzylguanidine (MBIG) Scan, Injected with MIBG radionuclide, isotope preferentially taken up in catecholamine-producing cells. 90% neuroblastoma cells take up isotope. Diagnosis is confirmed by biopsy, Evaluation of histology, Presence of n-myc amplification and Bone marrow biopsy for staging. The minimum criterion for a diagnosis of neuroblastoma is based on one of the following: an unequivocal pathologic diagnosis made from tumor tissue by light microscopy (with or without immunohistology, electron microscopy, or increased levels of serum catecholamines or urinary catecholamine metabolites) and the combination of bone marrow aspirate or biopsy containing unequivocal tumor cells and increased levels of serum catecholamines or urinary catecholamine metabolites as described earlier [30, 31].

Risk Determination

Stage (I: localized, IV: disseminated)

Histology

- n-myc amplification associated with aggressive disease.
- DNA ploidy of tumor.
- Chromosomal alterations.
- Age of patient

Favorable Prognosis

Age < 1 year.

Localized primary tumor: stage I or II.

Metastases limited to skin, liver, and bone marrow.

No poor prognostic indicators [33].

Treatment

Principal goal of surgery is to obtain at least 95% resection without compromising major structures, it includes Resection ± chemotherapy ± XRT.

High-risk Patients

Treat aggressively with Intensive chemotherapy, surgical resection, autologous stem cell transplant, Radiation, Immunotherapy [35].

Low-risk Patients

Surgical resection, less intensive chemotherapy, Observation.only when less than 50% of the tumor was resected or when symptoms developed that were life- or organ-threatening [34].

Table (6.2). International neuroblastoma staging system criteria [32].

Stage	Definition
1	Localized tumor with complete gross excision, with or without microscopic residual disease; representative ipsilateral lymph nodes negative for tumor microscopically (nodes attached to and removed with the primary tumor may be positive)
2A	Localized tumor with incomplete gross excision; representative ipsilateral nonadherent lymph nodes negative for tumor microscopically
2B	Localized tumor with or without complete gross excision, with ipsilateral nonadherent lymph nodes positive for tumor. Enlarged contralateral lymph nodes must be negative microscopically
3	Unresectable unilateral tumor infiltrating across the midline,* with or without regional lymph node involvement or Localized unilateral tumor with contralateral regional lymph node involvement or Midline tumor with bilateral extension by infiltration (unresectable) or by lymph node involvement
4	Any primary tumor with dissemination to distant lymph nodes, bone, bone marrow, liver, skin, or other organs (except as defined for stage 4S)
4S	Localized primary tumor (as defined for stage 1, 2A, or 2B), with dissemination limited to skin, liver, and bone marrow' (limited to infants younger than 1 year old)

*The midline is defined as the vertebral column. Tumors originating on one side and crossing the midline must infiltrate to or beyond the opposite side of the vertebral column 'Marrow involvement in stage 4S should be minimal (*i.e.*, <10% of total nucleated cells identified as malignant on bone marrow biopsy or on marrow aspirate). More extensive marrow involvement would be considered to be stage 4. The metaiodoberuylguanidine scan (if performed) should be negative in the marrow.

Stage 4S Neuroblastoma

Infant patient who typically had a single, small primary tumor, but had extensive metastatic disease in the liver, skin nodules ('blue berry muffin 'lesions), and small amounts of disease in the bone marrow (<10% of the mononuclear cells). Spontaneous regression and the good prognosis. Most of these patients are assigned to the low risk classification, and have a tumor with favorable biology (single copy MYCN, favorable Shimada histology, and DNA index>1). Limited chemotherapy, local irradiation, or minimal resection can be used to treat infants with life threatening symptoms of hepatomegaly. The rare infant with 4S disease and either unfavorable Shimada histology or a DNA index of 1 (or if the biology is not known) will be treated as intermediate risk disease. Those with 4S disease that is MYCN amplified will be treated as high risk disease [36].

Rhabdomyosarcoma

Primitive soft tissue tumor that arises from mesenchymal tissues and most common soft tissue sarcoma that accounting for 5% of all childhood cancers, it is the third most common pediatric extracranial solid tumor after Wilms tumor and neuroblastoma. Most cases of RMS are sporadic but have been associated with certain familial syndromes, such as neurofibromatosis type 1 (NF1) and Li-Fraumeni syndrome (other syndromes associated with RMS include Beck with wiedemann, Noonan, Costello, and hereditary retinoblastoma). The use of marijuana or cocaine during pregnancy has been linked to the development of RMS. Bimodal age of distribution with peak incidence is between 3-5 years and again at 12-18, but these tumor shave also been found inneonates, the male to female is 1·5: 1. Most common sites are Head and neck (36%), GU tract (2%) are ERMS. Extremities (19%) and trunk (9%) are ARMS which is more aggressive type [37].

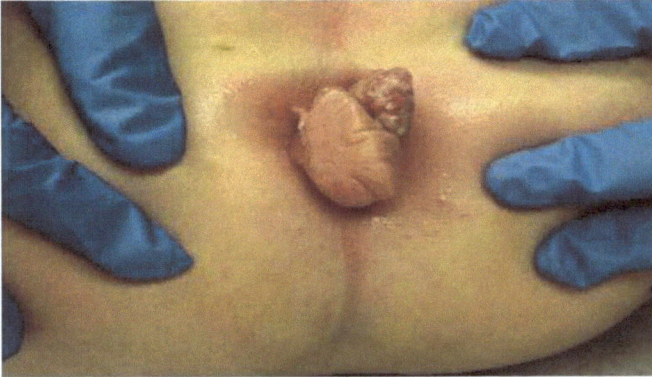

Fig. (6.11). Perianal rhabdomyosarcoma is seen in this young child.

Rhabdomyosarcoma is a small round blue cell tumor and must be distinguished from other common blue cell tumors of childhood (Fig. **6.11**). The hallmark of diagnosis is the presence of malignant skeletal muscle on histological examination. 25% of newly diagnosed cases have distant metastases with the lung being the most frequent site [38].

Clinical presentation of the tumor depends on the site of origin: asymptomatic Mass or signs and symptoms secondary to mass effect on adjacent structures and complications due to compression [39].

Diagnosis made by biopsy after evaluation by MRI (confirmed), CT scan of the affected area and the chest and bone marrow biopsy (Fig. **6.12**) [40].

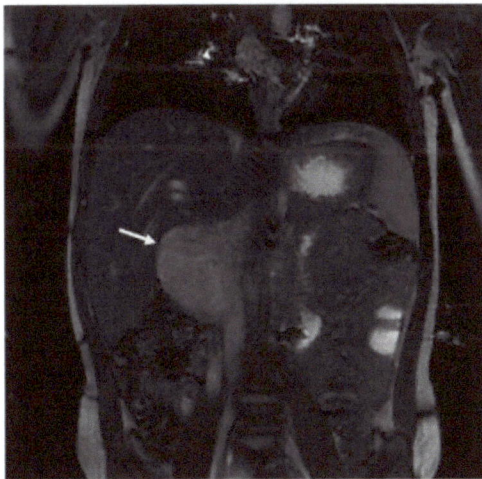

Fig. (6.12). MRI of patient with hepatobiliary embryonal rhabdomyosarcoma (arrow).

Table 6.3. Staging of rhabdomyosarcoma (TNM staging system).

Stage	Site	T	SIZE	N	M
1	Orbit, nonparameningeal head and neck, genitourinary (other than kidney, bladder, and prostate) and biliary	T1 OR T2	a or b	Any N	M0
2	Bladder\prostate, extremity, cranial parameningeal, others.	T1 OR T2	a	N0 or NX	M0
3	Bladder\prostate, extremity, cranial parameningeal, others.	T1 OR T2	a	N1	M0
			b	Any N	M0
4	All	T1 OR T2	a or b	Any N	M1

T1 = tumor confined to anatomic site of origin; T2 = tumor extension and/or fixed to surrounding tissues; a = ≤5 cm; b = >5 cm; N0 = regional nodes not clinically involved; N1 = regional nodes clinically involved; NX = regional node status unknown; M0 = no distant metastasis; M1 = metastasis present.
Clinical group:
Group 1: Localized disease, completely resected, no regional lymph node involvement.
Group 2: Localized disease, gross total resection but microscopic residual disease; or regional lymph nodes involved.
Group 3: Localized disease with gross residual disease after incomplete resection or biopsy only.
Group 4: Metastatic disease at diagnosis.

Treatment

If Resectable, do Surgical excision, ± chemotherapy and radiation therapy. if Unresectable give· him\her neoadjuvant chemo/XRT, then surgical excision. Radiation therapy benefit patients with group I tumors with alveolar or undifferentiated histology [41].

Site Specific Surgical Guidelines

In Head/Neck Tumors

Non parameningeal orbital and other head and neck RMS tumors are considered favorable sites and are classified as stage 1, regardless of size or nodal status. Operative management for orbital and other head and neck RMS tumors is largely restricted to biopsy followed by adjuvant chemotherapy and RT. Parameningeal tumors have slightly worse prognosis due to the presence of abundant lymphatics and a delay in diagnosis because of the hidden tumor.Metastatic disease to regional nodes is present in <3% of cases.An operative approach maybe justified with recurrent disease, and when there is evidence of persistent disease after adjuvant therapy [42].

TUMOR OF THE EXTREMITIES

Constitutes 15–20% of all pediatric RMS, Median age of 6 years, an unfavorable site, and 71% have alveolar histology. A high rate of regional lymph node involvement is found with extremity RMS.Initial staging of extremity RMS begins at stage 2 based on size, nodal involvement and metastasis. Evaluation of extremity RMS starts with; careful physical examination, CT to evaluate for bony erosion, MRI to determine tumor size and involvement of surrounding structures, FDG-PET is also helpful for clinically negative nodes or distant metastases that are equivocal by conventional CT or MRI.The operative goal for primary extremity tumors <5cm is to obtain circumferential disease-free margins while preserving form and function. After intensive multi agent chemotherapy and possibly RT, a second-look operation can be planned to resect residual disease. a 5mm circumference margin is currently recommended. Removal of tumor in a piecemeal fashion is considered group II even if the surgeon is confident all tumor is removed. For patients with larger tumors, or those in unfavorable anatomic sites involving neurovascular beds, an initial incisional biopsy is recommended. Definitive diagnosis and adequate tissue for biological studies is best obtained with an incisional biopsy rather than fine-needle or cone biopsies. Survival with multimodality therapy now approaches 75%, witha significantly lower rate for patients with nodal disease. Extremity RMS with microscopically positive or indeterminant margins, or after an initial resection was performed for presumed benign disease, PRE is recommended and has been shown to improve survival [43, 44].

Genitourinary Tumors

Accounted for 12% of all patients and >30% of nonmetastatic tumor patients. Bladder/prostate genitourinary primary tumors were most common.

Bladder/Prostate Tumors

RMS of the bladder and prostate occur in 2% and 4%, respectively.Ultrasound is usually performed at initial diagnosis, and serial CT or MRI are used to track the efficacy of primary chemotherapy.The initial operative approach is usually limited to biopsy, which can usually be obtained using endoscopy.Pelvic and retropertoneal lymph nodes also should be sampled for disease in these patients. Aggressive initial resection was performed with good local control rates, but with significant morbidity and low bladder salvage rates. Bladder salvage is now the primary goal in these patients.Complete resection may be feasible when the primary tumor involves only the dome of the bladder.Most bladder and prostate tumors are treated with chemotherapy and RT, followed by a more limited and conservative resection. More aggressive tumor resection including anterior or total pelvic exenteration. may be indicated to achieve local control if the tumor fails to respond to primary chemotherapy. The rate of exenterative cystectomy with current treatment is approximately 30%. Many patients will develop bladder dysfunction even with bladder salvage [45].

Vagina, Vulva, or Uterus, favorable site tumor. They have a 5-year OS>80% Comprise 3.5% all RMS tumors with half originating in the vagina. They are typically embryonal or botryoid histologic subtype and lymph node involvement is uncommon. Management begins with a biopsy, often transvaginally, and relies on effective chemotherapy as primary treatment. There is no role for initial aggressive resection such as vaginectomy or hysterectomy. Some physicians recommend avoidance of RT in group II and III vaginal RMS in patients <24 months old due to the high morbidity associated with external beam radiation. Followed with routine abdominal and pelvic MRI to document tumor response. A second-look operation with cystoscopy and re-biopsy is common. Relapsed or persistent disease is associated with a very poor outcome [46].

Paratesticular Tumors

Favorable site, with all paratesticular patients classified preoperatively as having stage 1 disease radical orchiectomy with proximal ligation of the spermatic cord at the internal inguinal ring *via* an inguinal incision is the recommended initial operative approach for para-testicular tumors. A trans-scrotal incision for biopsy or resection is contraindicated. If done, a subsequent hemiscrotectomy may be required to resect the contaminated tumor bed. Hemiscrotectomy is indicated when paratesticular tumors are fixed to the scrotal skin or invade the overlying scrotal skin. Paratesticular RMS has a high incidence (~30%) of spread to the retroperitoneal lymph nodes (RPLNs). All patients should have thin-cut (3.8–5.0mm) abdominal and pelvic CT scans to assess the retroperitoneum. The treatment guide lines vary by age since the outcome and the frequency of RPLN positivity with paratesticular RMS is partially age dependent. For patients younger than 10 years who are clinical group I, and do not have lymph node enlargement on CT scan, RPLN dissection or sampling is not recommended. These patients are followed with CT scans every 3 months. Suggestive or positive CT scans should prompt ipsilateral retroperitoneal node dissection with further therapy depending on the histologic findings. For all patients 10 years or older, or with tumor >5 cm, ipsilateral RPLN dissection is recommended up to the level of the renal hilum. Positive suprarenal nodes are considered metastatic. Thus, patients are considered group IV. A systematic approach is used to remove lymph nodes from the internal inguinal ring, along the iliac vessels and aorta, up to the renal hilum. RPLN dissection is associated with significant morbidity, including loss of ejaculatory function and lower extremity lymphedema [47].

Other Sites

Thorax, abdomen, pelvis, and perineum were found in only 12% of all IRS-IV patients. Truncal RMS tumors usually have an alveolar subtype. Primary resection is preferred in truncal tumors <5 cm when a negative operative margin can be realistically anticipated. For larger primary tumors, initial incisional biopsy is preferred. And postoperative reconstructive procedures may be necessary. Retroperitoneal and nongenitourinary pelvic tumors can be difficult to manage because of their relatively hidden location and subsequent late presentation. More than 90% present with large invasive tumors as clinical group III or IV. These patients generally undergo initial biopsy, aggressive multiple-agent chemotherapy, RT, and second-look operation, if indicated. Biliary RMS generally has a good prognosis without the need for aggressive resection. Most patients have botryoid RMS that responds well to chemotherapy. Biopsy followed by neoadjuvant chemotherapy frequently results in resolution of symptoms, including jaundice. Operative intervention is fraught with complications, including the inability to resect all disease in most cases and infections associated with external biliary drains. Perineal and perianal RMSs also are sites that have an overall poor outcome partially due to late presentation. More than one-third of patients are seen initially with presumed benign disease (usually infections). Improved survival is associated with tumors <5 cm, low clinical group and stage, negative nodes, and age younger than 10 years. Outcomes are not related to the tumor histology in this site. PRE frequently lowers the clinical group assignment, which improves outcome [48, 49].

Prognosis

Factors (site of origin, resectability, presence of metastases, number of metastatic sites, and histopathology.)Favorable characteristics include age <10 years at diagnosis, tumor size less 5 cm, embryonal fusion-negative tumor, orbit and nonparameningeal head/ neck primary, tumor completely excised prior to initiation of chemotherapy, and the lack of metastatic disease at diagnosis.HIPEC is a New strategy are being used to increase OS for patients with metastatic RMS and peritoneal sarcomatosis. Use in addition to chemotherapy and RT as a salvage therapy to improve the outcomes of these patients with advanced local disease. A recent report showed that HIPEC may offer improved OS in patients with complete cytoreduction [50].

Malignant Hepatic Tumors

Malignant liver neoplasms account for 1% of all pediatric malignancies and are the third most common intra-abdominal neoplasm after neuroblastoma and nephroblastoma. The two primary malignant neoplasms of the liver are hepatoblastoma and hepatocellular carcinoma. Survival has significantly improved for hepatoblastoma with the advent of new chemotherapy protocols and advances in liver surgery. The prognosis for hepatocellular carcinoma remains poor. Complete resection is required for cure.

Epidemiology

Most HBs present before the age of 3 years, with a median age of 18 months[51]. Approximately 4% of HBs are present at birth, 69% are present before age 3, and 90% develop before the age of 5 years. Only 3% of cases manifest in children older than 15 years. There is a male predominance of 1.7:1. 154 HBs are associated with a variety of clinical conditions, syndromes, and malformations (Box **6.2**). Beckwith–Wiedemann syndrome (BWS) is an overgrowth syndrome resulting in gigantism, macroglossia, omphalocele, hemihypertrophy, and neonatal hypoglycemia. Though BWS is associated with Wilms tumor, it is also linked to other tumors such as hepatoblastomas, gonadoblastomas, and adrenal carcinomas [54]. For children with BWS, ages 0–4 years, the rate of HB is elevated, and some protocols advocate serial AFP levels and an abdominal US every 3 months until the age of 4 years. However, there still is debate regarding the utility of such screening programs. Chromosomal abnormalities also have been documented in patients with HB. The most common defects are trisomy of chromosomes 2, 8, 18, or 20, individually or in combination. An accurate rate of HB in infants with trisomy 18 has not been determined since survival beyond 1 year is rare. Epidemiologic studies have revealed several factors associated with an increased risk for the development of neonatal HB, including: birth weight less than 1000 g, maternal age younger than 20 years, use of infertility treatment, maternal smoking and a higher pre-pregnancy body mass index (BMI of 25–29) (Box **6.2**).

Box 6.2. Conditions associated with hepatoblastoma.

Beckwith-wiedmann syndrome
Budd-Chiari syndrome
Gardner syndrome
Hemihypertrophy
Heterozygous alpha-1-antitrypsin deficiency
Isosexual precocity
Polyposis coli families
Triosomy 18
Type 1A glycogen storage disease
Very low birth weight

Biology and Cytogenetics

HB is thought to arise from unregulated proliferation of primary hepatoblasts and hepatic stem cells or human fetal liver multipotent progenitor cells (hHLMPCs). These hepatic precursor cells have potential for both proliferation and differentiation, which may in part explain the spectrum of histologic subtypes that characterizes HB. The development of HB is linked to dysregulation of the Wnt/β-catenin signaling pathway. The Wnt pathway mutations make up approximately 90% of genetic defects in HB tumors. Normally functioning Wnt/β-catenin signaling plays a critical role in embryonic development, including cell proliferation, migration, and fate determination, as well as body axis determination and organ system development. Most mutations associated with HB are the result of deletions or missense point mutations in exon 3 of CTNNB1, the gene that encodes β-catenin in humans. Such mutations change the serine/threonine phosphorylation site such that β-catenin cannot be phosphorylated and marked for degradation. It has been demonstrated that large deletions of exon 3 of CTNNB1 are associated with fetal histology HB, whereas those with point mutations in exon 3 of CTNNB1 are more frequent in embryonal and small cell undifferentiated (SCU) subtypes. In a comprehensive genomic analysis of 88 cases of HB tumors, three subgroups were identified as having distinct molecular and serum protein biomarker profiles that correlated with distinct clinical behaviors.Patients within the high-risk tumor group demonstrated upregulated nuclear factor and erythroid 2–like 2 (NFE2L2) activity, elevated lin-28 homolog B (LIN28B), high-mobility group AT-hook2 (HMGA2), spalt-like transcription factor 4 (SALL4), and AFP expression.

Tumors in this group also demonstrate coordinated expression of oncofetal proteins and stem cell markers.Intermediate-risk tumors demonstrate intermediate expression levels for hepatobiliary differentiation markers, low levels for stem cell markers, and lack activation of other cancer pathways. Low-risk tumors demonstrated stable cytogenomic analysis with little or no gain or loss in function mutations. They exhibit high levels of hepatic differentiation markers, low stem cell markers, and no mutations in metabolic or cancer pathways. Thrombocytosis is commonly observed in patients with HB and is associated with increases in serum levels of interleukin-6 (IL-6) and C-reactive protein (CRP). Elevated IL-1β levels (stimulates increased IL-6 production) also have been noted in hepatoblastoma cell lines. It is thought that these cytokines lead to increased thrombopoietin levels, which then stimulates thrombopoiesis and thrombocytosis.

Histology

The neoplastic transformation that occurs in HB is thought to occur at multiple points in the hepatocyte differentiation pathway, thereby leading to a diversity of histologic patterns and clinical behaviors. Individual HB tumors are typically made up of multiple cell types and histologic patterns. Interpreting HB pathology can be challenging due to this heterogeneity, the rarity of the tumor, and the architectural distortion produced by pre-biopsy chemotherapy. For these reasons, it is necessary to consult with an experienced pediatric pathologist in order to obtain a useful histologic assessment of HB tissue.Low-risk HB tumors often demonstrate fetal histology (Fig. **6.13**). Well-differentiated fetal (WDF) histology is an established histologic category that has the appearance of fetal hepatocytes with low levels of mitotic activity and accounts for 7% of all HB tumors. Patients with WDF typically experience better outcomes, and those without multifocal or metastatic disease can be effectively treated with resection alone. Intermediate-risk tumors demonstrate epithelial and mixed histology (Fig. **6.14**). In contrast, high-risk HB tumors most commonly demonstrate embryonal histology and demonstrate high-risk histologic features such as anaplasia, a macrotrabecular pattern, and cytologic features similar to those of HCC. The SCU histologic subtype is associated with low serum AFP, an attenuated response to chemotherapy, and worse survival. Hepatocellular neoplasm–not otherwise specified (HN-NOS) is a tumor that occurs in older children and has the features of both HCC and HB.Through international cooperation, it has been possible to achieve a consensus on an HB classification system.This international consensus classification system has Seven histologic subtypes, including both established and newly recognized histologies in Table **6.4**.

Table (6.4). Comparison of hepatoblastoma and hepatocellular carcinoma.

	Hepatoblastoma	Hepatocellular carcinoma
Incidence	1.2 cases per million	0.29 cases per million
Age distribution	6 months to 3 years	>5years
Risk factors	Bechwith-weidmann syndrome Familial adenomatous polyposis Hemihypertrophy Low birth weight	Hepatitis B virus Cirrhosis Liver disease
5-yr survival	52% to 75%	18% to 28%

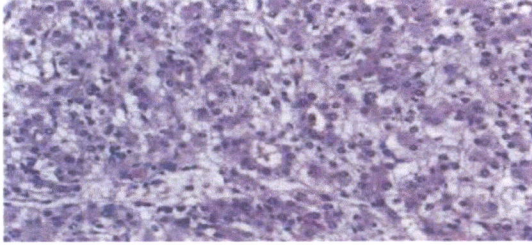

Fig. (6.13). Histology of a pure fetal hepatoblastoma. Note the hepa-tocytes have clear glycogen-rich cytoplasm and small, regular nuclei.

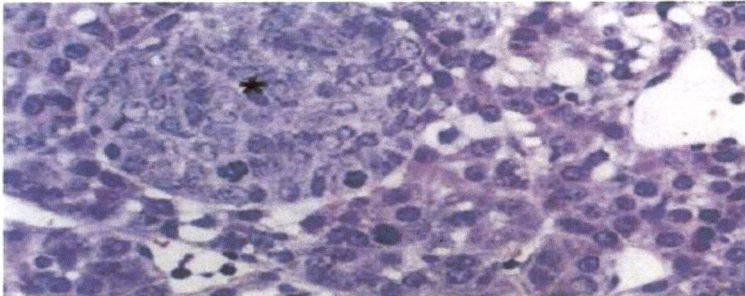

Fig. (6.14). Histology of a hepatoblastoma with mixedfetal and embry-onalelements. Note the large solidnest (asterisk) of poorlydifferentiat-ingcells (embryonal components).

Clinical Features and Laboratory Data

Most patients with liver tumors present with an abdominal mass, and more than two thirds of liver tumors are malignant". Although most patients are asymptomatic, some note abdominal distention, anorexia, weight loss, pain, nausea, and fatigue. Children with HB most commonly present with an asymptomatic right upper quadrant abdominal mass that may be noted incidentally by a parent, a relative, or the child's pediatrician. They can occupy a large portion of the abdomen, extending well across the midline or into the pelvis. Tumors of this size are often associated with anorexia and failure to thrive. Symptoms of acute or chronic liver dysfunction are rare in patients with HB, and liver function tests typically remain normal until the end stages of the disease. Tumor rupture can occur with hemoperitoneum and, at times, hemorrhagic shock. Sexual precocity can occur from tumor production of human chorionic gonadotropin.The most sensitive laboratory test for hepatoblastoma and hepatocellular carcinoma is serum AFP level. AFP is produced in the fetal liver and yolk sac, and levels decline to adult values during the first 6 months after birth. In contrast, note the surrounding trabeculae of the differentiating fetal hepatoblasts. Anemia and thrombocytosis (platelet count >500,000/ mm3) are often encountered in patients with HB [67]. The hallmark laboratory marker found in HB is, however, an elevated AFP level, which occurs in up to 90% of patients. The serum levels of AFP can sometimes exceed 1 million ng/mL.A patient with an extremely high AFP can sometimes have an inaccurately low AFP value due to the "hook" or "prozone" effect that occurs when the enzyme-linked immunosorbent assay (ELISA) detection antibodies become saturated with AFP antigen [68]. If there is suspicion for HB and a low AFP value is obtained, a request should be made to re-run the measurement using serial dilutions of the AFP sample. When considering a neonate with a hepatic mass, it is important to remember that neonates have a normally elevated AFP level (25–50,000 ng/ mL) at birth that does not decrease to "adult" levels until 6 months of age. AFP is used in postsurgical monitoring for tumor recurrence. Serum AFP has a half-life of 4–9 days, and the levels usually decrease to normal by 4–8 weeks after complete removal of the tumor.

Imaging

Abdominal US is the primary screening study for children with suspected liver pathology. US allows for the differentiation between a renal and hepatic mass as well as between a solid and cystic mass. HBs typically are unifocal masses: 50% are isolated to the right lobe, 15% are in the left lobe, and the rest are centrally located.HB staging is increasingly dependent on information from a high-quality axial imaging study, either abdominal MRI or CT. Abdominal CT with a liver enhancement protocol also can be helpful in making the diagnosis of HB, determining the stage of the tumor and its resectability. The CT appearance of HB is that of a well-defined, heterogeneous mass that is hypoattenuating relative to the surrounding liver parenchyma. CT studies can also reveal HB tumor necrosis, calcification, and hemorrhage, just as with MRI, CT allows the mass to be precisely located relative to the IVC, the hepatic veins, and the portal venous system (Fig. **6.15**). Since there are currently no imaging studies that can reliably differentiate between a benign and malignant liver mass, a biopsy should be considered if there is concern for a neoplasm. MRI angiography with gadolinium-based contrast is the most effective way to achieve full radiographic characterization of liver masses in children. MRI allows confirmation of the mass, determination of tumor type, and delineation of the tumor anatomy relative to the native hepatic vascular and biliary structures. In addition, information from the MRI enables determination of the tumor stage and resectability. Typically, HB appears as a heterogeneous hyperintense mass on T2-weighted MRI images and is hypointense on T1. Calcification appears in 40–50% of cases, and hemorrhage and necrosis also may be seen.

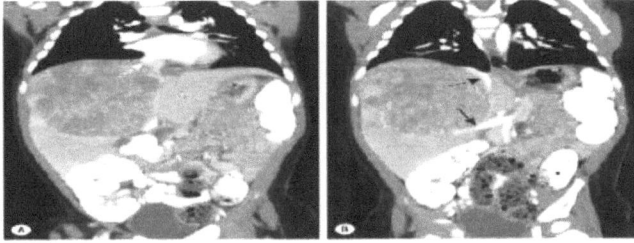

Fig. (6.15). (A) This CT scanobtained after intravenous administration of a contrast agent in a 1-year- old child shows a large mass in the righthepatic lobe. On other images, the mass appears to invade or compress the medial segment of the left lobe. The middle hepaticvein (dotted arrow) is beingcompressed by the tumor. (B) The inferiorvena cava (dotted arrow) is being displaced medially and anteriorly by the mass, and the portal vein (solid arrow) is marked lydis placed inferiorly.

Staging and Risk Stratification

The goals of therapy for HB involve two primary treatment modalities: complete surgical resection and cisplatin-based chemotherapy. The extent and relative timing of surgery as well as the chemotherapy protocol are determined for each patient based upon their risk stratification (Fig. **6.17**). The risk stratification is based upon radiographic staging (PRETEXT), tumor histology, AFP level, and the presence of distant metastasis (Fig. **6.16**). The treatment of HB requires a multidisciplinary approach that hinges on close cooperation between pediatric oncology, surgery, and radiology services. All HB cases should be managed within the framework of a protocol administered by a multicenter HB study group. The two largest multicenter study groups have historically used two distinct approaches to the relative timing of surgery and chemotherapy. The COG approach was based on the premise that all patients who present with HB should be considered for a primary resection. If this is not possible, the patient receives chemotherapy with the goal of shrinking the tumor to the point at which it is resectable. The intent of this approach is to limit the patient's exposure to chemotherapeutic drugs that carry significant side effects, including renal, cardiac, and ototoxicity. This is in contradistinction to the SIOPEL approach, in which all patients receive chemotherapy before surgical resection. The rationale for the SIOPEL approach is that chemotherapy will decrease the size, vascularity, and cellular viability of the tumor, thereby making surgical resection easier and more effective. The guidelines from the most recent SIOPEL 4 and 6 trials recommend that patients assigned to the standard group undergo six cycles of cisplatin (CDDP) before proceeding to surgery. Patients designated in the high-risk group are assigned to undergo eight weekly cycles of CDDP in addition to three weekly doses of doxorubicin before being re-imaged and evaluated for resection.

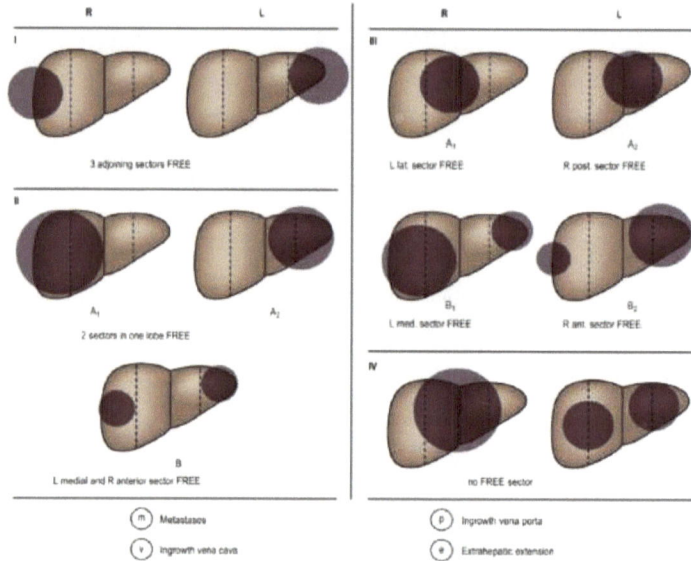

Fig. (6.16). Pretreatment Extent of Disease (PRETEXT) staging system. Stage is determined by the number of liver sectors free of tumor. IVC or hepatic vein.

Treatment

The goals of therapy for HB involve two primary treatment modalities: complete surgical resection and cisplatin-based chemotherapy. The extent and relative timing of surgery as well as the chemotherapy protocol are determined for each patient based upon their risk stratification. The risk stratification is based upon radiographic staging (PRETEXT), tumor histology, AFP level, and the presence of distant metastasis. The treatment of HB requires a multidisciplinary approach that hinges on close cooperation between pediatric oncology,surgery, and radiology services.All HB cases should be managed within the framework of a protocol administered by a multicenter HB study group.The two largest multicenter study groups have historically used two distinct approaches to the relative timing of surgery and chemotherapy. The COG approach was based on the premise that all patients who present with HB should be considered for a primary resection. If this is not possible, the patient receives chemotherapy with the goal of shrinking the tumor to the point at which it is resectable. The intent of this approach is to limit the patient's exposure to chemotherapeutic drugs that carry significant side effects, including renal, cardiac, and ototoxicity. This is in contradistinction to the SIOPEL approach, in which all patients receive chemotherapy before surgical resection. The rationale for the SIOPEL approach is that chemotherapy will decrease the size, vascularity, and cellular viability of the tumor, thereby making surgical resection easier and more effective. The guidelines from the most recent SIOPEL 4 and 6 trials recommend that patients assigned to the standard group undergo six cycles of cisplatin (CDDP) before proceeding to surgery.

Involvement (V), portal vein involvement (P), extrahepatic abdominal disease (E), tumor focality (F), tumor rupture (R), lymph node metastasis (N),

Caudate involvement (C), distant metastasis (M).

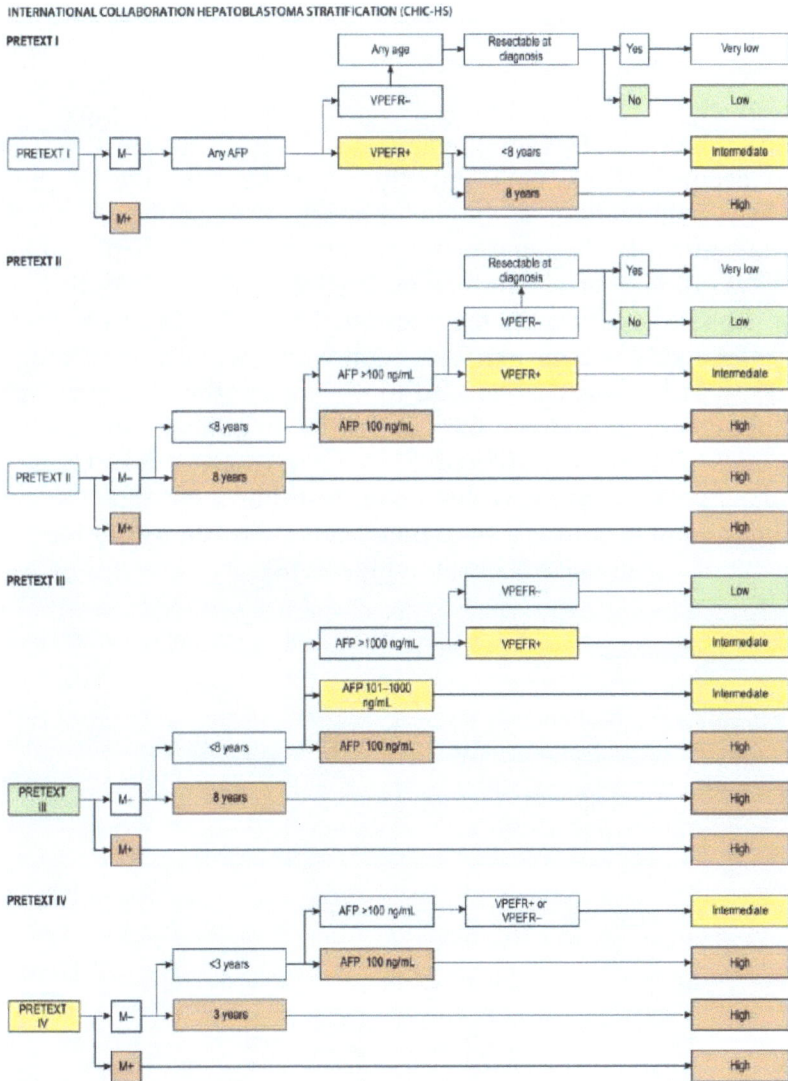

Fig. (6.17). Risk Stratification Trees for the Children's Hepatic Tumors.

Patients designated in the high-risk group are assigned to undergo eight weekly cycles of CDDP in addition to three weekly doses of doxorubicin before being re-imaged and evaluated for resection. In both COG and SIOPEL studies, the resection should be planned so that there is an anticipated clear margin of 2–3 mm of normal liver tissue around the tumor. If it is not possible to resect the tumor with a clear margin, in the COG protocols, the patient should undergo preoperative chemotherapy in an attempt to reduce the size of the tumor such that complete resection is possible.[72]CDDP is combined with VCR, doxorubicin, or 5-fluorouracil (5FU) and used in either an adjuvant or neoadjuvant fashion. The current COG recommended chemotherapy regimen for initially unresectable HB is doxorubicin, CDDP, 5FU, and VCR. The patients who have had complete resection of their tumor (without preoperative chemotherapy), four to six postoperative courses of chemotherapy are given. Children in whom the liver tumor was deemed unresectable initially, receive two rounds of chemotherapy, followed by repeat imaging. If the tumor appears resectable, resection should be done at this time. If the tumor is not resectable, the patient undergoes an additional two rounds of chemotherapy and should be referred to acenter with transplant capabilities. If, after the additional two rounds of chemotherapy, the tumor is resectable (total of four rounds), resection is performed. With chemotherapy and delayed or second-look surgery, the resection rate has been reported to increase to between 69% and 98%. In patients with stage IV d ease (initially unresectable), only 40% of these tumors were rendered resectable after four rounds of chemotherapy. If the tumor is still unresectable, the patient needs to be evaluated and listed for a liver transplant [73]. Algorithm for the diagnosis and treatment of a liver mass is given in Fig. (**6.18**).

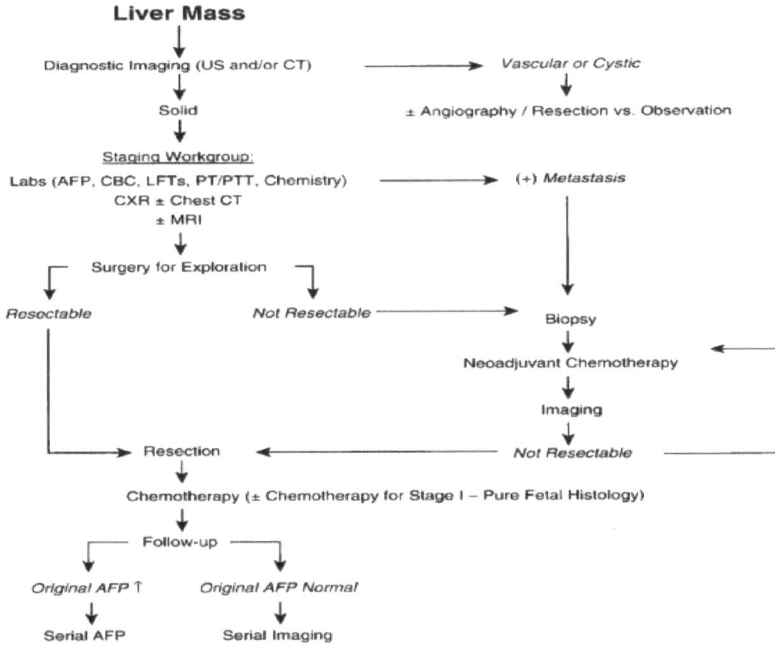

Fig. (6.18). Algorithm for the diagnosis and treatment of a liver mass. AFP, alpha fetoprotein; CBC, complete blood count; CT, computedtotnography; CXR, chest.

Radiograph; LFT, liver function tests; MRI, mag- neticrcsonance imaging; PT/PTT, prothrombin time/partialthrombo- plastin time; US, ultrasound.

Outcome

Outcomes for children with HB are based on the extent of the original tumor (PRETEXT), the tumor histology, and the tumor response to chemotherapy.Several studies has shown a good outcome with fetal histology and with complete resection of the tumor. Fetal tumors must have a histology in which the tumor has a mitotic activity of less than 2 per 10 high-power fields. Conversely, several studies have consistently reported a poor outcome for those patients who have SCU HB. Except for these data, no consistent correlation has been found with any of the other histologic patterns and patient outcomes.The AFP level at diagnosis has been found to have prognostic implications. Patients with an AFP level less than 100 ng/mL or greater than 1 million ng/mL have a worse prognosis.

PROGNOSIS AND FOLLOW-UP

The 5-year survival rate for hepatoblastoma has markedly improved from 35% 3 decades ago to 75% in some series. The prognosis for hepatocellular carcinoma remains dismal, with 5-year overall survival rates of less than 18% to 28%. lesions that are successfully resected have a better prognosis, with 91% to 100% 5-year survival in hepatoblastoma and 30% to 54% for hepatocellular carcinoma. The German Cooperative Pediatric Liver Tumor Study Group had similar results for disease-free survival in hepatoblastoma (mean follow-up 58 months): 89% (n = 27) for stage I, 100% (n = 3) for stage 11, 68% (n = 25) for stage 111, and 21% (n = 14) for stage 1V. a The primary predictor for poor prognosis in hepatoblastoma and hepatocellular carcinoma is metastatic disease.Multifocality, size, and lack of response to chemotherapy are also predictive of poor prognosis in hepatocellular carcinoma. Although metastatic disease portends a worse prognosis, some metastatic lesions have a complete response to chemotherapy. Pulmonary resection should be considered in selected patients with lung lesions that persist after chemotherapy. Following hepaticresection, most patients receivepostoperativechemotherapy. Patients should be followed closely to ensure that serum AFP levels return to normal and that the neoplasmdoes not recur. In those patients who present with normal AFP levels, serial ultrasonography or CT can be performed to screen for recurrence.

CONCLUSION

Advances in anesthesia, surgical technique, and chemotherapy have led to a significant improvement in the prognosis of children with hepatoblastoma. Outcomes for hepatocellular carcinoma remain poor. Liver transplantation is useful in patients with unrectable tumors. Continued cooperation of multi-institutional pediatric cancer study groups will be required to achieve additional advances in the treatment of malignant liver neoplasms.

Sacrococcygeal Teratoma

Sacrococcygeal teratoma is the predominant teratoma. It is the most common neoplasm of the fetus and newborn. Estimated incidence is 1 per 35,000–40,000 live births, female predominance ranging from 2:1 to 4:1 [74]. Most SCTs are histologically benign, approximately 17% exhibit malignant histologic or clinical features.Most cases of SCT occur sporadically, although 10% of patients have a family history of twinning. 10-20% of patients with SCT have coexisting anomalies such as tracheoesophageal fistula, imperforate anus, anorectal stenosis, spina bifida, genitourinary malformations, meningomyelocele, and anencephaly [74]. Also many patients have significant structural abnormalities of juxtaposed organs resulting from displacement by a large teratoma. SCTs account for

35–60% of teratomas (gonadal included) in large series.

Classification

A classification system developed by Altman *et al* divides SCTs into four distinct anatomic types that differ in the degree of intra- and extrapelvic extension.

Type I (46.7%) is predominantly external, with minimal pre-sacral extension.
Type II(34.7%) arises externally and has a significant intrapelvic component.
Type III(8.8%) is primarily pelvic and abdominal but is apparent externally.
Type IV(9.8%) is presacral and has no external manifestation.

These authors observed that the incidence of malignant components correlates not only with anatomic type (8% in type I *versus* 38% in type IV) but also with age at diagnosis and gender; however, the size of the tumor is unrelated.The rate of malignancy of tumors found in older infants (older than 6 months) and in children is significantly higher than that of the visible exophytic tumors seen in neonates. Malignant change appears to be more frequent in males, particularly those with solid *versus* complex or cystic tumors.The most common malignant elements identified within sacrococcygeal lesions are yolk sac tumor and embryonal carcinoma [75].

Deferential Diagnosis

Lumbosacral myelomeningocele is the most likely entity to be confused with SCT. This type of myelomeningocele and cystic SCT has similar findings on sonography. Because both are associated with elevated maternal levels of AFP, these levels are not helpful in distinguishing the two entities. Other critical information gained from sonography includes the possible presence of abdominal or pelvic extension, evidence of bowel or urinary tract obstruction, assessment of the integrity of the fetal spine, and documentation of fetal lower extremity function. Imaging of the fetal brain is helpful in establishing the diagnosis because most fetuses with lumbosacral myelomeningocele have cranial signs such as Arnold Chiarimalformation. When there is doubt, fetal MRI can be extremely valuable in clarifying fetal anatomy and making a definitive diagnosis. Other soft tissue tumors that may mimic SCT include neuroblastoma, hemangioma, leiomyoma, and lipoma.Tumors can grow at an unpredictable rate to tremendous dimensions and may extend retroperitoneally, displacing pelvic or abdominal structures. Large tumors can cause placentomegaly, nonimmune fetal hydrops, and the mirror syndrome. These conditions are thought to result from a hyperdynamic state induced by low-resistance vessels in the teratoma. Without fetal intervention, high-output cardiac failure and hydrops resulting in fetal demise are almost certain. Thus, in a select subset of fetuses that meet stringent criteria, restoring more normal fetal physiology may be achieved by surgical debulking of the SCT in utero. Neonatal death may occur due to obstetric complications from tumor rupture, preterm labor, or dystocia Impending preterm labor from polyhydramnios or uterine distention from tumor mass may require treatment by amnioreduction or cyst aspiration. Dystocia and tumor rupture can be avoided by planned cesarean section delivery for infants with tumors larger than 5 cm [76].

Prenatal Diagnosis

In recent decades, the diagnosis has often been made on prenatal US, especially when this examination is routinely performed in the second trimester. The site of the lesion, its complex appearance, and intrapelvic extension with or without urinary tract obstruction are easily recognized. Although most small teratomas do not adversely affect the fetus; the presence of a large solid vascular tumor is associated with a significant mortality rate, both in utero and perinatally [77]. Perinatal mortality is usually related to prematurity or tumor rupture with exsanguination (or both). Premature delivery may occur spontaneously from polyhydramnios or may be induced urgently because of fetal distress or maternal pre-eclampsia. Repeated US assessment of tumor size is important because the fetus should be delivered by cesarean section if the tumor is larger than 5 cm or larger than the fetal biparietal diameter [78]. Dystocia during vaginal delivery is associated with tumor rupture and hemorrhage and is an avoidable obstetric nightmare. The options in managing unexpected cases with dystocia include emergency cesarean section of the partially delivered fetus that has been intubated and ventilated after vaginal presentation of the head [78]. Polyhydramnios with larger tumors may lead to premature labor, and amnioreduction is often needed to decrease uterine irritability. Tumors that is larger than the fetal biparietal diameter at diagnosis, that grow faster than the fetus, or that grow faster than 150 mL/week are associated with a poor prognosis. As the tumor enlarges, the fetus may develop placentomegaly or hydrops, caused by high-output cardiac failure from vascular shunting within the tumor, with fetal anemia from intratumoral bleeding also playing a role. Early signs of cardiac failure can be recognized by Doppler US and fetal echocardiogram. Placentomegaly and hydrops are harbingers of impending fetal death and should lead to urgent cesarean delivery. Open fetal surgical excision/debulking is one option in fetuses considered too premature to deliver.Purely cystic teratomas occur in 10–15% of cases. Prenatal diagnosis allows percutaneous aspiration to facilitate delivery (Fig. **6.19**), decrease uterine irritability, or prevents tumor rupture at delivery [79]. Postnatally, the diagnosis is determined by clinical findings on physical examination, serum AFP and PHCG levels, and a number of radiographic imaging studies. Ninety percent of SCTs are noted at delivery, with a protruding caudal mass extending from the coccygeal region. Many larger SCTs manifest in utero and can be diagnosed prenatally. Although the diagnosis is usually made between 22 and 34 weeks' gestation, it has been made as early as 13 weeks. Uterine size larger than expected for gestational date (polyhydramnios or tumor enlargement) is the most common obstetric indication for performing a maternal-fetal ultrasound (US) examination.US may reveal an external mass arising from the sacral area of the fetus. This mass is composed of solid and cystic areas, with foci of calcification sometimes apparent. Most prenatally diagnosed SCTs are extremely vascular and can be seen on color-flow Doppler studies. Intrapelvic variants may have a delayed postnatal presentation. They are typically noted in infants and children between 4 months and 4 years of age. In contrast to the SCTs seen in neonates, these tumors are located in the pelvis and have no external component. More than one third is associated with malignancy. Clinical presentation may include constipation, anal stenosis, symptoms related to the tumor compressing the bladder or rectum, and a palpable mass. Presacral tumors are associated with sacral defects and anorectal malformations (Currarino's triad). Radiographs of the pelvis identify any sacral defects or tumor calcifications. Computed tomography (CT) with intravenous and rectal contrast material defines the intrapelvic extent of the tumor, identifies any nodal or distant metastases, and demonstrates possible urinary tract displacement or obstruction. CT also identifies liver metastasis and periaortic lymph node enlargement. MRI is useful when spinal involvement is suspected or if the diagnosis is in doubt. A chest radiograph is useful for revealing obvious pulmonary metastases, but because chest CT is more reliable in picking up smaller metastatic lesions, it should be performed when there is a high index of suspicion.The frequency of malignancy appears to correlate with age at diagnosis [3]. Approximately 8% of SCTs noted at birth is malignant. After 2 months of age, the frequency of malignant transformation rises sharply. By 6 months, 40% to 80% of SCTs are malignant, with the most common type of malignancy being yolk sac tumor. Because presacral (type IV) SCTs are often diagnosed at an older age, they have an increased rate of malignancy.

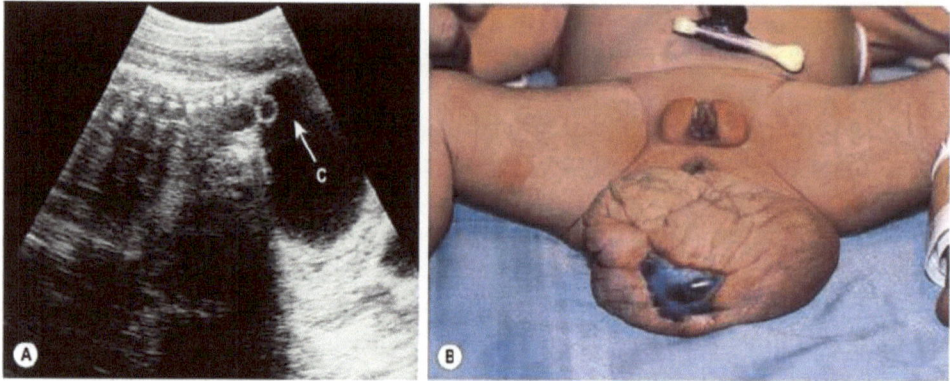

Fig. (6.19). (A) Ultrasound image of a female fetus at 38 weeks of gestation, showing a large cystic mass (C) attached to the coccyx, with tiny cysts anterior to the sacrum (arrow). An ultrasound evaluation at 18 weeks was normal. The cyst was gradually enlarging from an initial diameter of 9.5 cm at 31 weeks of gestation. The cyst was aspirated for 650 mL of fluid, permitting external rotation from breech to the vertex position. Two days later, when labor was induced, another 200 mL of fluid was removed to permit an uncomplicated vaginal delivery. (B) Twenty-four hours postnatally, the lesion remained floppy with an area of skin ulceration, likely a consequence of excessive in utero distention. A mature cystic teratoma was confirmed histologically.

Operative Approach

The treatment of choice for infants with SCT is complete surgical resection. With the exception of emergencies related to tumor rupture or hemorrhage that adversely affect the neonate's hemodynamic status; operative intervention can be undertaken on an elective basis early in the newborn period. The anatomic location of the tumor determines the operative approach. Tumors with extensive intrapelvic extension or a dominant abdominal component (type III or IV) are initiallyapproachedthrough the abdomen. A posterior sacral approach is sufficient for most type I and II tumors.

Operative goals include: complete and prompt tumor excision, resection of the coccyx to prevent tumor recurrence, reconstruction of the muscles of anorectal continence, and restoration of a normal perineal and gluteal appearance. A significant delay in performing surgery may result in serious complications, including pressure necrosis, tumor hemorrhage, and malignant degeneration. Adequate intravenous access, preferably in the upper extremities, and the availability of blood products should be ascertained before starting the operation, especially with large tumors. For most tumors, the major component is extrapelvic and the patient is placed in the prone position. If there is a significant intrapelvic or intra-abdominal component, or if the tumor is highly vascular and bleeding within the tumor is suspected, it may be wise to begin with a laparotomy or laparoscopy. Generally, most resections can be achieved completely in the prone position, especially if the internal portion is cystic. Although the chevron incision has been used by most surgeons, a vertical incision is sometimes possible. It is preferred for smaller teratomas because it leaves a nearly normal-looking median raphe.For patients with Currarino syndrome, the presacral mass can usually be resected through a posterior sagittal approach. The teratoma is often densely adherent to the rectal wall in such patients, and the surgeon should not be overly aggressive in the absence of malignancy. When an anterior meningocele or other anomaly of the terminal spinal cord is associated, a combined approach with a pediatric neurosurgeon is ideal.

Adjuvant Therapy

Detection of malignant elements warrants adjuvant multiagent chemotherapy. The most active antineoplastic drugs include cisplatin, etoposide, and bleomycin. Current reports indicate impressive survival rates in patients with both locally advanced and metastatic disease after the administration of intensive chemotherapy[80]. For patients in whom the primary malignant tumor is unresectable, a multiagent chemotherapy course is administered to facilitate subsequent resection. If a good tumor response is indicated by a diminishing serum AFP level and by CT and chest radiography, resection is undertaken after several cycles of chemotherapy.In patients with localized malignant recurrence, complete resection remains the cornerstone of salvage treatment. This is done in conjunction with adjuvant chemotherapy.Chemotherapy is also effective in the treatment of metastatic foci in the lungs and liver.

Prognosis

Fetuses with an SCT diagnosed in utero have a survival rate in excess of 90% if the tumors are small and discovered by routine prenatal US. If a complicated pregnancy is the indication for US evaluation, the mortality increases to 60%. Nearly 100% of patients die when hydrops or placentomegaly develops [79]. Dystocia and tumor rupture during delivery are likely underreported as a cause of mortality. In the absence of severe prematurity and perinatal complications, the prognosis depends on the presence of malignancy and is therefore related to age at operation and completeness of resection. When the tumor is benign and completely excised, the recurrence rate is low, unless the tumor is large and mostly solid. The recurrent tumor may be benign or malignant, and benign metastatic tissue may become evident in lymph nodes. Although immature or fetal elements in gonadal teratomas are associated with a higher risk of aggressive behavior, this is not considered true for SCTs. Patients whose tumors are resected after the newborn period have a higher risk of malignant recurrence, especially when an elevated AFP level is present at diagnosis. The elevated AFP likely signifies the presence of malignancy in the original tumor. It is important to monitor all patients with physical examination, including rectal examination and serum markers (AFP and CA 125) every 2 or 3 months for at least 3 years, because most recurrences occur within 3 years of operation [81]. Recurrent disease is usually local, but metastases to inguinal nodes, lung, liver, brain, and peritoneum can occur, including pseudomyxomaperitonei. Survival rates higher than 80–90% are now achieved, even in the presence of metastatic disease, but the risk of late recurrences or second malignancies persists. Older patients presenting with large malignant tumors usually undergo biopsy followed by chemotherapy before resection is attempted, in order to avoid sacrificing vital structures.Patients with Currarino syndrome, who often have a tethered cord in addition to the presacral tumor, appear to have an increased risk of bladder and bowel dysfunction [82]. A good outcome requires meticulous d section along the tumor capsule, preservation and reconstruction of muscular structures, and long-term follow-up. Many authors advocate early assessment of bladder, anorectal, and sexual function along with cosmetic results within a structured oncology follow-up program.

CONSENT FOR PUBLICATION

Not applicable.

CONFLICT OF INTEREST

The author declares no conflict of interest, financial or otherwise.

ACKNOWLEDGEMENTS

Declared none.

REFRENCES

[1]   Breslow N, Olshan A, Beckwith JB, Green DM. Epidemiology of Wilms tumor. Med Pediatr Oncol 1993; 21(3): 172-81.
        [http://dx.doi.org/10.1002/mpo.2950210305] [PMID: 7680412]

[2]   Coppes MJ, de Kraker J, van Dijken PJ, *et al.* Bilateral Wilms' tumor: long-term survival and some epidemiological features. J Clin Oncol 1989; 7(3): 310-5.
        [http://dx.doi.org/10.1200/JCO.1989.7.3.310] [PMID: 2537383]

[3]   Breslow NE, Norris R, Norkool PA, *et al.* Characteristics and outcomes of children with the Wilms tumor-Aniridia syndrome: a report from the National Wilms Tumor Study Group. J Clin Oncol 2003; 21(24): 4579-85.
        [http://dx.doi.org/10.1200/JCO.2003.06.096] [PMID: 14673045]

[4]   Beckwith JB, Kiviat NB, Bonadio JF. Nephrogenic rests, nephroblastomatosis, and the pathogenesis of Wilms' tumor. Pediatr Pathol 1990; 10(1-2): 1-36.
        [http://dx.doi.org/10.3109/15513819009067094] [PMID: 2156243]

[5]   Knudson AG Jr, Strong LC. Mutation and cancer: a model for Wilms' tumor of the kidney. J Natl

Cancer Inst 1972; 48(2): 313-24.
[PMID: 4347033]

[6]   Farber S. Chemotherapy in the treatment of leukemia and Wilms' tumor. JAMA 1966; 198(8): 826-36.
       [http://dx.doi.org/10.1001/jama.1966.03110210076025] [PMID: 4288581]

[7]   DeBaun MR, Tucker MA. Risk of cancer during the first four years of life in children from The
       Beckwith-Wiedemann Syndrome Registry. J Pediatr 1998; 132(3 Pt 1): 398-400.
       [http://dx.doi.org/10.1016/S0022-3476(98)70008-3] [PMID: 9544889]

[8]   Goldman M, Smith A, Shuman C, *et al.* Renal abnormalities in beckwith-wiedemann syndrome are
       associated with 11p15.5 uniparental disomy. J Am Soc Nephrol 2002; 13(8): 2077-84.
       [http://dx.doi.org/10.1097/01.ASN.0000023431.16173.55] [PMID: 12138139]

[9]   Chu A, Heck JE, Ribeiro KB, *et al.* Wilms' tumour: a systematic review of risk factors and meta-
       analysis. Paediatr Perinat Epidemiol 2010; 24(5): 449-69.
       [http://dx.doi.org/10.1111/j.1365-3016.2010.01133.x] [PMID: 20670226]

[10]   Khanna G, Rosen N, Anderson JR, *et al.* Evaluation of diagnostic performance of CT for detection of
       tumor thrombus in children with Wilms tumor: a report from the Children's Oncology Group. Pediatr
       Blood Cancer 2012; 58(4): 551-5.
       [http://dx.doi.org/10.1002/pbc.23222] [PMID: 21674767]

[11]   Grundy PE. JSD, Ehrlich PF, et al Renal tumors classification, biology and banking studies. Journal
       2016; pp. 18-33. [serial online]

[12]   Ehrlich PF, Ritchey ML, Hamilton TE, *et al.* Quality assessment for Wilms' tumor: a report from the
       National Wilms' Tumor Study-5. J Pediatr Surg 2005; 40(1): 208-12.
       [http://dx.doi.org/10.1016/j.jpedsurg.2004.09.044] [PMID: 15868587]

[13]   Drash A, Sherman F, Hartmann WH, Blizzard RM. A syndrome of pseudohermaphroditism, Wilms'
       tumor, hypertension, and degenerative renal disease. J Pediatr 1970; 76(4): 585-93.
       [http://dx.doi.org/10.1016/S0022-3476(70)80409-7] [PMID: 4316066]

[14]   Ritchey M, Daley S, Shamberger RC, *et al.* Ureteral extension in Wilms' tumor: a report from the
       National Wilms' Tumor Study Group (NWTSG). J Pediatr Surg 2008; 43(9): 1625-9.
       [http://dx.doi.org/10.1016/j.jpedsurg.2008.01.067] [PMID: 18778996]

[15]   Shamberger RC, Guthrie KA, Ritchey ML, *et al.* Surgery-related factors and local recurrence of
       Wilms tumor in National Wilms Tumor Study 4. Ann Surg 1999; 229(2): 292-7.
       [http://dx.doi.org/10.1097/00000658-199902000-00019] [PMID: 10024113]

[16]   Tournade MF, Com-Nougue C, de Kraker J, *et al.* Optimal duration of preoperative chemotherapy in
       unilateral non metastatic Wilms tumor in children older then six months. Results of the ninth
       International Society of Pediatric Oncology tumor trial. J Clin Oncol 2001; 19: 488-500.
       [http://dx.doi.org/10.1200/JCO.2001.19.2.488] [PMID: 11208843]

[17]   van den Heuvel-Eibrink MM, Grundy P, Graf N, *et al.* Characteristics and survival of 750 children
       diagnosed with a renal tumor in the first seven months of life: A collaborative study by the
       SIOP/GPOH/SFOP, NWTSG, and UKCCSG Wilms tumor study groups. Pediatr Blood Cancer 2008;
       50(6): 1130-4.
       [http://dx.doi.org/10.1002/pbc.21389] [PMID: 18095319]

[18]   Isaacs H Jr. Fetal and neonatal renal tumors. J Pediatr Surg 2008; 43(9): 1587-95.
       [http://dx.doi.org/10.1016/j.jpedsurg.2008.03.052] [PMID: 18778991]

[19]   Andrews PE, Kelalis PP, Haase GM. Extrarenal Wilms' tumor: results of the National Wilms' Tumor
       Study. J Pediatr Surg 1992; 27(9): 1181-4.
       [http://dx.doi.org/10.1016/0022-3468(92)90782-3] [PMID: 1331392]

[20]   Coppes MJ, Wilson PC, Weitzman S. Extrarenal Wilms' tumor: staging, treatment, and prognosis. J
       Clin Oncol 1991; 9(1): 167-74.
       [http://dx.doi.org/10.1200/JCO.1991.9.1.167] [PMID: 1845874]

[21]   Geller JI, Dome JS. Local lymph node involvement does not predict poor outcome in pediatric renal cell carcinoma. Cancer 2004; 101(7): 1575-83.
[http://dx.doi.org/10.1002/cncr.20548] [PMID: 15378495]

[22]   Virchow R. Hyperplasie der Zirbel und der Nebenniern. Die Krankhaften Geschwulste. Berlin: August Hirshwald 1865; Vol. 2: pp. 149-50.

[23]   Beckwith JB, Perrin EV. *In situ* neuroblastoma: A contribution to the natural history of neural crest tumors. Am J Pathol 1963; 43: 1089-104.
[PMID: 14099453]

[24]   Ambros IM, Zellner A, Stock C, Amann G, Gadner H, Ambros PF. Proof of the reactive nature of the Schwann cell in neuroblastoma and its clinical implications. Prog Clin Biol Res 1994; 385: 331-7.
[PMID: 7972228]

[25]   Russo C, Cohn SL, Petruzzi MJ, de Alarcon PA. Long-term neurologic outcome in children with opsoclonus-myoclonus associated with neuroblastoma: a report from the Pediatric Oncology Group. Med Pediatr Oncol 1997; 28(4): 284-8.
[http://dx.doi.org/10.1002/(SICI)1096-911X(199704)28:4<284::AID-MPO7>3.0.CO;2-E]   [PMID: 9078325]

[26]   Rudnick E, Khakoo Y, Antunes NL, *et al.* Opsoclonus-myoclonus-ataxia syndrome in neuroblastoma: clinical outcome and antineuronal antibodies-a report from the Children's Cancer Group Study. Med Pediatr Oncol 2001; 36(6): 612-22.
[http://dx.doi.org/10.1002/mpo.1138] [PMID: 11344492]

[27]   Shimada H, Chatten J, Newton WA Jr, *et al.* Histopathologic prognostic factors in neuroblastic tumors: definition of subtypes of ganglioneuroblastoma and an age-linked classification of neuroblastomas. J Natl Cancer Inst 1984; 73(2): 405-16.
[http://dx.doi.org/10.1093/jnci/73.2.405] [PMID: 6589432]

[28]   Shimada H, Ambros IM, Dehner LP, *et al.* The International Neuroblastoma Pathology Classification (the Shimada system). Cancer 1999; 86(2): 364-72.
[http://dx.doi.org/10.1002/(SICI)1097-0142(19990715)86:2<364::AID-CNCR21>3.0.CO;2-7] [PMID: 10421273]

[29]   Tsuchida Y, Honna T, Iwanaka T, *et al.* Serial determination of serum neuron-specific enolase in patients with neuroblastoma and other pediatric tumors. J Pediatr Surg 1987; 22(5): 419-24.
[http://dx.doi.org/10.1016/S0022-3468(87)80261-0] [PMID: 3585664]

[30]   Cheung NK, Kushner BH. Should we replace bone scintigraphy plus CT with MR imaging for staging of neuroblastoma? Radiology 2003; 226(1): 286-7.
[http://dx.doi.org/10.1148/radiol.2261020607] [PMID: 12511704]

[31]   Gelfand MJ. Meta-iodobenzylguanidine in children. Semin Nucl Med 1993; 23(3): 231-42.
[http://dx.doi.org/10.1016/S0001-2998(05)80104-7] [PMID: 8378796]

[32]   Brodeur GM, Pritchard J, Berthold F, *et al.* Revisions of the international criteria for neuroblastoma diagnosis, staging, and response to treatment. J Clin Oncol 1993; 11(8): 1466-77.
[http://dx.doi.org/10.1200/JCO.1993.11.8.1466] [PMID: 8336186]

[33]   Moroz V, Machin D, Faldum A, *et al.* Changes over three decades in outcome and the prognostic influence of age-at-diagnosis in young patients with neuroblastoma: a report from the International Neuroblastoma Risk Group Project. Eur J Cancer 2011; 47(4): 561-71.
[http://dx.doi.org/10.1016/j.ejca.2010.10.022] [PMID: 21112770]

[34]   Matthay KK, Lukens J, Haase GM, *et al.* Outcome and prognostic factors for 1008 children with neuroblastoma treated from 1989 1995 on Children's Cancer Group (CCG) protocols. Philadelphia: Advances in Neuroblastoma Research 1996.

[35]   Cohn SL, Pearson AD, London WB, *et al.* The International Neuroblastoma Risk Group (INRG) classification system: an INRG Task Force report. J Clin Oncol 2009; 27(2): 289-97.

[http://dx.doi.org/10.1200/JCO.2008.16.6785] [PMID: 19047291]

[36]　Nickerson HJ, Matthay KK, Seeger RC, *et al.* Favorable biology and outcome of stage IV-S neuroblastoma with supportive care or minimal therapy: a Children's Cancer Group study. J Clin Oncol 2000; 18(3): 477-86.
[http://dx.doi.org/10.1200/JCO.2000.18.3.477] [PMID: 10653863]

[37]　Crist WM, Anderson JR, Meza JL, *et al.* Intergroup rhabdomyosarcoma study-IV: results for patients with nonmetastatic disease. J Clin Oncol 2001; 19(12): 3091-102.
[http://dx.doi.org/10.1200/JCO.2001.19.12.3091] [PMID: 11408506]

[38]　Newton WA Jr, Soule EH, Hamoudi AB, *et al.* Histopathology of childhood sarcomas, Intergroup Rhabdomyosarcoma Studies I and II: clinicopathologic correlation. J Clin Oncol 1988; 6(1): 67-75.
[http://dx.doi.org/10.1200/JCO.1988.6.1.67] [PMID: 3275751]

[39]　Wiener ES, Anderson JR, Ojimba JI, *et al.* Controversies in the management of paratesticular rhabdomyosarcoma: is staging retroperitoneal lymph node dissection necessary for adolescents with resected paratesticular rhabdomyosarcoma? Semin Pediatr Surg 2001; 10(3): 146-52.
[http://dx.doi.org/10.1053/spsu.2001.24695] [PMID: 11481652]

[40]　Rodeberg D, Paidas C. Childhood rhabdomyosarcoma. Semin Pediatr Surg 2006; 15(1): 57-62.
[http://dx.doi.org/10.1053/j.sempedsurg.2005.11.009] [PMID: 16458847]

[41]　Cecchetto G, Carli M, Sotti G, *et al.* Importance of local treatment in pediatric soft tissue sarcomas with microscopic residual after primary surgery: results of the Italian Cooperative Study RMS-88. Med Pediatr Oncol 2000; 34(2): 97-101.
[http://dx.doi.org/10.1002/(SICI)1096-911X(200002)34:2<97::AID-MPO4>3.0.CO;2-8]　[PMID: 10657868]

[42]　Crist W, Gehan EA, Ragab AH, *et al.* The Third Intergroup Rhabdomyosarcoma Study. J Clin Oncol 1995; 13(3): 610-30.
[http://dx.doi.org/10.1200/JCO.1995.13.3.610] [PMID: 7884423]

[43]　Kumar R, Shandal V, Shamim SA, Halanaik D, Malhotra A. Clinical applications of PET and PET/CT in pediatric malignancies. Expert Rev Anticancer Ther 2010; 10(5): 755-68.
[http://dx.doi.org/10.1586/era.10.12] [PMID: 20470007]

[44]　Leaphart C, Rodeberg D. Pediatric surgical oncology: management of rhabdomyosarcoma. Surg Oncol 2007; 16(3): 173-85.
[http://dx.doi.org/10.1016/j.suronc.2007.07.003] [PMID: 17689957]

[45]　Ferrer FA, Isakoff M, Koyle MA. Bladder/prostate rhabdomyosarcoma: past, present and future. J Urol 2006; 176(4 Pt 1): 1283-91.
[http://dx.doi.org/10.1016/j.juro.2006.06.019] [PMID: 16952614]

[46]　Finelli A, Babyn P, Lorie GA, Bägli D, Khoury AE, Merguerian PA. The use of magnetic resonance imaging in the diagnosis and followup of pediatric pelvic rhabdomyosarcoma. J Urol 2000; 163(6): 1952-3.
[http://dx.doi.org/10.1016/S0022-5347(05)67607-0] [PMID: 10799238]

[47]　Dasgupta R, Rodeberg DA. Update on rhabdomyosarcoma. Semin Pediatr Surg 2012; 21(1): 68-78.
[http://dx.doi.org/10.1053/j.sempedsurg.2011.10.007] [PMID: 22248972]

[48]　Blakely ML, Lobe TE, Anderson JR, *et al.* Does debulking improve survival rate in advanced-stage retroperitoneal embryonal rhabdomyosarcoma? J Pediatr Surg 1999; 34(5): 736-41.
[http://dx.doi.org/10.1016/S0022-3468(99)90366-4] [PMID: 10359174]

[49]　Raney RB, Stoner JA, Walterhouse DO, *et al.* Results of treatment of fifty-six patients with localized retroperitoneal and pelvic rhabdomyosarcoma: a report from The Intergroup Rhabdomyosarcoma Study-IV, 1991-1997. Pediatr Blood Cancer 2004; 42(7): 618-25.
[http://dx.doi.org/10.1002/pbc.20012] [PMID: 15127417]

[50]　Hill DA, Dehner LP, Gow KW, *et al.* Perianal rhabdomyosarcoma presenting as a perirectal abscess:

A report of 11 cases. J Pediatr Surg 2002; 37(4): 576-81.
[http://dx.doi.org/10.1053/jpsu.2002.31613] [PMID: 11912514]

[51] Spector LG, Birch J. The epidemiology of hepatoblastoma. Pediatr Blood Cancer 2012; 59(5): 776-9.
[http://dx.doi.org/10.1002/pbc.24215] [PMID: 22692949]

[52] Exelby PR, Filler RM, Grosfeld JL. Liver tumors in children in the particular reference to hepatoblastoma and hepatocellular carcinoma: American Academy of Pediatrics Surgical Section Survey--1974. J Pediatr Surg 1975; 10(3): 329-37.
[http://dx.doi.org/10.1016/0022-3468(75)90095-0] [PMID: 49416]

[53] Howlander N, Noone AM, Krapcho M, *et al.* SEER Cancer Statistics Review. National Cancer Institute.

[54] Trobaugh-Lotrario AD, Venkatramani R, Feusner JH. Hepatoblastoma in children with Beckwith-Wiedemann syndrome: does it warrant different treatment? J Pediatr Hematol Oncol 2014; 36(5): 369-73.
[http://dx.doi.org/10.1097/MPH.0000000000000129] [PMID: 24608075]

[55] Kalish JM, Doros L, Helman LJ, *et al.* Surveillance recommendations for children with overgrowth syndromes and predisposition to Wilms tumors and hepatoblastoma. Clin Cancer Res 2017; 23(13): e115-22.
[http://dx.doi.org/10.1158/1078-0432.CCR-17-0710] [PMID: 28674120]

[56] Mussa A, Ferrero GB. Screening hepatoblastoma in BeckwithWiedemann syndrome: a complex issue. J Pediatr Hematol Oncol 2015; 37(8): 627.
[http://dx.doi.org/10.1097/MPH.0000000000000408] [PMID: 26241723]

[57] Oda H, Imai Y, Nakatsuru Y, Hata J, Ishikawa T. Somatic mutations of the APC gene in sporadic hepatoblastomas. Cancer Res 1996; 56(14): 3320-3.
[PMID: 8764128]

[58] Giardiello FM, Offerhaus GJA, Krush AJ, *et al.* Risk of hepatoblastoma in familial adenomatous polyposis. J Pediatr 1991; 119(5): 766-8.
[http://dx.doi.org/10.1016/S0022-3476(05)80297-5] [PMID: 1658283]

[59] Rumbajan JM, Maeda T, Souzaki R, *et al.* Comprehensive analyses of imprinted differentially methylated regions reveal epigenetic and genetic characteristics in hepatoblastoma. BMC Cancer 2013; 13: 608.
[http://dx.doi.org/10.1186/1471-2407-13-608] [PMID: 24373183]

[60] Spector LG, Puumala SE, Carozza SE, *et al.* Cancer risk among children with very low birth weights. Pediatrics 2009; 124(1): 96-104.
[http://dx.doi.org/10.1542/peds.2008-3069] [PMID: 19564288]

[61] Spector LG, Johnson KJ, Soler JT, Puumala SE. Perinatal risk factors for hepatoblastoma. Br J Cancer 2008; 98(9): 1570-3.
[http://dx.doi.org/10.1038/sj.bjc.6604335] [PMID: 18392049]

[62] Ikeda H, Hachitanda Y, Tanimura M, Maruyama K, Koizumi T, Tsuchida Y. Development of unfavorable hepatoblastoma in children of very low birth weight: results of a surgical and pathologic review. Cancer 1998; 82(9): 1789-96.
[http://dx.doi.org/10.1002/(SICI)1097-0142(19980501)82:9<1797::AID-CNCR28>3.0.CO;2-Z] [PMID: 9576303]

[63] Maruyama K, Ikeda H, Koizumi T, *et al.* Case-control study of perinatal factors and hepatoblastoma in children with an extremely low birthweight. Pediatr Int 2000; 42(5): 492-8.
[http://dx.doi.org/10.1046/j.1442-200x.2000.01287.x] [PMID: 11059537]

[64] Shew SB, Keshen TH, Jahoor F, Jaksic T. Assessment of cysteine synthesis in very low-birth weight neonates using a [13C6]glucose tracer. J Pediatr Surg 2005; 40(1): 52-6.
[http://dx.doi.org/10.1016/j.jpedsurg.2004.09.011] [PMID: 15868558]

[65]   Bell D, Ranganathan S, Tao J, Monga SP. Novel advances in u ing of molecular pathogenesis of hepatoblastoma: a Wnt/β-catenin perspective. Gene Expr 2017; 17(2): 141-54.
[http://dx.doi.org/10.3727/105221616X693639] [PMID: 27938502]

[66]   Sato Y, Kokubu A, Fukushima K, *et al.* Fluctuations in C-reactive protein in a hepatoblastoma patient with thrombocytosis. Clin Pract 2011; 1(3): e56.
[http://dx.doi.org/10.4081/cp.2011.e56] [PMID: 24765317]

[67]   López-Terrada D, Alaggio R, de Dávila MT, *et al.* Towards an international pediatric liver tumor consensus classification: proceedings of the Los Angeles COG liver tumors symposium. Mod Pathol 2014; 27(3): 472-91.
[http://dx.doi.org/10.1038/modpathol.2013.80] [PMID: 24008558]

[68]   Roy RD, Rosenmund C, Stefan MI. Cooperative binding mitigates the high-dose hook effect. BMC Syst Biol 2017; 11(1): 74.
[http://dx.doi.org/10.1186/s12918-017-0447-8] [PMID: 28807050]

[69]   Meyers AB, Towbin AJ, Geller JI, Podberesky DJ. Hepatoblastoma imaging with gadoxetate disodium-enhanced MRI--typical, atypical, pre- and post-treatment evaluation. Pediatr Radiol 2012; 42(7): 859-66.
[http://dx.doi.org/10.1007/s00247-012-2366-6] [PMID: 22419052]

[70]   Zsiros J, Brugieres L, Brock P, *et al.* Dose-dense cisplatin-based chemotherapy and surgery for children with high-risk hepatoblastoma (SIOPEL-4): a prospective, single-arm, feasibility study. Lancet Oncol 2013; 14(9): 834-42.
[http://dx.doi.org/10.1016/S1470-2045(13)70272-9] [PMID: 23831416]

[71]   Czauderna P, Haeberle B, Hiyama E, *et al.* The Children's Hepatic tumors International Collaboration (CHIC): Novel global rare tumor database yields new prognostic factors in hepatoblastoma and becomes a research model. Eur J Cancer 2016; 52: 92-101.
[http://dx.doi.org/10.1016/j.ejca.2015.09.023] [PMID: 26655560]

[72]   Trobaugh-Lotrario AD, Meyers RL, O'Neill AF, Feusner JH. Unresectable hepatoblastoma: current perspectives. Hepat Med 2017; 9: 1-6.
[http://dx.doi.org/10.2147/HMER.S89997] [PMID: 28203111]

[73]   Meyers RL, Tiao G, de Ville de Goyet J, Superina R, Aronson DC. Hepatoblastoma state of the art: pre-treatment extent of disease, surgical resection guidelines and the role of liver transplantation. Curr Opin Pediatr 2014; 26(1): 29-36.
[http://dx.doi.org/10.1097/MOP.0000000000000042] [PMID: 24362406]

[74]   Bale PM. Sacrococcygeal developmental abnormalities and tumors in children. Perspect Pediatr Pathol 1984; 8(1): 9-56.
[PMID: 6366733]

[75]   Hawkins EP, Perlman EJ. Germ cell tumors in childhood: Morphology and biology. In: Parham DM, Ed. Pediatric Neoplasia: Morphology and Biology. New York: Raven Press 1996; p. 297.

[76]   Shamberger RC. Teratomas and germ cell tumors. 2004.

[77]   Holterman AX, Filiatrault D, Lallier M, Youssef S. The natural history of sacrococcygeal teratomas diagnosed through routine obstetric sonogram: a single institution experience. J Pediatr Surg 1998; 33(6): 899-903.
[http://dx.doi.org/10.1016/S0022-3468(98)90670-4] [PMID: 9660225]

[78]   Flake AW. Fetal sacrococcygeal teratoma. Semin Pediatr Surg 1993; 2(2): 113-20.
[PMID: 8062028]

[79]   Hedrick HL, Flake AW, Crombleholme TM, *et al.* Sacrococcygeal teratoma: prenatal assessment, fetal intervention, and outcome. J Pediatr Surg 2004; 39(3): 430-8.
[http://dx.doi.org/10.1016/j.jpedsurg.2003.11.005] [PMID: 15017565]

[80]   Hawkins EP, Perlman EJ. Germ cell tumors in childhood: Morphology and biology. In: Parham DM, Ed. Pediatric Neoplasia: Morphology and Biology. New York: Raven Press 1996; p. 297.

[81]   Pauniaho SL, Heikinheimo O, Vettenranta K, *et al.* High prevalence of sacrococcygeal teratoma in Finland - a nationwide population-based study. Acta Paediatr 2013; 102(6): e251-6.
       [http://dx.doi.org/10.1111/apa.12211] [PMID: 23432104]

[82]   Lee NG, Gana R, Borer JG, Estrada CR, Khoshbin S, Bauer SB. Urodynamic findings in patients with Currarino syndrome. J Urol 2012; 187(6): 2195-200.
       [http://dx.doi.org/10.1016/j.juro.2012.01.128] [PMID: 22503009]

CHAPTER 7

Neurosurgery

Sultan M. Ghanim[1,*] and **Asalah T. Gumer**[2]

[1] *ME Unit, Medical College, Faculty of Medicine, University of Kufa, Iraq*

[2] *6th Grade Medical College, Faculty of Medicine, University of Kufa, Iraq*

Abstract: This chapter will provide a broad overview of the more common pediatric neurosurgical conditions seen in a children's hospital setting, with the exception of trauma. Emphasis will be placed on conditions in which the pediatric surgeon and neurosurgeon interface in the care of the child. Also, tips on what to do when a neurosurgeon is not available will be discussed. Extra effort will be spent explaining the various devices pediatric neurosurgeons implant that can very well complicate anticipated or unanticipated general surgical procedures.

Keywords: Implant, Neurosurgeon, Neurosurgical.

HYDROCEPHALUS

Cerebrospinal fluid (CSF) is produced constantly. Although the volume produced is likely proportional to the size of the brain and the child and hence less in infants compared with older children, the volume is substantial regardless of age or size. By the age of 5 years, the brain has already achieved 90% of the adult size.2 in the full-sized or near full-sized brain; CSF production averages approximately 20 mL/h or 480 mL/day. Under normal circumstances, the majority of CSF is produced by the choroid plexus within the ventricular system. The brain, however, can still produce CSF *via* bulk flow. This bulk flow is thought to be extracellular fluid within the brain parenchyma that moves centripetally toward the ventricular system. Hence, removing the choroid plexus cannot eliminate or even reduce CSF production. The failure to circulate or absorb even a small percentage of the CSF produced can cause problems of ventricular distention and/or raised ICP. An obstruction within the ventricular system, its outlets, or the subarachnoid cisterns or a failure of absorption at normal CSF pressures into the venous system can lead to ventricular distention and/or enlarged subarachnoid spaces. Causes of hydrocephalus can be divided into congenital and acquired.

* **Corresponding author Sultan M. Ghanim:** ME Unit, Medical College, Faculty of Medicine, University of Kufa, Iraq; Tel: +9647816669997; E-mail: sultanmalsaadi@uokufa.edu.iq

Common congenital causes of hydrocephalus are congenital aqueduct stenosis and in association with myelomeningoceles. Acquired causes are intraventricular hemorrhage most often in association with prematurity, post-meningitis or post-traumatic status, and from brain tumors. An infant with raised ICP may present with a history of irritability, emesis, poor feeding, and lethargy. In addition to these the child may present with complaints of headache, visual disturbance, and loss of developmental milestones, impaired academic performance, and clumsiness. Hydrocephalus is rarely a cause of seizures, and a seizure in a child with raised ICP may actually be posturing (flexor or extensor) from impending herniation and not an electrical seizure. Posturing from raised ICP is an urgent matter. Although seizure disorders commonly coexist in the child with hydrocephalus, they are generally regarded as not being caused by hydrocephalus. On examination of the infant, the occipital-frontal circumference (OFC), character of the fontanels, separation of the cranial sutures, scalp vein distention, eye position, heart rate, blood pressure, and respiratory rate are important factors to assess, as a rule of thumb in the neonatal setting, OFC growth greater than a centimeter per week serves as a possible indication of raised ICP in the neonate. Prominence of scalp veins can serve as a possible indication of elevated ICP. "Sun-setting" eyes with lid retraction is a downward deviation of the eyes with impaired upgaze (Fig. **7.1**).

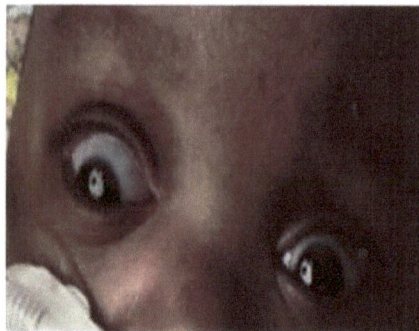

Fig. (7.1). This infant exhibits "sun-setting" eyes with downward deviation of the eyes. The upper sclera is unnaturally visible.

The upper sclera becomes unnaturally visible and is a sign of elevated ICP or midbrain abnormality. Esotropia, medial deviation of one or both eyes because of weakness in the abductor muscle supplied by the sixth cranial nerve, also can be a sign of raised ICP. Elevated ICP can cause vital sign changes referred to as Cushing's triad of bradycardia, hypertension, and irregular respirations. In the monitored setting, trends of any one vital sign such as a slowing heart rate, an increasing blood pressure, or a reduced respiratory rate can signal a possible elevation in ICP. The whole triad does not need to be present when ICP is elevated. A more in-depth examination is possible in an older child. With the exception of the fontanels and cranial suture examination, many of the same signs are looked for when examining a child beyond infancy. In addition, a funduscopic examination may be possible to look for papilledema or optic pallor. If the child is cooperative, tests of memory, coordination, balance, and gait are helpful in trying to detect impaired brain function from elevated ICP. Cranial imaging of the child with possible hydrocephalus can involve plain radiographs, ultrasound (US), computerized tomography (CT), and magnetic resonance imaging (MRI) (Fig. **7.2 A**). Plain radiographs are not recommended but may show the effects of chronically elevated ICP on the inner table of the skull causing a "copper beaten" appearance. An open fontanel is required for cranial US. The US can nicely show the lateral ventricles, but extra-axial spaces and the posterior fossa contents as well as fourth ventricle are usually incompletely visualized at best. However, the US can be performed at the bedside and without the need for transport or sedation. A cranial CT gives more information with very good visualization of all ventricles, the extra-axial spaces, and skull anatomy.

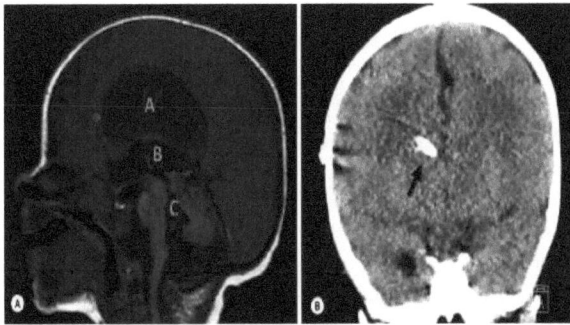

Fig. (7.2). (A) This neonate has untreated congenital hydrocephalus. Note the enlarged lateral A, third B, and fourth C ventricles. (B) Cranial CT in the coronal plane following placement of a shunt. The ventricles are completely collapsed, and the catheter (arrow) resides in the right frontal horn of the lateral ventricle.

MRI sequences that take only a few minutes have been developed to simply assess the ventricular anatomy in the setting of known hydrocephalus to avoid or minimize sedation; however, there remains a higher likelihood of the need for sedation and reduced patient access when they are in the bore of the magnet compared with CT. The endoscopic approach to the third ventricle with or without choroid plexus coagulation has been used with greater regularity in recent years5 and serves a role in very select patient populations, though the mainstay of treatment for hydrocephalus remains the ventriculoperitoneal shunt (VPS) (See Fig. **7.2 B**). A common clinical scenario is the timing of gastrostomy and VPS placement in the premature intraventricular hemorrhage neonatal intensive care unit population as well as some children with malignant tumors in whom either the neurologic sequela or the chemotherapy impede adequate nutritional intake.

Skull Masses

It is not uncommon for a pediatric surgeon to be asked to excise lumps or bumps on the skull of a young child. Most of these masses will be dermoid cysts. A general rule is not to touch anything in the midline without intracranial imaging or neurosurgical input. Dermoid cysts can extend intracranial and intradural. They are nontender, firm, rubbery lesions to palpation that inevitably enlarge. Rupture and drainage through a sinus tract are possible in all locations Fig. (**7.3**). Often diagnosed in the infant, they also can manifest later in life. Midline lesions are associated with the higher likelihood of intracranial extension, particularly in the occipital region.

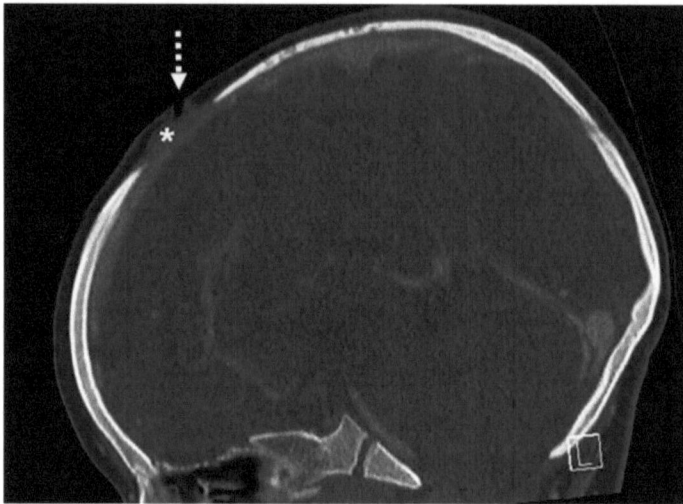

Fig. (7.3). Dermoid cyst (asterisk) is shown overlying the anterior fontanel in an infant. Air (dotted arrow) is seen within a draining dermal sinus tract.

Langerhans cell histiocytosis (LCH) is second in frequency. Solitary LCH is usually present after infancy, and the lesions are characteristically tender and mushy to palpation. They are associated with bony destruction. They can have a far-ranging natural history from spontaneous regression of a single skull lesion to being associated with infantile disseminated progressive multiorgan disease (Letterer-Siwe disease). For isolated skull lesions, curettage is often curative. Larger lesions can be associated with dural erosion and significant vascularity. Involvement of a pediatric oncologist is important with LCH to help exclude the more severe varieties of multisite disease and to guide adjuvant therapy.

Neural Tube Defects

Defects in closure of the neural tube during development can be divided into two broad categories: myelomeningoceles and encephaloceles. Meningoceles differ from myelomeningoceles in that the spinal cord is not involved in a Meningoceles. Meningoceles are not commonly encountered. Although myelomeningoceles, also commonly referred to as spina bifida, can involve any level of the spinal cord, the lumbar region is the most common. Encephaloceles are commonly categorized as either anterior or posterior (Fig. **7.4**). Myelomeningoceles represent a failure of primary neurulation. When the tube fails to completely close at a spinal level, the anatomic result can be a myelomeningoceles (Fig. **7.5**). The causes of myelomeningoceles are poorly understood, but folic acid in the diet of the mother prior to conception reduces their incidence. Genetic and teratogenic influences likely play roles as well. With the exception of cervical myelomeningoceles, the site of the defect dictates the level of neurologic function. With cervical myelomeningoceles, there remains spinal cord function caudal to the lesion. On the other hand, a baby with an upper lumbar myelomeningoceles (at approximately L2) may be expected to have hip flexor function (iliopsoas, L1-2) and impaired bowel and bladder function (S2-4) but no knee extension (quadriceps, L3-4) or motion at the ankle or toes (L5–S2). The defect in the spine leads to more than just functional problems. The entire neural axis is affected both during and after development. The egress of CSF into the spinal defect allows mechanical changes to occur more rostrally, resulting in descent of the posterior fossa structures (both brain stem and cerebellum) into the cervical canal, which is known as the Chiari type II malformation. The anatomic abnormalities that lead to the Chiari II malformation occur almost exclusively in children with a myelomeningoceles. Lower cranial nerve dysfunction can be life threatening early in the life of these children and can occur due to maldevelopment of the brain stem or compression of the medulla as hydrocephalus transmits further pressure into the Chiari II anomaly. Also, the supratentorial brain is not immune from injury, and hydrocephalus, polymicrogyria, enlarged thalamic adhesion, beaked midbrain tectum, and interdigitated falx are often seen. The neonatal management is straightforward. The defect should be kept covered with a sterile, moist dressing. Prophylactic antibiotics are often administered following birth and continued through the postoperative period. Surgical closure is not an emergency but should be performed in the first 72 hours of life to reduce the incidence of infection. The treatment of any hydrocephalus in regard to timing and technique varies greatly by surgeon and institution. Prenatal closure has resulted in a significant reduction in the development of the Chiari II malformation and hydrocephalus.

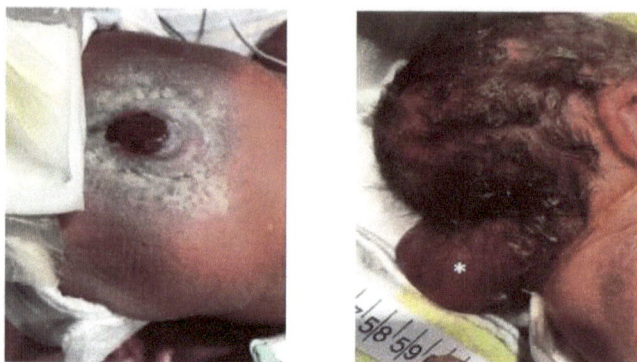

Fig. (7.4). On the left this newborn was born with a lumbar myelomeningoceles. Figure 7.5 on the right a posterior encephaloceles (asterisk) is seen in this newborn. This encephaloceles contained critical vascular structures from the deep venous system and was repaired in stages.

Craniosynostosis

Only in the setting of multiple fused sutures and life-threatening increased ICP is there ever urgency for treatment. However, early diagnosis is important because the treatment options diminish with age. Skull shape abnormalities also can be acquired in the infant. The most common acquired skull shape abnormality is labeled as "positional molding," "positional plagiocephaly," or "posterior plagiocephaly." This acquired deformation is best understood by considering the neonatal skull as a parallelogram with all corners being hinges, compression and flattening of one posterior side leads to advancement or protrusion of the ipsilateral anterior side of the cranial vault and base. Whether the skull shape abnormality is truly Craniosynostosis or acquired, the diagnosis and differentiation is best done by a physician expert in pediatric craniofacial abnormalities. Because some forms of Craniosynostosis are best treated early in infancy, immediate referral to a specialist is important when Craniosynostosis is suspected. The need for radiographic confirmation or refutation of a diagnosis is rarely necessary.

Vascular Malformations of the Brain

Four subtypes of intracranial vascular malformations warrant discussion: arteriovenous malformations (AVMs), cavernous malformations (CMs), arteriovenous fistula (AVF), and developmental venous anomalies (DVAs). These entities are not unique to the intracranial space and can occur in other organ systems. However, it is important to remember that a 5-mL hemorrhage in the brain can be lethal when compared with a 5-mL hemorrhage in the liver.

AVMs are thought to represent a persistence of fetal circulation with the failure of development of an intervening capillary network. The arterialized blood flow enters the venous side directly, which results in the thin-walled venous system being subjected to arterial pressures. Also, the reduced vascular resistance can create a local steal phenomenon as blood flow preferentially courses through the low-resistance AVM (Fig. **7.6 A**). Although the vascular pathophysiology can cause headaches, neurologic deficits, and chronic seizures, the most feared sequelae is hemorrhage. Mortality and major morbidity from a single bleed is likely more than 10%. The annual bleed rate for all AVMs is approximately 3%. AVMs that have bled have a higher recurrent hemorrhage rate than those that have never bled. AVMs represent the single most likely cause of spontaneous intracranial hemorrhage in a child. Any child presenting with a spontaneous intraparenchymal hemorrhage (Fig. **7.6 B**) should be assumed to have an AVM until proven otherwise. Other causes of spontaneous intracranial hemorrhage in children are neoplasms, aneurysms, cysts, and coagulopathy. CMs are slow-flow lesions and infrequently associated with catastrophic hemorrhage unless located in the brain stem. They can slowly expand over time like a slow-growing neoplasms. The "leakage of blood" more than frank rupture, results in iron deposition in the surrounding brain parenchyma. Hence, these lesions often manifest with seizures (Fig. **7.7**). When familial, they are often associated with multiple intracranial CMs. CMs have a very characteristic appearance on MRI and rarely represent a diagnostic quandary after appropriate imaging has been obtained Angiography is not indicated when the MRI studies are diagnostic. For lesions that are causing problems such as neurologic deficit or seizures or associated with multiple hemorrhages or expanding in size on surveillance imaging, resection is indicated if the lesion is accessible. The experience with SRS is not as robust with CMs as with AVMs; however, there is some evidence that SRS. Can favorably alter the rebleed rate in lesions that would be considered too high risk for operative resection? However, microsurgical resection remains the optimal treatment to eliminate the bleeding risk and favorably influence seizure outcomes. In the pediatric age group, the AVF that occurs with some frequency is the so-called vein of Galen aneurysm. This is a misnomer because aneurysms occur on the arterial side and varices on the venous side. Nevertheless, the fistula inputs directly into the deep venous system resulting in a compensatory dilatation of the vein of Galen and/or other components of the deep venous system in this region. These are often high-flow lesions that can be associated with enough of a shunt that an infant may present initially with high-output cardiac failure. Because of intracranial venous hypertension, hydrocephalus is often sequelae of such lesions. Microsurgery is not a realistic option for these children. This entity is best managed with aggressive medical management for any cardiac issues and then staged embolization to slowly reduce the arteriovenous shunt. DVAs are not pathologic entities but represent an anatomic variant of necessary venous drainage because of an aberration in normal venous development. They are not the cause of intracranial hemorrhage or seizures. They have a classic appearance of "caput Medusa" on MRI. The finding often triggers a neurosurgical evaluation that results in simply providing reassurance and education about the benign nature of the finding. CMs can be associated with DVA.

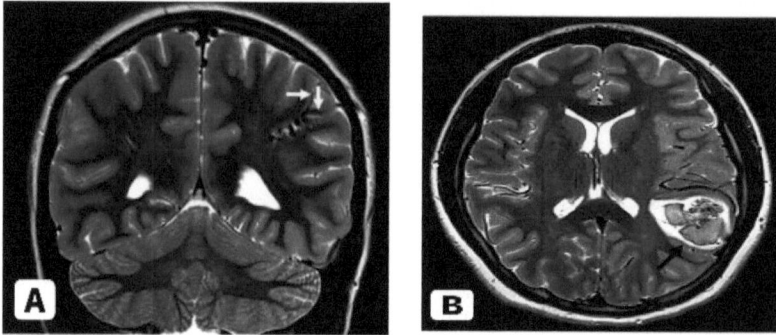

Fig. (7.6). A) T2-weighted coronal MR image of the brain in a 12-year-old boy presenting with a seizure. It shows an unruptured arteriovenous malformation with the horizontal arrow indicating a feeding artery and the vertical arrow indicating the enlarged draining vein. B) T2-weighted axial MR image showing a ruptured arteriovenous malformation (AVM) (arrow) in a bilingual (Mandarin and English) teenager with hemorrhage involving the primary speech area. English was her second language and was more affected by the hemorrhage than her native language. Surgical removal of the hematoma and AVM resulted in markedly improved language function.

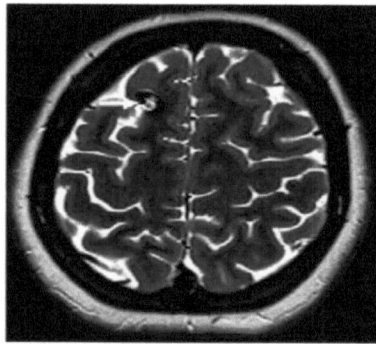

Fig. (7.7). T2-weighted axial MR image of the brain showing a right frontal cavernous malformation (arrow) in a teenager with epilepsy. Her seizures were cured with microsurgical resection of the lesion.

Tethered Spinal Cord

The pediatric surgeon caring for children with the VACTERL syndrome, cloacal abnormalities, or sacral agenesis needs to be aware of the association with a tethered spinal cord, though most children with a tethered spinal cord do not have an accompanying identifiable syndrome. A tethered spinal cord represents a spinal cord considered at risk for being under tension from an anatomic abnormality. This tension is thought to cause neurologic dysfunction from injury to, or impedance of, function within the spinal cord. Clinically this can result in bowel or bladder dysfunction, neurologic deficits of the lower extremities, scoliosis, and back pain. In neonates, neurologic deficits are often not recognizable. However, a club foot may represent neurologic dysfunction and is a not an infrequent finding with a tethered cord presenting in infancy. The examination of these infants should include inspection of the back for any cutaneous markers of a tethered spinal cord or scoliosis. These cutaneous signs include a midline hemangioma, subcutaneous lipoma (Fig. **7.8 A**), dimples or tracts above the gluteal cleft (Fig. **7.8 B**), and midline appendage, such as a vestigial tail, hairy patch (Fig. **7.8 C**), or any midline skin abnormality. An examination with attention to foot deformities, motor function, and grimace or cry to pin prick in the lumbosacral dermatomes is important. Rarely is a tethered spinal cord a clinical emergency. Spinal US before 3 months of age can provide clinically useful information, but it also can provide inaccurate or confusing information. A spinal MRI in the early neonatal period is predictably of poor quality. If the clinical scenario allows, an MRI delayed until 3–6 months of age is a reasonable strategy when assessing an infant for a tethered spinal cord (Fig. **7.9**). The one scenario in which earlier intervention is indicated is in the setting of a dermal sinus tract with intraspinal connection. These children are thought to be at risk for bacterial meningitis because of the potential communication and should be explored for sinus tract excision and spinal cord release when diagnosed. As a general statement, neurologic decline during infancy from a tethered spinal cord would be an exceedingly rare event. Intracranial neoplasms in children are the most common solid tumors in children. The histopathology, size, and locations of these brain tumors vary widely. Accordingly, the clinical presentation, management, and outcomes of children harboring brain tumors vary widely.

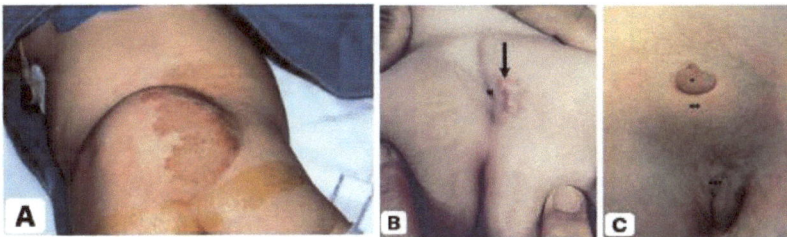

Fig. (7.8). (A) sizable lipomyelomeningocele is seen with a cutaneous hemangioma. (B) Photograph of the lumbosacral region in an infant with a lipomyelomeningocele. Note the abnormal hemangiomatous skin (arrow) and irregular dimpling above the gluteal cleft (asterisk). (C) This photograph of the lumbosacral region in an infant shows a lipomyelomeningocele with a midline skin appendage (*), subcutaneous lipoma (**), and hairy patch with deviated crease above the gluteal cleft (***).

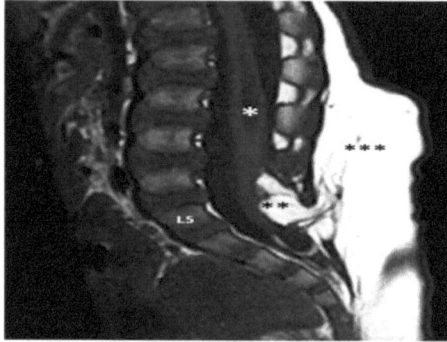

Fig. (7.9). T1-weighted MR image of the lumbar spine in the sagittal plane in an infant presenting with a foot deformity that shows a syrinx in the lumbar spinal cord (*), an intraspinal lipoma (**) tethering the cord at the L5 level, and the clinically obvious subcutaneous lipoma (***) often seen with these lesions. L5, fifth lumbar vertebral body.

Pilocytic Astrocytoma

Often referred to as juvenile Pilocytic astrocytoma (JPA), this is histopathological the most benign tumor, being a World Health Organization (WHO) grade I. These tumors are often, though not always, well circumscribed and brightly enhancing on contrast imaging. There is commonly an associated cyst with minimal surrounding edema, and they are often located in noncritical locations. Because of a low proliferative index, most JPAs are slow growing and can therefore reach tremendous size before coming to clinical attention (Fig. **7.10**). Those in the cerebellum will commonly manifest because of symptoms caused by obstructive hydrocephalus. Surgical excision remains the standard therapy. However, because of location or involvement of critical structures, complete excision often can cause significant morbidity.

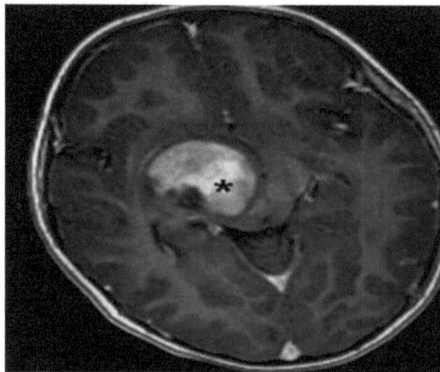

Fig. (7.10). T1-weighted MR image with gadolinium in the axial plane shows a large circumscribed enhancing tumor (asterisk) involving the brain stem in a toddler presenting with a mild hemiparesis. This was found to be a Pilocytic astrocytoma.

Medulloblastoma

Molecular sub typing of this small, round, blue cell tumor involving the cerebellum has made the label "medulloblastoma" almost obsolete. By definition, this tumor occurs in the posterior fossa. In children, medulloblastoma most commonly involves the midline of the cerebellum and fourth ventricle with variable invasion of the brain stem and is almost always associated with obstructive hydrocephalus by the time of clinical presentation. Dissemination throughout the CSF can occur at presentation and should be screened for with craniospinal contrasted MRI preoperatively, if possible (Fig. **7.11**). As with most cerebella and fourth ventricular tumors, complete resection is the goal. Small amounts of residual tumor, however, do not affect prognosis. Adjuvant therapy is always necessary and guided by the molecular subtype.

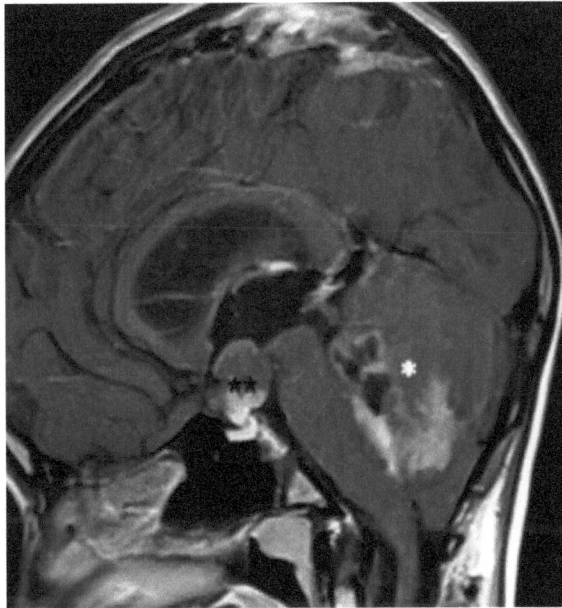

Fig. (7.11). T1-weighted MR image with gadolinium in the sagittal plane shows a medulloblastoma of the fourth ventricle (*) presenting with dissemination of the tumor into the third ventricle (**).

EPENDYMOMA

Thought to have its origin from ependymal cells that line the ventricular surface, this tumor is often found within or abutting a ventricle. Ependymomas can be found in either the supratentorial or infratentorial spaces. The histopathology can be anaplastic or not anaplastic. However, a lack of anaphase does not qualify this tumor as benign. Recent molecular sub typing has identified two groups that carry different prognostic expectations. When these tumors involve the fourth ventricle, they can extrude through the fourth ventricular outlets and wrap around the lower cranial nerves and arteries of the cerebellopontine angle all the way to include the basilar artery (Fig. **7.12**). Complete resection is very important to achieve the best prognosis but can come at a price if critical structures are involved. There is no defined role yet for chemotherapy with these tumors. It is not clear if radiation therapy helps prevent recurrence in tumors that appear completely resected.

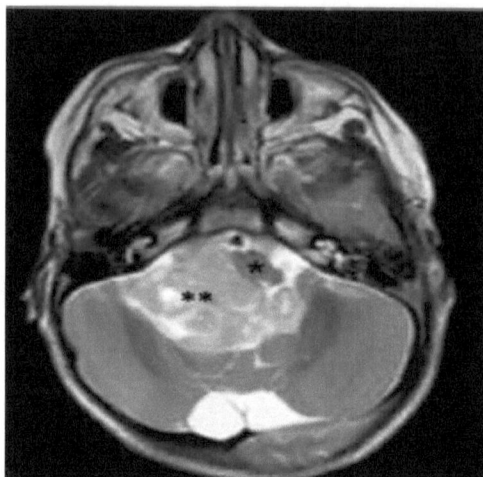

Fig. (7.12). This T2-weighted MR image in the axial plane was taken in a toddler with worsening gait. The signs were found to be due to an anaplastic Ependymomas. Note the brain stem (asterisk) distortion by the tumor (double asterisk) as it fills and exits the fourth ventricle.

Complete resection is very important to achieve the best prognosis but can come at a price if critical structures are involved. There is no defined role yet for chemotherapy with these tumors. It is not clear if radiation therapy helps prevent recurrence in tumors that appear completely resected.

Choroid Plexus Tumours

Tumors of the choroid plexus can be benign (choroid plexus papilloma) (Fig. **7.13**) or very malignant (choroid plexus carcinoma). They most often manifest in infants and toddlers, though delayed presentation into the teenage years also can occur. At times they will even present as incidental lesions. The mode of clinical presentation is often secondary to hydrocephalus. The tumor is located intraventricular and is brightly enhancing on contrasted MRI. Carcinomas are associated with parenchymal invasion and edema and are highly vascular, making them surgically treacherous in a small child with a limited blood volume. Mortality rates are high with the malignant form of this neoplasm.

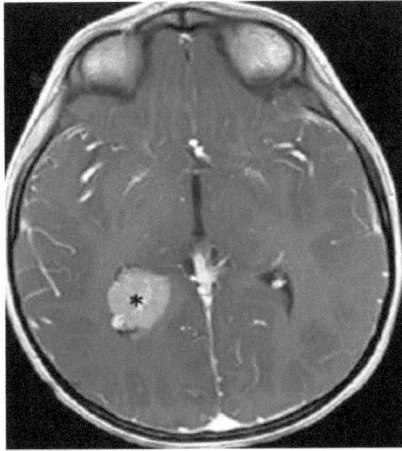

Fig. (7.13). T1-weighted MR with gadolinium in axial plane shows a right intraventricular choroid plexus papilloma (asterisk).

Germ Cell Neoplasms

These neoplasms also range from benign to highly malignant. They are thought to originate from pluripotent cells early in development. The most benign would be a teratoma without malignant characteristics, a pure germinoma, although malignant and requiring adjuvant therapy has an extremely high cure rate. Mixed malignant germ cell tumors, with components of choriocarcinoma, endodermal sinus tumor, or embryonal carcinoma, are highly malignant tumors and require intensive adjuvant therapy. Many of these lesions manifest in the pineal region. A primary suprasellar location is often associated with germinoma and is associated with diabetes insipid us. No part of the brain, however, is immune from germ cell neoplasms and thalamic and basal ganglia locations are possible as well. Whereas teratoma requires resection, the malignant germ cell tumors respond very nicely to adjuvant therapy, though the response may not be enduring. Diagnosis can sometimes be achieved without tissue confirmation through a combination of imaging and CSF or serum tumor markers for α-fetoprotein and human chorionic Gonadotropin.

DIFFUSE INTRINSIC PONTINE GLIOMA

Diffuse intrinsic pontine glioma represents the most malignant of pediatric brain tumors in that it is essentially universally fatal. This tends to be a tumor that manifests in school-age children, though the preschool and teenage years are not immune. These children present with ataxia, cranial neuropathies, and occasionally raised ICP. The diagnosis is made by imaging on MRI without the need for biopsy. The imaging shows a hyper intense signal on T2 sequences that is centered within and expands the pons (Fig. **7.14**). Enhancement is variable following injection of contrast. Hydrocephalus is not usually significant at presentation. Biopsy is currently being advocated to obtain material for scientific investigation, but not necessarily to help the particular child undergoing the biopsy. Fractionated radiation is effective at reducing tumor size and temporarily improving neurologic deficits. No role for chemotherapy has been defined.

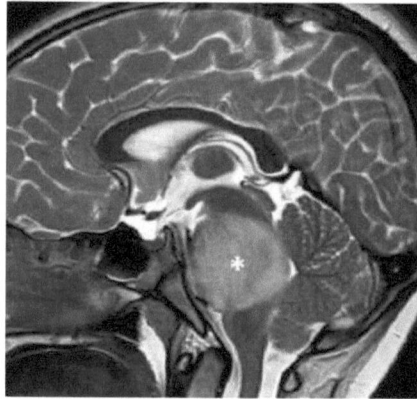

Fig. (7.14). This T2-weighted sagittal MR image shows a hyper intense expansible lesion (asterisk) diagnostic for a diffuse intrinsic pontine glioma.

Intracranial Infections

An intracranial infectious process requiring immediate neurosurgical intervention is subdural emphysema. The typical child is a preadolescent or teenage boy with sinusitis that presents with worsening headache, fever, a neurologic deficit, encephalopathy, or seizure. No age group or gender is immune. These subdural emphysemas should not be confused with extra-axial spinal fluid collections associated with infantile meningitis. Intracranial imaging even with contrast may be subtle regarding the extra-axial collection in the subdural space caused by subdural emphysema. It is the subtlety of the imaging that makes this such a confusing and dangerous entity.

Mild degrees of mass effect with minimal extra-axial collections can be incorrectly interpreted as not representing a critical condition. It is absolutely critical to perform an immediate craniotomy upon diagnosis of subdural emphysema. The mortality rate is extremely high without prompt neurosurgical intervention. It is also important to involve an otolaryngologist for debridement or drainage of the paranasal sinuses that represent the original source of the infection. The need for repeat craniotomy is very real with this disease as it can recur or develop in a new area even while on appropriate antibiotics. Although streptococcal species are the most frequent causative organisms, broad-spectrum coverage to include anaerobes is necessary until all cultures have returned.

Anticonvulsants should be administered because the seizure-inducing nature of this disease, from both inflammation and cortical venous thrombosis, is significant. Short-term repeat imaging is critical in management as the collections of pus can recur or parenchymal involvement with frank brain abscess can develop. Brain abscesses can be bacterial or fungal. In children, congenital heart disease may be an underlying cause, though more often the abscesses are complications of sinusitis as just described. Fungal abscesses can be seen in survivors of near-drowning events in fresh water. Treatment is driven by the need for identifying the organism, relief of any mass effect or elevated ICP, and clearance of infection. Stereotactic techniques allow for safe needle aspiration of an abscess located almost anywhere within the cranium.

CONSENT FOR PUBLICATION

Not applicable.

CONFLICT OF INTEREST

The author declares no conflict of interest, financial or otherwise.

ACKNOWLEDGEMENTS

Declared none.

REFRENCES

[1]   Yasuda T, Tomita T, McLone DG, Donovan M. Measurement of cerebrospinal fluid output through external ventricular drainage in one hundred infants and children: correlation with cerebrospinal fluid production. Pediatr Neurosurg 2002; 36(1): 22-8.
[http://dx.doi.org/10.1159/000048344] [PMID: 11818742]

[2]   Dekaban AS, Sadowsky D. Changes in brain weights during the span of human life: relation of brain weights to body heights and body weights. Ann Neurol 1978; 4(4): 345-56.
[http://dx.doi.org/10.1002/ana.410040410] [PMID: 727739]

[3]   Sato O, Yamguchi T, Kittaka M, Toyama H. Hydrocephalus and epilepsy. Childs Nerv Syst 2001; 17(1-2): 76-86.
[http://dx.doi.org/10.1007/s003810000381] [PMID: 11219629]

[4]   Boyle TP, Paldino MJ, Kimia AA, *et al.* Comparison of rapid cranial MRI to CT for ventricular shunt malfunction. Pediatrics 2014; 134(1): e47-54.
[http://dx.doi.org/10.1542/peds.2013-3739] [PMID: 24918222]

[5]   Weil AG, Fallah A, Chamiraju P, Ragheb J, Bhatia S. Endoscopic third ventriculostomy and choroid plexus cauterization with a rigid neuroendoscope in infants with hydrocephalus. J Neurosurg Pediatr 2016; 17(2): 163-73.
[http://dx.doi.org/10.3171/2015.5.PEDS14692] [PMID: 26517057]

[6]   Yavuz C, Demırtas S, Calıskan A, *et al.* Reasons, procedures, and outcomes in ventriculoatrial shunts: A single-center experience. Surg Neurol Int 2013; 4: 10.
[http://dx.doi.org/10.4103/2152-7806.106284] [PMID: 23493480]

[7]   Bui CJ, Tubbs RS, Pate G, *et al.* Infections of pediatric cerebrospinal fluid shunts related to fundoplication and gastrostomy. J Neurosurg 2007; 107: 365-7.

[8]   Handler MH, Callahan B. Laparoscopic placement of distal ventriculoperitoneal shunt catheters. J Neurosurg Pediatr 2008; 2(4): 282-5.
[http://dx.doi.org/10.3171/PED.2008.2.10.282] [PMID: 18831665]

[9]   Vender JR, Hester S, Waller JL, *et al.* Identification and management of intrathecal baclofen pump complications: a comparison of pediatric and adult patients. J Neurosurg 2006; 104: 9-15.

[10]   Elliott RE, Rodgers SD, Bassani L, *et al.* Vagus nerve stimulation for children with treatment-resistant epilepsy: a consecutive series of 141 cases. J Neurosurg Pediatr 2011; 7(5): 491-500.
[http://dx.doi.org/10.3171/2011.2.PEDS10505] [PMID: 21529189]

[11]   Bui CJ, Tubbs RS, Shannon CN, *et al.* Institutional experience with cranial vault encephaloceles. J Neurosurg 2007; 107(1) (Suppl.): 22-5.
[PMID: 17644916]

[12]   Adamo MA, Pollack IF. Current management of craniosynostosis. Neurosurg Q 2009; 19: 82.
[http://dx.doi.org/10.1097/WNQ.0b013e3181a32e1e]

[13]   Virchow R. Uber den Cretinismus, namentlich in Franken, und uberpathologische Schadelformen. Verhandl Phys-Med Gessellschr Wurz-burg 1851; 2: 241.

[14]   Laughlin J, Luerssen TG, Dias MS. Prevention and management of positional skull deformities in infants. Pediatrics 2011; 128(6): 1236-41.
[http://dx.doi.org/10.1542/peds.2011-2220] [PMID: 22123884]

[15]   El-Ghanem M, Kass-Hout T, Kass-Hout O, *et al.* Arteriovenous malfor- mations in the pediatric population: review of the existing literature. Intervent Neurol 2016; 5(3-4): 218-25.
[http://dx.doi.org/10.1159/000447605] [PMID: 27781052]

[16]   DeSouza RM, Jones BRT, Lowis SP, Kurian KM. Pediatric medulloblastoma - update on molecular classification driving targeted therapies. Front Oncol 2014; 4: 176.
[http://dx.doi.org/10.3389/fonc.2014.00176] [PMID: 25101241]

[17]   Ramaswamy V, Hielscher T, Mack SC, *et al.* Therapeutic impact of cyto- reductive surgery and irradiation of posterior fossa ependymoma in the molecular era: a retrospective multicohort analysis. J Clin Oncol 2016; 34(21): 2468-77.
[http://dx.doi.org/10.1200/JCO.2015.65.7825] [PMID: 27269943]

[18]   Siegfried A, Morin S, Munzer C, *et al.* A French retrospective study on clinical outcome in 102 choroid plexus tumors in children. J Neurooncol 2017; 135(1): 151-60.
[http://dx.doi.org/10.1007/s11060-017-2561-2] [PMID: 28677107]

[19]   Huang X, Zhang R, Mao Y, Zhou LF, Zhang C. Recent advances in molecular biology and treatment strategies for intracranial germ cell tumors. World J Pediatr 2016; 12(3): 275-82.
[http://dx.doi.org/10.1007/s12519-016-0021-2] [PMID: 27351562]

[20]   Clark AJ, Cage TA, Aranda D, Parsa AT, Auguste KI, Gupta N. Treatment-related morbidity and the management of pediatric craniopharyngioma: a systematic review. J Neurosurg Pediatr 2012; 10(4): 293-301.
[http://dx.doi.org/10.3171/2012.7.PEDS11436] [PMID: 22920295]

[21]   Cohen M, Bartels U, Branson H, Kulkarni AV, Hamilton J. Trends in treatment and outcomes of pediatric craniopharyngioma, 1975-2011. Neuro-oncol 2013; 15(6): 767-74.
[http://dx.doi.org/10.1093/neuonc/not026] [PMID: 23486689]

[22]   Hamisch C, Kickingereder P, Fischer M, Simon T, Ruge MI. Update on the diagnostic value and safety of stereotactic biopsy for pediatric brainstem tumors: a systematic review and meta-analysis of 735 cases. J Neurosurg Pediatr 2017; 20(3): 261-8.
[http://dx.doi.org/10.3171/2017.2.PEDS1665] [PMID: 28621573]

[23]   Quraishi H, Zevallos JP. Subdural empyema as a complication of sinusitis in the pediatric population. Int J Pediatr Otorhinolaryngol 2006; 70(9): 1581-6.
[http://dx.doi.org/10.1016/j.ijporl.2006.04.007] [PMID: 16777239]

CHAPTER 8

Breast Surgery

Nada R. Alharis[1], Najah R. Hadi[2,*] and Sultan M. Ghanim[3,*]

[1] *Faculty of Medicine University of Kufa, Iraq*

[2] *Faculty of Medicine University of Kufa, Iraq*

[3] *ME Unit, Medical College, Faculty of Medicine, University of Kufa, Iraq*

Abstract: At the end of week 4 of human embryonic development, paired thickenings appear in the ectoderm on the ventral aspect of the torso. Extending from the axilla to the inguinal region, they form the mammary ridges or "milk lines." Subsequently they regress and leave a pair of primary mammary buds at the level of the fourth and fifth inter- costal spaces. The primary buds thicken into lens-shaped mammary placodes. Epithelial cells invade the underlying mesenchyme during weeks 7 and 8 to form the primitive mammary disk. In week 9, a surge of mesenchymal proliferation occurs, coincident with a thinning of the overlying epithelium. A dense mesenchymal stroma then coalesces around the bud. Between weeks 10 and 12, epithelial buds form, begin to branch, and extend into the epithelial–mesenchyme bound- ary. By the first half of the second trimester (weeks 13–20), there are 15–20 solid epithelial cords that converge at the nipples. Ramification processes continue to week 32, when the cords undergo apoptosis to establish tubules and alveoli. At birth, male and female mammary glands are equally formed. There are 20 lactiferous ducts draining into the dimple. In later stages of the final trimester, the mesoderm underlying the dimple changes it into a true nipple with an areola. Placental estrogens during the final weeks of gestation cause breast buds to enlarge to create a true breast nodule at birth, about 1 cm in size, in both genders.

Keywords: Breast, Buds, Mammary.

DEVELOPMENT, ANATOMY, AND PHYSIOLOGY

At the end of week 4 of human embryonic development, paired thickenings appear in the ectoderm on the ventral aspect of the torso. Extending from the axilla to the inguinal region, they form the mammary ridges or "milk lines" Subsequently they regress and leave a pair of primary mammary buds at the level of the fourth and fifth intercostal spaces. The primary buds thicken into lens-shaped mammary placodes. Epithelial cells invade the underlying mesenchyme during weeks 7 and 8 to form the primitive mammary disk. In week 9, a surge of

---

* **Corresponding author Sultan M. Ghanim:** ME Unit, Medical College, Faculty of Medicine,University of Kufa, Iraq; Tel: +9647816669997; E-mail: sultanmalsaadi@uokufa.edu.iq

mesenchymal proliferation occurs, coincident with a thinning of the overlying epithelium. A dense mesenchymal stroma then coalesces around the bud.

Table (8.1). Causes of breast enlargement in female patient.

Bilateral	Unilateral
INFANCY **Normal breast bud** **Neonatal hypertrophy**	Normal breast bud Normal hypertrophy
CHILDHOOD **Premature thelarche** **Precocious puberty**	Asynchronous thelarche Simple cyst
ADOLESCENT **Virginal hypertrophy**	Giant fibroadenoma Phyllodes tumor Leukemia Lymphoma Metastatic cancer Primary breast cancer

Between weeks 10 and 12, epithelial buds form, begin to branch, and extend into the epithelial–mesenchyme boundary. During the first half of the second trimester or between 13-20 weeks, 15-20 solid epithelial cords approach towards an intersection point that is nipple. Ramification process in the epithelial cords leads to apoptosis to establish tubules and alveoli till week 32. At birth, male and female mammary glands are equally formed, each consisting of about 20 lactiferous ducts that open into a dimple. Late in the final trimester, proliferation of the mesoderm beneath the dimple transforms it into a true nipple with an areola. Placental estrogens during the final weeks of gestation cause breast buds to enlarge to create a true breast nodule at birth, about 1 cm in size, in both genders. The first sign of puberty in girls, thelarche, is the appearance of a breast bud. The appearance of pubic and axillary hair, pubarche, is a process that is dependent on the adrenal production of androgens and generally appears within a year after thelarche. Menarche, the final event of puberty, occurs a little more than 2 years after thelarche [2]. Marshall and Tanner formally described the development of the mature female breast in five stages, a process that takes about 4.5 years [3]:

Stage 1: Preadolescent ; This indicates the time when papilla elevates
Stage 2: Breast bud stage ; breast and areola eleavtes and areola diameter increases
Stage 3: Further enlargement period of breast and areola,
Stage 4: Projection of the areola and papilla to form a secondary mound above the level of the breast

Stage 5: Mature stage: Projection of papilla only.

Pathophysiology

An aberration of normal development and involution (ANDI) leads to benign diseases in the female breast. ANDI organizes benign breast disorders and diseases into a framework of normal events of breast development: fibroadenoma, a disorder related to normal lobular development ; juvenile hypertrophy, stroma development; cysts and ductal ectasia, involution. The breast in early infancy goes through similar events during the mini-puberty, so some of the same categories of disorders can also be found during infancy and early childhood [4]. ANDI is a useful framework that organizes benign breast disorders with commonsense therapeutic strategies [5]. Breast cancer is rarely present in pediatric stage of life, late adolescence is the age when it is usually diagnosed. Dysregulation of genetic controls of breast embryogenesis, such as homeobox genes, may play a role in the development of adult breast cancer [1].

Disorder of Development and Growth Neonatal Hypertrophy

As discussed previously, the newborn breast bud enlarges during the mini-puberty of early infancy (Fig. **8.1**). This phase seldom lasts longer than a few months. Infant breast enlargement involutes spontaneously within a few weeks without specific treatment.

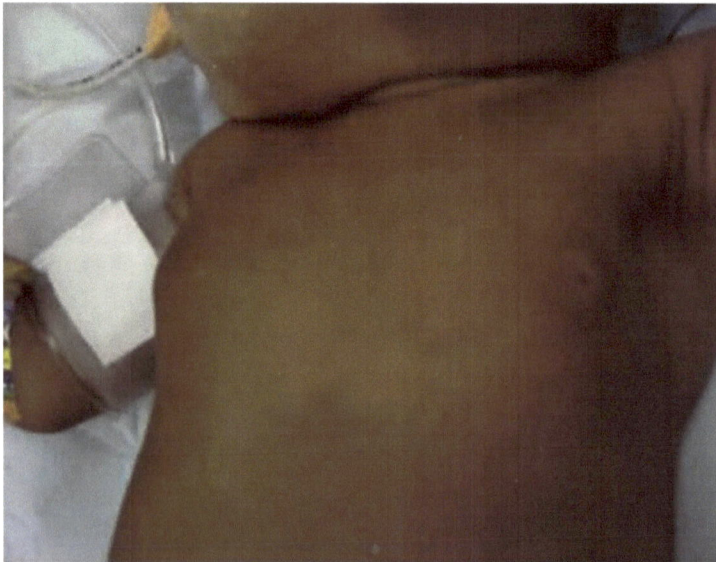

Fig. (8.1).   This 3-month-old girl with neonatal hypertrophy is undergoing an operation for another indication. Breast enlargement in early infancy is normal and regresses without treatment.

Polythelia

This is associated with the the presence of supernumerary nipples. It is a condition in which areolae develops anywhere along the milk line from axilla to pubis in up to 5% of children, mostly it appears below the actual breast (Fig. **8.2**). An auxiliary breast is rarely encountered as a discrete mass, with or without a nipple, most commonly in the axilla. Unsightly structures should be removed by surgery or liposuction [6, 7].

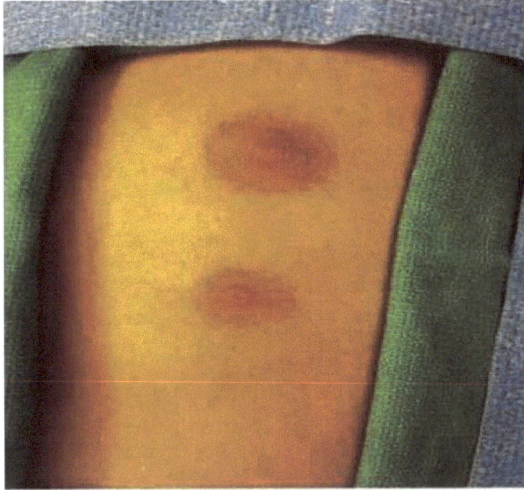

Fig. (8.2). This 6-year-old girl has polythelia. The accessory areola is inferior to the normal areola.

Hypoplasia and Aplasia

Breast asymmetry is common (Fig. **8.3**). Profound differences in size may lead to cosmetic surgery, including augmentation of the smaller breast with implant, and reduction and mastopexy of the larger breast, once both breasts are fully developed at age 17–18. Use of tissue expanders may be necessary if differences are extreme, or combining augmentation of the smaller breast with reduction of the larger one [7]. Breast development is affected by Poland's syndrome, a range of malformations characterized by varying degrees of hypoplasia and aplasia of the breast and nipple, pectoralis major and sternocleidomastoid muscles, thorax, and hand. Reconstruction strategies depend on the extent of breast hypoplasia and the degree of pectoral and thoracic maldevelopment. The most profound defects will require reconstruction with a prosthesis and chest wall augmentation using a variety of flap techniques [6]. Incisions for a central venous catheter, chest tube, and drainage of a breast abscess may interfere with later breast growth and development [8]. This is a matter of extra care to make incisions in premature infants, as the breast bud is not developed and visible. Thoracotomy and chest wall reconstruction for pectus deformities may interfere with breast development in older children.9 Bilateral hypoplasia suggests delayed puberty, defined clinically by the absence or incomplete development of secondary sexual characteristics by age 13 in girls and age 14 years in boys [2]. Hypogonadism is the absence of physical signs of puberty by age 18 in both genders. Delayed puberty requires evaluation by a pediatric endocrinologist for ovarian failure. There are some other assessments also to be made in case of delayed puberty and these include gonadal dysgenesis, congenital adrenal hyperplasia, varieties of intersex disorders, and hypogonadotrophism [10].

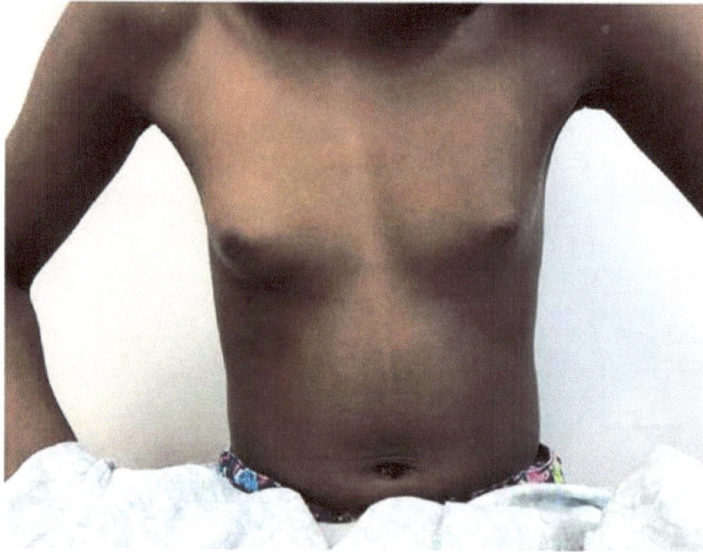

Fig. (8.3). An 11-year-old was referred for right breast enlargement. On clinical exam, both breasts were normal, but the right one was larger. Endocrinological evaluation was also normal. Asymmetric breast development and size is not unusual.

Gynecomastia

Gynecomastia is also a benign condition in male resulting from the proliferation of glandular tissue of breast resembling to that of a female. This proliferation of male breast may occur in the neonate, adolescent, and elderly. Gynecomastia that occurs after infancy and before puberty warrants an urgent referral to a pediatric endocrinologist to evaluate for feminizing adrenal and testicular tumors, an array of endocrine and metabolic disorders that end with excess estrogen or deficient androgen, and chromosomal defects that have feminized phenotypes. Review of medications and possible exogenous sources of environmental agents is mandatory, because of the long list of drugs associated with gynecomastia Table **8.2** [12]. Pubertal status and testicular size are a necessary part of the physical examination. Laboratory indices include appropriate tests for hypogonadism, thyroid, liver, and kidney disease. Specific hormone levels include morning serum testosterone and LH, FSH, prolactin estrogen, and human chorionic gonadotropin (hCG) [12]. Up to 70% of boys exhibit physiologic or pubertal gynecomastia, often associated with pain and tenderness. This condition first appears in males of age 10 and 12 years, and boys of age 13–14 years are more prone to this condition, corresponding to Tanner stage 3 or 4. Within 1–3 years, up to 90% of boys have regression of their breast enlargement and resolution of discomfort [11].

Table (8.2). Drugs associated with gynecomastia.

Drug	Examples
Hormones	Androgens, anabolic steroids, estrogens, estrogen agonists and human chorionic gonadotropin
Antiandrogens\inhibitors of androgen synthesis	Bicalutamide, flutamide, nilutamide, cyproterone and gonadotropinreleasing hormone agonists (leuprolide and goserelin)
Antibiotic	Metronidazole, ketoconazole, β-minocycline, isoniazid
Anti-ulcer	Cimetidine, ranitidine, omeprazole
Abuse	Alcohol, heroin, amphetamines
Chemotherapy	Methotrexate, alkylating agents, Vinca alkaloids, cyclophosphamide
Cardiovascular	Digoxin, furosemide, spironolactone, angiotensin-converting enzyme inhibitors (captopril and enalapril), calcium channel blockers (diltiazem, nifedipine, verapamil), reserpine, amiodarone, α-methyldopa, spironolactone, and minoxidil
Psychiatric\neurologic	Anxiolytic agents (*e.t.*, diazepam), tricyclic antidepressants, phenothiazines, haloperidol, phenytoin, risperidone, clonidine, selective serotonin reuptake inhibitors
Others	Antiretroviral therapy for HIV, metoclopramide, penicillamine, phenytoin, sulindac, cyclosporine

True gynecomastia can be palpated as a disc of rubbery tissue concentrated under and around the nipple and areola. There is another condition known as pseudogynecomastia, which is the result of prominence of adipose tissue under the breast. During palpation both the conditions can be easily differentiated. True gynecomastia is evaluated by the family history of the patient and examination of testes in adolescence. Usually the follow-up evaluations are conducted after 6 months and this condition may take 1 year untill it is totally resolved. If the condition is not resolved it may lead to rapid increase in the size of breast > 4 cm in diameter, known as macrogynecomastia and the other condition is known as or pubertal gynecomastia. An endocrine and oncological workup is the key treatment. If the condition prevails even after one year, imaging of the testes and adrenals is conducted for the evaluation of tumor [11]. In case of severe pain, tenderness, or embarrassment interfering patient's activities, a surgery may be required. Subcutaneous mastectomy through a periareolar incision and liposuction are both acceptable [23].

INFLAMMATORY LESIONS

Breast Trauma and Fat Necrosis

Fat necrosis in childhood almost always arises from trauma. In about half of cases the child does not recall an injury. Hemorrhage in fat leads to cystic degeneration and scarring, a process that may resolve completely or leave a cyst, a nodular mass, or a lesion that may mimic breast carcinoma on exam. A hyperechoic lesion on ultrasonography (US) in the setting of recent injury is almost always benign fat necrosis [13]. Magnetic resonance imaging (MRI) is helpful when internal signal characteristics are identical to adjacent fat and no evidence of enhancement is seen after intravenous contrast. The diagnosis is difficult when fat necrosis leaves calcification detectable on mammography; when surrounding inflammation creates contrast enhancement on computed tomography (CT), positron emission tomography–computed tomography (PET–CT), and MRI; or if the area creates indistinct and speculated scarring [14]. The rarity of malignancy in adolescent girls is reassuring, but biopsy is necessary to exclude malignancy.

MASTITIS AND ABSCESS

Infections of the breast of a neonate primarily affect the neonatal breast before ductal involution later in infancy. Peak incidence is in the fourth and fifth weeks of life and affects girls more often than boys, in a 1.7:1 ratio. Staphylococcus, a genus of Gram-positive bacteria is associated with 90% of cases and other causative organisms may include Streptococcus, Enterobacter, Salmonella, and *Escherichia coli* [28]. The skin and nipple are red in simple mastitis with swelling and edema surrounding the area. Erythema and swelling are seen in nearly all cases. Deep discoloration and edema suggest the presence of an abscess beneath the fascia. Fluctuance is diagnostic of an abscess. Discharge may occur from the involved area, and sometimes from the nipple. Fever, irritability, and refusal to feed may be present in 14–43% [15]. One-fourth of the patients has pustular skin lesions elsewhere, often in the inguinal region. Infants receive additional laboratory studies, including serum C-reactive protein (CRP) levels (elevated in 51%), and blood, urine, and cerebrospinal fluid (CSF) cultures. Sonography may be useful in distinguishing abscesses from areas of inflammation [16]. In almost all cases, mastitis in neonates responds to antibiotics and warm packs to the affected breast. Initial antibiotic therapy must cover methicillin-resistant Staphylococcus aureus (MRSA). If the inflammation even with the antibiotics, it indicates the presence of pus that requires drainage or an organism besides MRSA.15 Drainage of an abscess must avoid damage as it may lead to breast deformity later in adolescence. Needle aspiration is a usually the first step, with repeated aspirations if signs of inflammation improve. Somtimes it may require incision to ensure the drainage in an area away from the developing breast bud.

BREAST MASSES

Evaluation of Breast Masses

While making a diagnosis for breast masses, the age of the patient is the key factor (Boxes **8.1** and **8.2**) and the requirements for this may include Patient age, history, and physical examination. Traditional terms such as fibrocystic disease lack pathologic and clinical precision. An accurate diagnosis based on histology defines the risk for malignancy so that appropriate risk reduction interventions may be initiated. US is the appropriate initial imaging modality in children. It distinguishes cysts from solid masses and mastitis from abscess, clinically important distinctions. US gives sufficient detail to diagnose duct ectasia, hematoma, fat necrosis, infantile hemangioma, duct ectasia, juvenile papillomatosis, and fibroadenoma. Diagnostic mammography, because of the particularly high sensitivity of the developing breast to ionizing radiation, is rarely used in children and adolescents. CT is not used in the assessment of pediatric breast masses for the same reason. MRI is also not the first modality used in the assessment of breast cancer. It is appropriate for imaging vascular and lymphatic malformations that involve multiple anatomic compartments and may be close to major vessels and nerves [17]. Fludeoxyglucose (18F) positron emission tomography (FDG–PET) and PET-CT are not used for primary breast cancer detection because of the high false-negative and false-positive rates [18]. Fine-needle aspiration (25 or 22 gauge) will drain simple cysts and allow cytologic diagnosis of ductal ectasia. Core needle biopsy (14 to 9 gauge) with vacuum or automated devices provides larger samples with architectural detail. Small adolescent breasts may not accommodate a core biopsy needle. Lack of cytologic criteria and sampling issues limit the use of both fine and core needle techniques in the diagnostic assessments of fibroadenoma and phyllodes tumor. Open biopsy becomes necessary when cytology and core biopsy results yield high-risk lesions [19].Clinical evidence indicates that breast self-examination may not affect breast cancer outcome, with one national task force recommending against its use [20].

Benign Breast Diseases

Juvenile papillomatosis is a rare variant of epithelial hyperplasia, with a histologic appearance that would be considered premalignant in adults. Some patients develop breast cancer later in adulthood. Histology includes duct stasis and apocrine cysts that give it a descriptive pathologic term, "Swiss cheese disease" One-fourth has a family history of breast cancer. The age range, 12–48 years, includes adolescents [21]. Complete surgical excision is recommended to prevent relapse and the later development of cancer [22]. Tubular adenomas have prominent adenosis-like epithe- lial proliferation with sparse intervening stroma.

Box 8.1. Breast masses in children.

Physiologic
Normal breast bud
Premature thelarche
Pathologic
Inflammatory
Mastitis
Breast abscess
Fibrosis
Fat necrosis
Benign neoplasms
Hemangioma
Cyst Lipoma
Papilloma
Malignant neoplasms
Metastatic(*e.t.*, rhabdomyosarcoma,lymphoma)
Secretory carcinoma

Box 8.2. Breast masses in adolescent.

Physiologic
Thelarche
Unilateral hypertrophy
Pathologic
Inflammatory
Mastitis
Breast abscess
Fibrosis
Fat necrosis
Benign neoplasms
Fibroadenoma
Phyllodes tumor
Cyst
Fibrocystic disease
Neurofibroma
Malignant neoplasms
Primary breast cancer
Metastatic (*e.t.*, lymphoma)

Generally affecting young women of childbearing age, they rarely affect adolescents. Presenting as a well-circumscribed breast lump clinically indistinguishable from a fibroadenoma, they require needle or excisional biopsy for tissue diagnosis [23]. Pseudoangiomatous stromal hyperplasia (PASH) is a benign mesenchymal proliferation of stromal myofibroblasts. Although primarily affecting pre- and perimenopausal adult women, they can occur in adolescents. They present as well-circumscribed, rubbery, round or oval masses that clinically are indistinguishable from a simple fibroadenoma. Fixation artifacts create slit-like spaces that make the lesion appear like a low-grade angiosarcoma. Not being true vascular spaces, they contain no red blood cells, in contrast to a true angiosarcoma of the breast where vascular channels in the lesion contain blood. Patients not at increased risk for breast cancer can be observed [24].

SIMPLE CYSTS

These benign cysts may occur inchildhood, and most commonly with thelarche. They are soft and painless, range in size from 1–10 mm in diameter, and are not fixed to the surrounding breast tissue. They are thought to arise when acini or terminal ductules dilate and untwist to form a unilocular cyst. Those close to the skin may appear blue-tinged. The columnar epithelium that lines simple cysts have apocrine-like features and may form papillary tufts. Some believe that the apocrine changes represent metaplasia, but cysts do not have increased cancer risk if they are free from other proliferative lesions of higher risk. Needle aspiration of the cyst leads to its disappearance. Its fluid may be serous or brown. Biopsy is required if the cyst has suspicious features, such as internal hypoechoic areas and solid areas, or if the mass persists after aspiration [25].

FIBROEPITHELIAL TUMORS

Fibroadenomas

It is the most common breast mass among adolescent girls [26]. Three categories exist, based on presentation. Simple adenomas are most common, comprising 70–90% of cases. They are found as a single mass, painless, smooth, mobile, rubbery mass with distinct borders (Fig. **8.4**). They generally are about 1–3 cm in size, but occasionally they reach 10 cm in diameter. The remaining 25–30% are multiple, either in the same or both breasts. Giant fibroadenoma is a rare variant, about 1% of cases. Characterized by rapid growth, diagnostic criteria include size ≥ 5 cm in diameter, weight >500 g, and involvement of more than four-fifths of the breast. Venous engorgement and skin ulceration may occur. It is the most common cause of unilateral breast enlargement of the breast in adolescence [27].

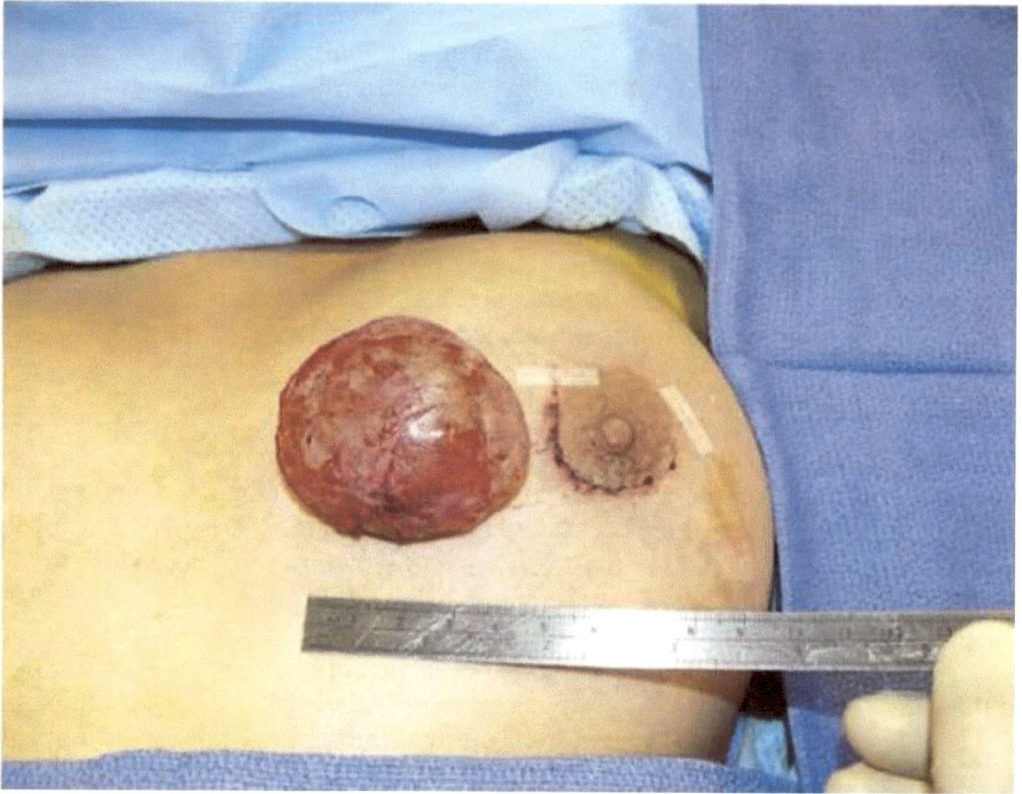

Fig. (8.4). An enlarged, painful fibroadenoma in her left breast shown by a 16 year old patient. The lesion measured 7 cm × 5 cm × 4 cm on ultrasound examination.

A fibroadenoma does not have a true capsule but a well- demarcated stromal interface. This is the place where the tumor may touch the normal tissue. Focal hemorrhage sometimes may be present, that could possibly be the cause of pain and rapid enlargement. Microscopic examination reveals a rich cellular stroma and a prominent glandular epithelium. Fibroadenomas are benign, but their presence doubles the risk for breast cancer. While a fibroadenoma rarely may harbor a carcinoma in an adult woman, such an association has not been reported in an adolescent [27]. Practical decisions regarding the diagnosis and manage ment of simple fibroadenomas are guided by three facts: A clinical diagnosis of a simple fibroadenoma can be made on history, physical examination, and US. Many of them will resolve, and in an adolescent girl, there is almost no risk of malignancy. Most painless, mobile, well-circumscribed breast lumps will be a benign simple fibroadenoma. US findings are characteristic but not specific, and are shared with phyllodes tumor and PASH36, both entities that can safely undergo a prolonged period of observation. Criteria for excision include size > 5 cm in diameter, rapid increase in size, painful lesions, those that distort the shape of the breast, multiple and bilateral lesions, stromal hypercellularity on US, and patients with a high risk for malignancy. Often patients and families will insist on removal of small tumors. Most can be convinced to wait at least 3–4 months before excision [27].

Phyllodes Tumors

Because their histology is similar, fibroadenomas may be related to phyllodes tumors. Phyllodes tumors, first called cystosarcoma phyllodes by Johannes Müller in his original report in 1838, are rare benign fibroepithelial tumors with a 40% risk for local recurrence) or malignant (with rapid growth and metastasis). The younger women of age below 20, are less affacted by this (10%); the usual age range is 33–55 years. The breast mass rapidly grows more than 6cm, with a range of 1–40 cm. Like a fibroadenoma, a phyllodes tumor may appear well circumscribed, but it, too, lacks a true capsule. Fibrous areas interspersed with soft, fleshy areas and cysts filled with clear or semisolid bloody fluid are the features that distinguish Phyllodes tumors from fibroadenoma. Stromal cell atypia, interstitial cell hyperplasia, mitotic activity, and whether the tumor boundary is infiltrated determine whether a phyllodes tumor is malignant. Fibroadenomas in adolescents tend to have increased stromal cellularity and increased mitotic activity, features that must be interpreted with caution. The mea nage of the patients is another factor that may distinguish Phyllodes tumors from fibroadenoma. (Mean age, 28.5 years in fibroadenoma, 44 years in phyllodes tumor). This tumor tends to be larger (>4 cm in diameter) compared with a fibroadenoma. On sonography, cysts within an otherwise solid mass are indicative of phyllodes tumor. Fine-needle aspiration is done if dimorphic pattern of stromal elements and benign epithelial tissue is detected. The diagnosis of phyllodes tumor can be made from core needle biopsy specimens in most cases with sufficient certainty to avoid surgery in >80% of cases. When preoperative workup cannot distinguish between a fibroadenoma and a phyllodes tumor, excisional biopsy may be necessary. Tumor grade correlates poorly with recurrence risk and metastatic potential. Benign, borderline, and malignant phyllodes tumors have 10–17%, 14–25%, and 2–30% risk of recurrence after excision, respectively. For each grade, the risk of metastasis is 0.13%, 1.62%, and 16.7%, respectively, illustrating the difficulty in distinguishing benign from malignant behavior on histologic criteria alone. There is exciting recent molecular evidence of a common mutation of MED [12] among fibroadenomas and both benign and malignant phyllodes tumors. Still, there are no molecular markers that predict malignant behavior. The nonaggressive behavior of benign phyllodes tumor warrants a conservative surgical approach. Wide local excision with 1-cm margin of normal breast tissue has been the mainstay recommendation for phyllodes tumor. Margin width does not correlate with recurrence, however, so less radical excision with narrower margins may be appropriate, especially if aggressive surgery will deform the remaining breast. Re-excision may not be required for benign tumors that had been enucleated without margins. Wide margins, with re-excision if necessary, may be a priority in a subgroup of small tumors (<50 mm in diameter) with high mitotic activity (>10 mitoses per 10 high-power fields), a group that was found to be associated with a particularly high rate of recurrence in a recent study (55.6%). Recurrent and malignant tumors should undergo excision with negative margins. Malignant phyllodes tumors are treated with simple mastectomy. Only 5% have pathologically confirmed axillary lymph node metastasis ; however, when it does occur, prognosis is poor. The application of sentinel lymph node biopsy has not been addressed. The role of radiation therapy and adjuvant chemotherapy has not been determined by randomized clinical trials.

Breast Cancer

In children, Malignancies of the breast can be divided into three groups: primary malignancies, metastatic tumors involving the breast, and secondary malignancies. Malignant phyllodes tumor has been discussed previously. Primary breast cancer although very less prevalent in children, has been reported in children <5 years, in both boys and girls. The lesion usually presents as a painless, firm, poorly circum- scribed breast mass, whose margins are irregular or microlobulated. Historically the histology generally associated with primary breast cancer in childhood has been secretory carcinoma, an unusual histologic tumor type among adult breast cancer. Secretory breast carcinoma is a relatively slow-growing tumor with a typically good prognosis, although about 20% have nodal involvement at the time of diagnosis. Most cases are in young women, with a median age of 25 years, although men occasionally can have the disease as well. The youngest patient reported is a 3-year-old boy. The typical clinical presentation is a painless, well-circumscribed, mobile, palpable mass. Any part of the breast can be involved, including ectopic tissue in the axilla. Prepubertal patients have subareolar mass because of the small size of the breast. Nipple discharge can be present, so cytology is indicated if a suspicious lesion is encountered. Standard treatment for secretory carcinoma is simple mastectomy. Recently there have been recommendations for breast-conserving therapy, given the indolent growth of the tumor, even though the recommendation remains unsupported by formal clinical study. Sentinel lymph node biopsy has been recommended, with axillary node dissection if nodes are clinically involved. Radiation therapy is not performed. In the absence of systemic disease, chemotherapy is not given. Using a large population-based cancer registry, the Surveillance, Epidemiology, and End Results (SEER) program of the National Cancer Institute, infiltrating ductal carcinoma was found to occur more commonly among the 11- to 19-year age group than secretory carcinoma. Infiltrating ductal carcinoma probably represents the leading edge of the prevalence distribution for adult primary breast cancer. Patients aged 11–19 present with less differentiated tumors and more often at a higher clinical stage (stages II, III, and IV) than adult patients. Stage for stage, survival among children is the same as adults. Its treatment course is similar to that of adults having primary breast cancer. The most common cause of malignant breast mass is involvement by a hematologic malignancy (leukemia and lymphoma) and metastatic disease (rhabdomyosarcoma, neuroblastoma, retinoblastoma, and osteosarcoma). The breast is a common site for an acute leukemic relapse. Alveolar rhabdomyosarcoma usually leads to the breast cancer. A major risk factor for primary breast cancer in young patients is prior mantle field radiation for Hodgkin disease. The American College of Radiology suggests that after 8-10 years of the completion of therapy and adjunct breast MRI screening such patients should undergo screening mammography. Familial cancer syndromes such as BRCA1 and BRCA2 may also increase the risk for breast cancer in adolescents.

CONSENT FOR PUBLICATION

Not applicable.

CONFLICT OF INTEREST

The author declares no conflict of interest, financial or otherwise.

ACKNOWLEDGEMENTS

Declared none.

REFRENCES

[1]   Musumeci G, Castrogiovanni P, Szychlinska MA, *et al*. Mammary gland: From embryogenesis to adult life. Acta Histochem 2015; 117(4-5): 379-85.
       [http://dx.doi.org/10.1016/j.acthis.2015.02.013] [PMID: 25800977]

[2]   Abreu AP, Kaiser UB. Pubertal development and regulation. Lancet Diabetes Endocrinol 2016; 4(3): 254-64.
       [http://dx.doi.org/10.1016/S2213-8587(15)00418-0] [PMID: 26852256]

[3]   Marshall WA, Tanner JM. Variations in pattern of pubertal changes in girls. Arch Dis Child 1969; 44(235): 291-303.
       [http://dx.doi.org/10.1136/adc.44.235.291] [PMID: 5785179]

[4]   Hughes LE, Mansel RE, Webster DJ. Aberrations of normal development and involution (ANDI): a new perspective on pathogenesis and nomenclature of benign breast disorders. Lancet 1987; 2(8571): 1316-9.
       [http://dx.doi.org/10.1016/S0140-6736(87)91204-9] [PMID: 2890912]

[5]   Kaur N, Agarwal N, Panwar P, Mishra K. Clinicopathologic profile of benign breast conditions in Indian women: prospective study based on aberrations of normal development and involution classification. World J Surg 2012; 36(9): 2252-8.
       [http://dx.doi.org/10.1007/s00268-012-1671-4] [PMID: 22744217]

[6]   Caouette-Laberge L, Borsuk D. Congenital anomalies of the breast. Semin Plast Surg 2013; 27(1): 36-41.
[http://dx.doi.org/10.1055/s-0033-1343995] [PMID: 24872738]

[7]   Kulkarni DD, Dixon JD. Congenital abnormalities of the breast. Wom- ens Health (Lond) 2012.
[http://dx.doi.org/10.2217/WHE.11.84]

[8]   Eidlitz-Markus T, Mukamel M, Haimi-Cohen Y, Amir J, Zeharia A. Breast asymmetry during adolescence: physiologic and non-physiologic causes. Isr Med Assoc J 2010; 12(4): 203-6.
[PMID: 20803877]

[9]   Glicksman CA, Ferenz SE. The etiologies of chest wall and breast asymmetry and improvement in breast augmentation. Clin Plast Surg 2015; 42(4): 519-30.
[http://dx.doi.org/10.1016/j.cps.2015.06.009] [PMID: 26408441]

[10]   Loomba-Albrecht LA, Styne DM. The physiology of puberty and its disorders. Pediatr Ann 2012; 41(4): e1-9.
[http://dx.doi.org/10.3928/00904481-20120307-08] [PMID: 22494212]

[11]   Ma NS, Geffner ME. Gynecomastia in prepubertal and pubertal men. Curr Opin Pediatr 2008; 20(4): 465-70.
[http://dx.doi.org/10.1097/MOP.0b013e328305e415] [PMID: 18622206]

[12]   Narula HS, Carlson HE. Gynaecomastia--pathophysiology, diagnosis and treatment. Nat Rev Endocrinol 2014; 10(11): 684-98.
[http://dx.doi.org/10.1038/nrendo.2014.139] [PMID: 25112235]

[13]   Pellegrin MC, Naviglio S, Cattaruzzi E, Barbi E, Ventura A. A teenager with sudden unilateral breast enlargement. J Pediatr 2017; 182: 394.
[http://dx.doi.org/10.1016/j.jpeds.2016.11.044] [PMID: 27956018]

[14]   Kerridge WD, Kryvenko ON, Thompson A, Shah BA. Fat necrosis of the breast: a pictorial review of the mammographic, ultrasound, CT, and MRI findings with histopathologic correlation. Radiol Res Pract 2015; 2015: 613139.
[http://dx.doi.org/10.1155/2015/613139] [PMID: 25861475]

[15]   Montague EC, Hilinski J, Andresen D, Cooley A. Evaluation and treatment of mastitis in infants. Pediatr Infect Dis J 2013; 32(11): 1295-6.
[http://dx.doi.org/10.1097/INF.0b013e3182a06448] [PMID: 24145956]

[16]   Borders H, Mychaliska G, Gebarski KS. Sonographic features of neonatal mastitis and breast abscess. Pediatr Radiol 2009; 39(9): 955-8.
[http://dx.doi.org/10.1007/s00247-009-1310-x] [PMID: 19506847]

[17]   Valeur NS, Rahbar H, Chapman T. Ultrasound of pediatric breast masses: what to do with lumps and bumps. Pediatr Radiol 2015; 45(11): 1584-99.
[http://dx.doi.org/10.1007/s00247-015-3402-0] [PMID: 26164440]

[18]   Adejolu M, Huo L, Rohren E, Santiago L, Yang WT. False-positive lesions mimicking breast cancer on FDG PET and PET/CT. AJR Am J Roentgenol 2012; 198(3): W304-14.
[http://dx.doi.org/10.2214/AJR.11.7130] [PMID: 22358030]

[19]   Neal L, Sandhu NP, Hieken TJ, *et al.* Diagnosis and management of benign, atypical, and indeterminate breast lesions detected on core needle biopsy. Mayo Clin Proc 2014; 89(4): 536-47.
[http://dx.doi.org/10.1016/j.mayocp.2014.02.004] [PMID: 24684875]

[20]   Nelson AL. Controversies regarding mammography, breast self-examination, and clinical breast examination. Obstet Gynecol Clin North Am 2013; 40(3): 413-27.
[http://dx.doi.org/10.1016/j.ogc.2013.05.001] [PMID: 24021250]

[21]   Rosen PP, Holmes G, Lesser ML, Kinne DW, Beattie EJ. Juvenile papillomatosis and breast carcinoma. Cancer 1985; 55(6): 1345-52.

[http://dx.doi.org/10.1002/1097-0142(19850315)55:6<1345::AID-CNCR2820550631>3.0.CO;2-B] [PMID: 3971303]

[22] Lad S, Seely J, Elmaadawi M, *et al.* Juvenile papillomatosis: a case report and literature review. Clin Breast Cancer 2014; 14(5): e103-5.
[http://dx.doi.org/10.1016/j.clbc.2014.03.003] [PMID: 24997851]

[23] Salemis NS, Gemenetzis G, Karagkiouzis G, *et al.* Tubular adenoma of the breast: a rare presentation and review of the literature. J Clin Med Res 2012; 4(1): 64-7.
[http://dx.doi.org/10.4021/jocmr746w] [PMID: 22383931]

[24] Bowman E, Oprea G, Okoli J, *et al.* Pseudoangiomatous stromal hyperplasia (PASH) of the breast: a series of 24 patients. Breast J 2012; 18(3): 242-7.
[http://dx.doi.org/10.1111/j.1524-4741.2012.01230.x] [PMID: 22583194]

[25] Berg WA, Sechtin AG, Marques H, Zhang Z. Cystic breast masses and the ACRIN 6666 experience. Radiol Clin North Am 2010; 48(5): 931-87.
[http://dx.doi.org/10.1016/j.rcl.2010.06.007] [PMID: 20868895]

[26] Knell J, Koning JL, Grabowski JE. Analysis of surgically excised breast masses in 119 pediatric patients. Pediatr Surg Int 2016; 32(1): 93-6.
[http://dx.doi.org/10.1007/s00383-015-3818-5] [PMID: 26590129]

[27] Lee M, Soltanian HT. Breast fibroadenomas in adolescents: current perspectives. Adolesc Health Med Ther 2015; 6: 159-63.
[PMID: 26366109]

Abbreviations

ACTH	adrenocorticotropic hormone
ADP	adenosine diphosphate
AFP	alpha fetoprotein
ANDI	aberration of normal development and involution
ASD	atrial septal defect
AVF	arteriovenous fistula
AVM	arteriovenous malformation
BMI	body mass index
BWS	beckwith-wiedmann syndrome
BWT	bilateral wilms tumors
CAH	congenital adrenal hyperplasia
CAIS	complete androgen insensitivity Syndrome
CBAVD	congenital bilateral absence of vas Deferens
CBD	common bile duct
CC	choledochal cyst
CCAM	congenital cystic adenomatoid Malformation
CDH	congenital diaphragmatic hernia
CF	cystic fibrosis
CFTR	CF transmembrane regulator
CIS	carcinoma in situ
CM	cavernous malformations
CRL	crown rump length
CRP	C-reactive protein
CSF	cerebrospinal fluid
CT	computed tomography
DHT	dihydro testosterone
DISDIA	diisopropyl iminodiacetic acid
DSD	disorders of sex development
DVA	develpmental venous anomalies
ECG	electrocardiography
ECMO	extracorporal membrane oxygenation
ELISA	enzyme linked immunosorbent assay

ERCP endoscopic retrograde Cholangiopancreatography

FDG PET fludeoxyglucose positron emission Tomography

FEF forced expiratory flow

FEV forced expiratory volume

FSH follicle stimulating hormone

GDNF glial cell line- derived neurotropic factor

GI gastrointestinal

HAEC hirschsprung associated Enterocollitis

HB hebatoblastoma

HCC hepatocellular carcinoma

hCG human chorionic gonadotrophin

HFOV high frequency oscillatory ventilation

HN-NOS hepatocellular neoplasm – not otherwise specified

HPS hypertrophic pyloric stenosis

HVA homovanillic acid

ICC interstitial cell of cajal

INPC international neuroblastoma Classification pathology

IO interosseous

KUB kidney, ureter, bladder

LCH Langerhans cell histiocytosis

LFT liver function test

LH luteinizing hormone

MEN multiple endocrine neoplasia

MGD mixed gonadal dysgenesis

MI meconium ileus

MIBG metaiodobenzylguanidine

MRCP magnetic resonance Cholangiopancreatography

MRI magnetic resonance imaging

MRSA methicillin resistance ataphylococcus Aureus

NEC necrotizing enterocolitis

NF1 neurofibromatosis

NG nasogastric

NGCT nongerm cell tumor

NPO nil per os

PASH pseudoangiomatous stromal Hyperplasia

PDA patent ductus arteriosus

PNET primitive neuroectodermal tumours

PSARP posterior sagittal anorectoplasty

RCC renal cell carcinoma

RMS rhabdomyosarcoma

RPLND retroperitoneal lymph node dissection

SBRCT small blue round cell tumour

SCT sacrococcygeal tumour

SEER surveillance, epidemiology and end Result

SMA superior mesenteric artery

SRS stereoactic radiosurgery

TPN parenteral nutrition

UDT undescended testis

UGI upper gastrointestinal

US vertical expandable prostheticTitanium ribs

VLBW very low birth weight

VMA ventriculoperitoneal shunt

VSD ventricular septal defect

WDF well differentiated fetal

WT wilms tumour

YST yolk sac tumour

SUBJECT INDEX